FROM PSYCHOANALYSIS TO GROUP ANALYSIS

NEW INTERNATIONAL LIBRARY OF GROUP ANALYSIS

Series Editor: Earl Hopper

Other titles in the Series

Contributions of Self Psychology to Group Psychotherapy
by Walter N. Stone

Difficult Topics in Group Psychotherapy: My Journey from Shame to Courage
by Jerome S. Gans

Resistance, Rebellion and Refusal in Groups: The 3 Rs
by Richard M. Billow

The Social Unconscious in Persons, Groups, and Societies. Volume 1: Mainly Theory
edited by Earl Hopper and Haim Weinberg

Trauma and Organizations
edited by Earl Hopper

Small, Large, and Median Groups: The Work of Patrick de Maré
edited by Rachel Lenn and Karen Stefano

The Dialogues In and Of the Group
Macario Giraldo

FROM PSYCHOANALYSIS TO GROUP ANALYSIS

The Pioneering Work of Trigant Burrow

Edited and with an Introductory Essay by

Edi Gatti Pertegato and Giorgio Orghe Pertegato

Foreword by

Malcolm Pines

Routledge
Taylor & Francis Group
LONDON AND NEW YORK

First published 2013 by
Karnac Books Ltd.

Published 2019 by Routledge
2 Park Square, Milton Park, Abingdon, Oxon OX14 4RN
52 Vanderbilt Avenue, New York, NY 10017

First issued in hardback 2019

Routledge is an imprint of the Taylor & Francis Group, an informa business

British Library Cataloguing in Publication Data

A C.I.P. for this book is available from the British Library

ISBN 13: 978-0-367-10099-5 (hbk)
ISBN 13: 978-1-78049-028-1 (pbk)

Edited, designed and produced by The Studio Publishing Services Ltd
www.publishingservicesuk.co.uk
e-mail: studio@publishingservicesuk.co.uk

CONTENTS

To the fond remembrance of Dr Franco Pertegato, whose discreet but meaningful and learned support and collaboration accompanied us during the entire adventure of this book in its Italian and English versions. He will live on through it as well as in our hearts.

ACKNOWLEDGEMENTS

To the late Alfreda Sill Galt, Burrow's collaborator and last pioneer of group analysis, who, in 1926, took part in one of the first "Lifwynn Camp" summer sessions of experimental community and group analysis, we address our thankful and affectionate recollection for her availability, tenacity, and enthusiasm in encouraging and supporting the publication of this book. Just shortly before her death, she wanted dictate from her hospital bed the foreword here published for the Italian version of the book. We are very grateful also to Lloyd Gilden, who, in succeeding Alfreda as President of the Lifwynn Foundation, promptly offered us his collaboration. We also thank him for his permission to include Burrow's unpublished paper "Psychoanalysis and life" (1913), which Alfreda Galt gave us in April 1993.

Special thanks to Max Rosenbaum, who was so generous in sending us plenty of material about significant figures who wrote on Burrow and outstanding members of the Lifwynn Foundation, including a tape-recorded interview with Hans Syz, one of Burrow's co-workers, who pioneered group analysis with him.

Heartfelt thanks to Malcolm Pines, who kept abreast of our research on Burrow and, through the years, allowed us to rely on his mine of historical facts, and to Harold Behr for the interesting exchange of views, his sympathy, and suggestions for problematic issues. We also enjoyed their humour in our correspondence. Additionally, we derived much pleasure from the exchange of views with Kevin Power on the correspondence between Burrow and D. H. Lawrence.

We express our thanks to Diego Napolitani, who, twenty years ago, entrusted us with the task of outlining the history of group analysis, which, in turn, led us to Burrow's tracks. We feel particularly indebted to both Giusy Cuomo and Gemma Corradi Fiumara, dearest friends and colleagues, who, in the course of the years, made themselves available to discuss with us the shades of meaning of some of Burrow's psychoanalytic and group analytic terms, as well as some crucial paragraphs.

Our warm thanks to Alberto Lampignano for his encouragement during the vicissitudes we met with in the realisation of this book; to Adriano Verdecchia for his keen observations and deep interest in the undoing of censorship of Burrow's thinking; to Rachele Gatti for her translation of the editors' essay, and to Wendy Russel for her suggestions about stylistic issues.

We have fond memories of Juan Campos who, in distant 1993, helped us find the way to the Lifwynn Foundation and, through the years, warmly encouraged us in our effort to bring Burrow's work to light. We would like to express a deep-felt recollection of Leonardo Ancona, who was awaiting the publication of this book with great interest and curiosity; we deeply regret the loss of an enthusiastic supporter of Burrow's work, in which, a few years ago, he had rediscovered its original and remarkable value for psychoanalysis and group analysis.

Furthermore, we want to extend particular thanks to Oliver Rathbone, Karnac's Managing Director, who caught the importance and topicality of Burrow's thinking by promptly accepting the proposal of its publication. Many thanks also to Lucy Shirley, Karnac's Publishing Assistant, for her competent support, and to Rod Tweedy, Editorial Assistant, who continued to give us his very helpful and clever collaboration, and to Constance Govindin, Karnac's Publicity and Digital Content Manager, for her perspicacious interventions.

And last, but not least, we nourish loving memories and deep gratitude to Franco Pertegato, respectively editors' husband and father, who suddenly left us a year ago. After having spent forty years as a hospital doctor, through his suggestions and the reconsideration of all the material and essays, he constituted a sort of litmus test (*cartina di tornasole*) to ensure the comprehension of the text by non-specialist but interested readers from related fields. We also fondly remember his frequent Greek and Latin quotations, which he used to connote peculiar aspects of human behaviour.

We could say, indeed, that the publication of this book represents the result of a demanding and involving *group event*: we hope it will be welcome and fruitful.

ABOUT THE EDITORS

Edi Gatti Pertegato, PsyD, trained in psychoanalysis and group analysis, with particular interest in precocious developmental processes, the role of the environment, and research on psychoanalytic and group analytic history. She used to deal with expert reports for the Italian law courts and was responsible for the Foreign Section of the *Rivista Italiana di Gruppo Analisi*. She is a founder member of the *European Journal of Psychoanalysis*, former fellow and supervisor of the Italian Group Analytic Society, a full member of the Group Analytic Society International, member of the American Group Psychotherapy Association and the International Association of Group Psychotherapy, and author of a number of articles and books on psychoanalysis and group analysis.

Giorgio O. Pertegato, MD, is a psychiatrist trained in psychoanalysis and group analysis integrated in the phenomenological approach. He also worked in family psychotherapy and with people with drug addiction, and, from 2000 onwards, has worked in the Mental Health Department of ULSS 12 of Venice, where he deals specifically with rehabilitation and self-help promotion of psychotic patients through group techniques, including the conducting of a group of "voices' hearers". In addition, he collaborated on a number of articles and books on psychoanalysis and group analysis.

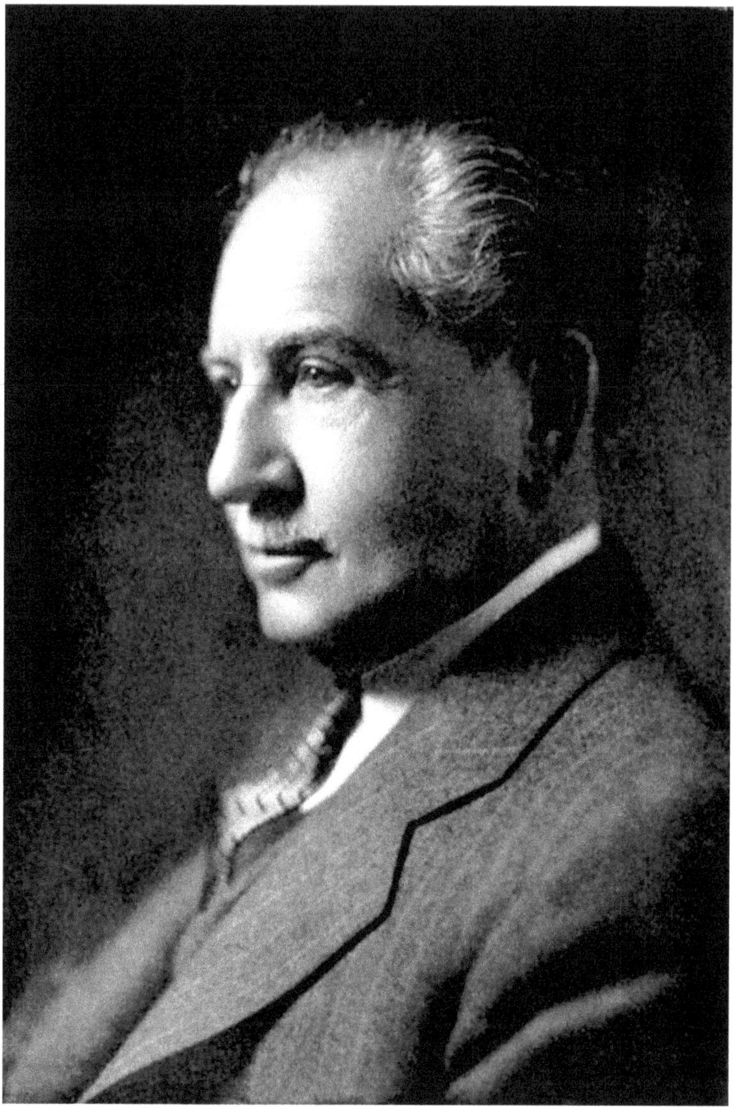

SERIES EDITOR'S FOREWORD

The authors of books in the New International Library of Group Analysis take several aspects of the social unconscious as both axiomatic and problematic: socialisation processes, relationships involving the creation and maintenance of self and other, the collective mind of various kinds of groupings and their social systems, and the collective mind of groupings and social systems associated with territory. Although colleagues vary in their emphasis and focus on these phenomena, they all agree that such phenomena are overlapping and intertwining, and that their specification is a matter of the gestalt and frame of reference of the observer's perception of them. The magna is always both one and primary, and the specification of elements of it is always secondary. This overarching perspective informs the actual practice of group analysis and other forms of psychoanalytical group therapy, as well as consultation to natural groupings, such as organisations (Hopper & Weinberg, 2011).

The study of intellectual ancestry can help in creating and maintaining intellectual, professional and personal "identity". It can help in avoiding the proverbial reinvention of the wheel, and in revitalising the study of particular themes in our work and variations on them. However, the positioning and contextualising of an intellectual and professional ancestor and our relationship to him/her and their work always involves a narrative of the political life of our profession, concerning the emphasis given to certain aspects of a problem and ways of defining it. Our ancestors in the study of the social unconscious, on whose shoulders we stand, are many and various, ranging from the founders of the social sciences in general to the socio-cultural revisionists of Freudian thinking in psychoanalysis and its many applications. Of course, special attention must be given to the work of the founders of the study of group dynamics and group analysis, in particular, Moreno, Pichon-Rivière, Bion, and Foulkes. However, it is often overlooked that to this list must be added many of the members of the Group of Independent Psychoanalysts of the British Psychoanalytical Society (Hopper, 2003). It is relevant that all the group analysts who were psychoanalysts were also members of the Group of Independent Psychoanalysts, although, alas, I am the last of the Mohicans.

It is now obvious that to this list of founders and more contemporary colleagues who were interested in the social unconscious, and who have contributed to the development of our thinking about it, must be added the name of Trigant Burrow. In fact, our professional identity has been structured by many of the processes described by him. It is fascinating to read and study his many papers, articles, and books, mostly written in English but also in German, in parallel with reading the work of Freud and perhaps that of his early disciples and colleagues in Europe and the USA. In both agreement and in polemic with them, Burrow explored the social, cultural, and political factors and forces, interest in which was repressed and split off, and perhaps suppressed the psychoanalytical project. Especially in the USA, psychoanalysis had become regulated by psychiatry and the use of the medical model, not only in treatment, but also in theorising human development. These scotoma must be understood in the context of the sociology and psychoanalysis of knowledge and professionalisation, including defensive processes against the anxiety aroused by curiosity and knowing about the external world.

The work of Trigant Burrow shows many of the problems that confront the study of the social unconscious and his work is coloured by many of the qualities and assumptions of late nineteenth-century and early twentieth-century social sciences, philosophy, and biology. None the less, it cannot be denied that Burrow was ahead of his time in his attempts to integrate psychoanalysis with sociology. It was he who coined the term "Group Analysis", later used by Foulkes without acknowledgement, perhaps not entirely unlike Foulkes' study of "persons" as opposed to the abstractions of either "individuals" or "groups", an approach developed by Norbert Elias, more or less in parallel with Burrow. Although, previously, I have myself credited Erich Fromm with having first used the term "social unconscious", I have now learnt that actually Burrow introduced it in 1924 in *Social Images Versus Reality.*

Edi and Giorgio Pertegato, the editors of this book, are aware of, and empathetic with, the personal and professional position in which Burrow found himself. Although he continued to identify with the Freudian psychoanalytical project, albeit one that gave much more attention to sociological considerations, the psychoanalytical establishment refused to include him in their widening circle. His work is very rarely cited in the bibliographies of training courses in the Institutes that comprise the American Psychoanalytical Association, as well as those in other countries. Similarly, although he contributed to the development of group analysis through his many books and articles, and he conducted a large correspondence with members of the international community of scientists, his work is almost never included in the curricula of Institutes of group analysis and psychoanalytical group psychotherapy. Several of us can identify with this multiple marginalisation involving an interpersonal and intellectual "location" which is not entirely of our own making. Personally, I doubt whether Burrow's difficulties can be traced to his own personal and intellectual style as much as to the socio-cultural and political dynamics of the society within which his work was spawned. However, psychoanalysts throughout the world continue to have difficulties in recognising and understanding the sociality of human nature.

I am most grateful to the Pertegatos for their perseverance in their labour of love, through which they have brought to our attention the work of Trigant Burrow. Trained in psychology and literature, Edi Pertegato was influenced by the late Professor Renata Gaddini, who, along with her husband, Eugenio Gaddini, shared many of the ideas of the Group of Independent Psychoanalysts (Gaddini, 1992). Edi trained in group analysis with Diego Napolitani, who was a member of the international network of group analysts. Having faced many personal challenges whose mastery required dedication and resilience, she extended her intellectual and cultural horizons through international travel. Although born and bred in Milan, she married Franco Pertegato, who was from the Veneto region. He qualified in medicine, specialising in radiology and respiratory system diseases at Padua University. Edi and Franco Pertegato shared many interests and activities and they relished their family life. Their son, Giorgio Pertegato, who is the co-editor of this book, qualified in medicine and specialised in psychiatry. Trained in psychoanalysis in Padua and in group analysis in Rome, Giorgio works in the Venice Mestre Department of Psychiatry of the NHS.

This book has been a long time in the making, and not without many challenges to its preparation and publication, perhaps analogous to those that characterised Burrow's gaining acceptance for his attempts to modify the theory and practice of psychoanalysis and to create both for group analysis. It is ironic that it is our colleagues from Italy who have brought the work of Trigant Burrow to the renewed attention of an English-speaking audience. Although language difficulties have inhibited the cross-translation of much contemporary work, we are fortunate in our mutually supportive personal and professional relationships, which have extended across geographical borders, in the context of the Group Analytic Society International and the International Association for Group Psychotherapy and Group Process.

References

Gaddini, E. (1992). *A Psychoanalytic Theory of Infantile Experience.* London: Tavistock/Routledge.

Hopper, E. (2003). *The Social Unconscious: Selected Papers.* London: Jessica Kingsley.

Hopper, E., & Weinberg, H. (Eds.) (2011). *The Social Unconscious in Persons, Groups and Societies, Volume 1: Mainly Theory.* London: Karnac.

FOREWORD: "BURROW LIVES AGAIN!"

From Darwin's notebooks: "Origin of man now proved.—Metaphysic must flourish.—He who understands a baboon would do more towards metaphysic than Locke" (2008, p. 257). By metaphysic, in his time, he meant the increase of knowledge.

Now we have a book, *Baboon Metaphysics: The Evolution of a Social Mind* (Cheney & Seyfarth (2008). In baboon groups, social pressures change constantly, rapidly, and unpredictably. Their social world is inherently dynamic and they possess a limited ability to recognise the mental states of others. However, what are, possibly, their rich causal narratives remain private, with no ways of sharing with others; there is no gossip. They live in the present and cannot engage in the human thought activity of "what if". Here we have a complex society that operates without language, only with signs, or only with evidence of theory of mind—that is, knowing that what is in the mind of the other is understood by my sharing in that way of understanding myself.

Darwin said,

> as man advances in civilisation, and small tribes are united in the larger communities, the simplest reason will tell each individual that he ought to extend his social instincts and sympathies to all the

> members of the same nation, though personally unknown to him. This point being once reached there is only an artificial barrier to prevent his sympathies extending to the men of all nations and races. (2008, p. 251)

What wonderful days these would be were Burrow alive! This book of his papers, researched and edited by Edi and Giorgio Pertegato and introduced by his loyal co-workers Alfreda Galt and Lloyd Gilden of the Lifwynn Foundation, presents and preserves his group analytic work, which began over ninety years ago. Burrow lives again! And what an era this would be for Burrow the researcher: the rise of neuro-Darwinism, brain sciences, primatology (which deals with the social life of primates) (Hrdy, 2009), and the new knowledge and understanding of the central value of co-operation which exists in balance with competition in the biological sciences. Burrow the dedicated researcher would today find so many avenues for exploration in connection with these new models.

Among the panoply of explorers of the "social unconscious", Goldstein, Schilder, Foulkes, Moreno, Slavson, now also the current editor of this new series, nearly all had pioneered studies in brain sciences and how this knowledge could be applied to the new group therapies. Freud must be included, for, though he fiercely denied the value of Burrow's "experimental studies", Freud made great contributions to group psychology, as did the great neurologist Wilfred Trotter, whose ideas were a foundation for those of his pupil, Wilfred Bion, though at that time a surgeon.

Burrow's collected papers, edited and presented together here for the first time, show his very acute thinking about the primary union of infant and mother, then an unheard aspect of psychoanalysis which was then based upon Freud's drive theory and its Oedipal manifestations. Ferenczi, Balint, Klein, Bowlby, Winnicottt, Anna Freud, and René Spitz were yet to be heard as was, much later, Heinz Kohut. Yet, Burrow's writings resonated with D. H. Lawrence, Herbert Read, and others outside the psychoanalytic community. There was an exchange of letters with D. H. Lawrence which commenced in 1925. "I am in entire sympathy with your ideas of social images." In 1926, Lawrence wrote, "Many thanks for the paper 'Psychoanalysis in Theory and Life' . . . It is true, the essential self is so simple – and nobody lets it be. But I wonder if you ever get anyone to listen to you" (Huxley, 1932, p. 634).

In 1927, he wrote,

> It is really funny – resistances – that we are all of us existing by resisting – and that . . . a p.-a. [psycho-analyst] doctor and his patient only come to hugs in order to offer a perfect resistance to mother or father or Mrs Grundy – sublimating one existence into another existence – each man his own nonpareil, and spending his life secretly or openly resisting the nonpareil pretensions of all other men – a very true picture of us all, poor dears. All bullies, or being bullied.
>
> Men will *never* agree – can't in their *"subjective sense perception"*. Subjective sense perceptions are individualistic, *ab ovo*. But do tell them to try! (Huxley, 1932, p. 615)

Burrow's writings had immediate deep meaning for D. H. Lawrence, for the psychoanalytic community, agitations and dismissal. Burrow's challenge was that the psychoanalytic community shared in a social cover-up; the fact that we all disguise is that neurosis is social and that a social neurosis can only be met through a social analysis. History was repeated when, similarly, Bion and Rickman challenged the British army at Northfield Military Hospital. They were dismissed.

Burrow's education was in the America of pragmatic psychology, of Cooley, Dewey, James, and George Herbert Mead.[1] His primary group work was conducted as an experimental science, which, for him, had either to be confirmed or rebutted. The psychoanalysis of his days, principally the 1920s and 1930s, was based on the writings and methods of Freud, so Burrow's words fell on stony ground, and this book challenges why he has remained, to a very large extent, unheard. For myself, as a historian of Foulkesian group analysis, I have had to reconsider why he has remained "one of the Forgotten Pioneers" of whom I have written. The pivotal moment for the recognition of group methods as essential to a broad-based response to the challenges of wartime and post war psychiatry began at Northfield Military Hospital, where both Bion and Foulkes were seminal figures. Bion was dismissed, Foulkes educated and listened to with respect. The psychiatric world had moved on and was able now to listen.

Why was Foulkes heard, whereas Burrow was not? Foulkes had impeccable European psychoanalytic credentials: training in Vienna, and work at the Frankfurt Institute of Psychoanalysis. For Burrow's background and psychoanalytic training, please see "The psychoanalytic period: from drives to relationships" (p. xxxix). Less obvious was his sociological education through his friendship with Norbert Elias, a peripheral member of the Frankfurt School of Marxist sociologists. Foulkes gained and retained his status as a training analyst for the Anna Freud Group of the British Psychoanalytical Society, which included Bowlby and Fairbairn as members, later James Anthony and myself. Foulkes was influential as a teacher of group psychotherapy at the Maudsley Hospital, which was the centre of British postgraduate education. He immersed himself in the creation, with Moreno, of The International Association of Group Psychotherapy. He founded the London Group Analytic Society from which the Institute of Group Analysis (London) developed and which has had a major role in the development of group analysis throughout Europe.

Foulkes was a gradualist who charmed and retained his audience; Burrow held on to his fundamental principles and, thus, his words did not compromise. Now he must again be listened to.

I hope that this book, which is part of the New International Library of Group Analysis, will have wide readership, and that Trigant Burrow regains his rightful place in the pantheon of group analysis and group psychotherapy.

Malcolm Pines

Editors' note

1. For Burrow's background and psychoanalytic training, see the section headed "The psychoanalytic period: from drives to relationships" (p. xxxix.

FOREWORD

In this volume, with a significant selection of Burrow's papers, Edi Gatti Pertegato of the SGAI Milano (Italian Group Analytic Society) and Giorgio Pertegato, psychiatrist and group analyst, have performed a valuable service for Italian readers and particularly for those concerned with psychoanalysis and the procedure called group analysis. They have undertaken to elucidate the origins of group analysis, which we refer to at the Lifwynn Foundation as social self-enquiry. The Lifwynn Foundation involves an egalitarian group of researchers who are attempting to investigate further the mechanisms of what Trigant Burrow identified as social neurosis.

A student of Jung in 1909–1910, Burrow practised psychoanalysis at the Phipps Clinic of the Johns Hopkins Medical School. He practised there for some ten years before concluding that, as he wrote to Adolf Meyer, director of the clinic in August of 1921, "the basic occasion of the failure of analysis (is) our exclusive emphasis on the personal to the utter neglect of inherent social factors". Burrow came to believe that it was only through examination of the social factors in the patient's situation that his or her needs could be fully encompassed. As described in the papers, which Giorgio Pertegato has so carefully translated, this required a certain approach, which developed in the course of Burrow's mutual analysis with an unusual patient, Clarence Shields, who remained his closest collaborator throughout their lives. Together, they undertook to enquire into the authoritarianism that lies behind the position of the analyst, and also that of the ordinary human being, with our sense of rightness and defensiveness.

Edi Gatti Pertegato and Giorgio Pertegato have returned to the original roots of Burrow's writings in his formulation of what he referred to as the "principle of primary identification" or "the preconscious". The infant's identification with the maternal organism was, in his view, the prototype for every human being of our connection with the phylic organism and our oneness with the species as a whole. The volume begins with an unpublished presentation given in 1913 that is well worth consideration.

The editors have chosen to concentrate on this very early aspect of Burrow's pioneering studies and to postpone for a possible later volume examination of Burrow's major studies of the 1930s and 1940s, which focus on the internal discrimination of two contrasting modes of attention he identified as "cotention" and "ditention", and their relationship to the fragmentation of our species and alienation from each other and the environment.

I look forward to further consideration of these significant later aspects of Burrow's innovative studies and, in the meantime, I want to recommend serious consideration of this volume by all those concerned with the study of human behaviour and group analysis.

Alfreda Sill Galt
President of the Lifwynn Foundation, June 1998

FOREWORD

Trigant Burrow put forth a view of the human species, which was unique in his era, beginning in the early years of the twentieth century. His first book, *The Social Basis of Consciousness*, published in 1927, was inspired, in part, by Einstein's theory of relativity. A precursor to the book is included in this book in the paper "Relative concept of consciousness: an analysis of consciousness in its ethnic origin".

Burrow draws a distinction between the absolutistic form of consciousness analogous to Newtonian physics and organic consciousness, analogous to Einstein's relativity physics.

> As in the intrinsic principle of absolutism comprising the Newtonian system of gravitation, so in the self-determined principle of absolutism comprising our present system of psychology a dimensional factor has been left out of account the inclusion of which completely shifts the basis of former calculations and so distorts our habitual reckonings as to demand the fundamental reconstruction of accepted values . . .
>
> It is worthy of note that between the objective or mathematical theory of relativity of Einstein and the subjective or organismic[1] theory of relativity here envisaged there is to be traced, however inconclusively, a philosophical parallelism that is significant . . . this cosmological parallel between the subjective and objective spheres of relativity marks a

> concomitance that is consistent throughout . . . the subjective and objective spheres of life, embodying the bipolar aspects of the phenomenal world, represent but obverse phases of one and the same universe. The analogy that interests me here, however, has to do with the feature that is equally the basis of the two modes of relativity, namely, the feature which entails the abrogation of absolute standards of evaluation and the recognition of the kinetic factor that is organic to both.

Burrow went on to correlate the absolutistic mode of thinking with social neurosis in his paper "Our mass neurosis". In that paper, he says, "nervous disorder and insanity are not restricted alone to the isolated individual . . . the actual presence of demonstrable disordered mental states exists unrecognized within the social organizations that form our present day civilization".

He then points out that disordered mental states are manifested in conflicts between religious groups, for example, Protestants and Catholics, and political groups, for example, Republicans and Democrats, etc. In these and many other conflicts

> each disputant claims on the authority of his personal system that he is right . . . As long as our criterion rests upon the dual standard of an unconscious absolutism we are embroiled in the inaccessible conflict of the absolute alternative . . .

The developmental step by which we arrive at our tendency for social conflict involves social conditioning, first in our relationships with our parents and family, then with the community at large. In "Social images versus reality", Burrow suggests that

> what is called the mother image is but the sum of the impressions reflected by the mother from the social environment about her, and that these impressions are again transmitted by us to others through their reflection with ourselves.

Our parental experiences are generalised to our social relationships. Just as we sought the safety and satisfaction of approval from our parents, we seek "approbation of the community".

> As in our individual fixation upon the image of the mother, our constant affect oscillates between the issues of fear or favour, praise or blame, so in the social fixation upon our cherished image of the

> community, as it exists under our various institutions, economic, political, social, and personal, our constant preoccupation vacillates perpetually between the dual issues represented by our success or failure, our private profit or private loss. . . .
>
> To form a conception of our unconscious mass mind and its social condensations, it is required that we forego our present absolute basis of evaluations residing in the private judgement of the individual and that instead we assume a basis which, being relative to, and inclusive of, our mental and social processes, will envisage both on the basis of a more universal and encompassing evaluation.

The autonomy of the "I"

In order to adopt a more relativistic perspective, it is necessary that we confront our tendency to assume we are separate, autonomous individuals, which we label as "I".

As Burrow states in *The Basis of Group Analysis*: "A social group or community consists of persons each of whom is represented under the symbol he calls "I", or "I, myself".

The "I" assumes undisputed authority "based upon private images and connotations, every one of which may be flatly and quite as authoritatively contradicted by another individual or "I" who happens to be under the influence of an opposite system of images or prejudices" (Autonomy of the "I" from the standpoint of group analysis).

Some examples of "I" statements are: "I don't like John"; "I just can't stand a crowd"; "I possess the truest religion and the only country worth while"; "My children possess exceptional talent"; "That man is not favourably disposed toward me and I have no use for him".

These are the kinds of assumptions that foment conflict. Within social groups on all levels, from families to local communities, to international communities, the assumption of autonomy and authority of one's views creates a sense of opposition and alienation. We develop antagonism, when someone holds a different belief or opinion, and steadfastly hold on to what our "I" believes is right.

Group analysis

Burrow created group analysis as a medium for addressing the societal forces that create our separative, alienated sense of "I".

> This over-evaluation in each individual of the self-image symbolised as "I", this image of oneself which one tends to carry about with him, comparing himself with the mental image he carries of others and which others carry of him, is again and again brought to open group awareness. But always emphasis is upon the common, socially pervasive character of what the individual presumes are quite privately cherished and secretly guarded images, so that the immediate recourse of the isolated individual to elaborations of the self-image called "I", or "I, myself", is viewed not as specific to the individual, but as generic to the group, and not to any particular group, but to the community as a whole.

Over the years, group analysis has evolved into a specific technique called social self-enquiry. The process involves exploration of the group members' self-image, referred to as the "I"-persona. The authoritarian sense of rightness is identified subjectively by participants, and, in their exchanges, they share these observations with each other. The whole spectrum of emotions that arise with group interactions (anger, anxiety, sentimentality, elation, depression, etc.) and their related behaviours (aggressiveness, defensiveness, manipulativeness, self-aggrandisement, ingratiation, etc.) are the subject of study.

When enquiry is directed within and attention is paid to the bodily sensations that accompany such self-biased beliefs and emotions, awareness of localised tensions associated with the different mood states develops. Over time, as participants gain experience in self-enquiry, they might become aware of a broader frame of reference: the organism-as-a-whole. This provides a new perspective on conflictual behaviour. The connections between thoughts and feelings, which Burrow referred to as "affect", is recognised. Emotions are recognised as conditioned reactions that are triggered by social images.

Ultimately, awareness of one's own organismic reactions leads to recognition of the commonality of all human organisms. There is the realisation that beyond our separative, self-righteous view of others, we are members of the same species with similar needs; and, with that, a feeling of solidarity.

Lloyd Gilden
President of the Lifwynn Foundation

Note

1. "By organismic, I mean the feelings and reactions common to the social body regarded as a coherent, integral organism. The term organismic, as I use it in its social application, is identical with the term organic in its individual application; so that the connotations organic and organismic are here used interchangeably."

PARABLE

The Madman

It was in a garden of a madhouse that I met a youth with a face pale and lovely and full of wonder.

And I sat beside him upon the bench, and I said, "Why are you here?"

And he looked at me in astonishment, and he said, "It is an unseemly question, yet I will answer you. My father would make me a reproduction of himself; so also would my uncle. My mother would have me the image of her illustrious father. My sister would hold up her seafaring husband as the perfect example for me to follow. My brother thinks I should be like him, a fine athlete.

"And my teachers also, the doctor of philosophy, and the music-master, and the logician, they too were determined, and each would have me but a reflection of his own face in a mirror.

"Therefore I came to this place. I find it more sane here. At least, I can be myself."

Then of a sudden he turned to me and he said, "But tell me, were you also driven to this place by education and good counsel?"

And I answered, "No, I am a visitor."

And he said, "Oh, you are one of those who live in the madhouse on the other side of the wall."

(Kahlil Gibran, *The Wanderer*, 1932)

INTRODUCTORY ESSAY

Trigant Burrow's psychoanalytic and group analytic research on man's social nature through censorship and subterranean ransacking

Edi Gatti Pertegato & Giorgio Orghe Pertegato
(Translated by Rachele M. Gatti)

> "No man is an island, entire in itself; every man is a piece of a continent, a part of the main. . . . any man's death diminishes me, because I am involved in mankind; and therefore never send to know for whom the bell tolls; it tolls for thee"
>
> (Donne, 1624, in Meditation XVII)

This volume gathers a significant selection of psychoanalytic and group analytic essays by Trigant Burrow (1875–1950), who was a co-founder of the American Psychoanalytic Association (APA) and founder of group analysis. They show the development of the relational orientation in psychoanalysis and the origin and evolution of group analysis, meant primarily as a social conception of the human being, as well as a therapeutic means, applicable both to dual and group settings.

Given the overcoming of so many obstacles the editors met with in their twenty years of research, the publication of this present volume represents a great relief and a deep satisfaction, first of all in that it brings to light the historical truth about Burrow's work; second, because it affords an extraordinary contribution both to group analysis and group therapy in general, and to those professionals who work in the fields of human behaviour and its distortions, as well as in educational, training, and institutional contexts.

After a persistent censorship, which began in the 1920s and continued until recent years, both Italy (in a translated volume) and, later, the UK have dared to publish these selective writings that show how innovative Burrow's research was.

This research that, at first sight, might appear as a sort of historical find to be consigned to the past, or a significant trophy to be exhibited, is instead distinguished because of its novelty and its marked originality. Besides "throwing open the window" to the brand new elaboration of themes of great topicality, such as, for example, the individual and social conflict that is more and more affecting our times, as well as the questioning of so-called "normality", it takes us to the inception of both psychoanalysis and group analysis, whose history—as we will see—is insistently asking for reconsideration and rewriting. And, certainly, we are all aware of how essential it is to have knowledge of one's own history in order to avoid its unconscious repetition by re-examining it through a critically reflexive attitude and learning to distinguish the "good from evil". This enables us creatively to go beyond the mere reproduction of the induced models that overwhelm one's authenticity either in individual, interpersonal, group, community, or institutional contexts.

The publication of the present book represents the onerous, yet very exciting, effort started in 1993 to unearth Burrow's work, with the aim of getting rid of the thick layer of silence which, in several ways and with the complicity of some distorted historiography, has somehow prevailed in Europe and the USA until a few years ago.

The unexpected unearthing of Burrow's work

Which were the events that brought us to the discovery of Burrow and to the finding of his writings?

The unveiling of such an "eminent unknown man" (E. Gatti Pertegato, 1994a) happened in a quite unusual, unexpected way and, due to many difficulties that arose, both in the beginning and along the way, it seemed to assume the form of an obstacle course or some sort of "adventure" just to find out something more about Burrow directly through his writings. Here, we show some of the stages of that adventure.

This book represents the completion of a long and difficult research, originating in the Italian Group Analytic Society with the inception of a specific study group led by Diego Napolitani, who, in January 1993, charged Edi Gatti Pertegato with the task of writing down a brief historical profile of group analysis that could be a reference for the research.

At first, it seemed an easy task that could be accomplished quickly. However, the lack of material about Trigant Burrow, whom we knew had introduced the term "group analysis" and around whom there was an air of mystery, with vague and contradictory references to only a couple of works, along with the impossibility of finding his original writings, created numerous unanswerable questions, which impelled a trip to the USA in order to search for his tracks.

Following these tracks turned into an investigation which resulted in a vast gathering of psychoanalytic and group analytic writings whose existence was unsuspected. In truth, they were very difficult to consult, as most of them were published in out of print books, or disseminated in old journals, while others were located at Lifwynn Foundation[1] (E. Gatti Pertegato & G. O. Pertegato, 2006a) and at Yale University in New Haven, Connecticut.

These findings changed the study group's objectives, conveying it directly to the years 1910 and 1920 when, inside psychoanalysis, the importance of the relationship between the individual and his environment emerged through the original formulations of Burrow's thinking, and, from there, led to the beginning of group analysis.

From that moment on, the group's work focused on the periodic reports that E. Gatti Pertegato made, along with fruitful discussions on the articles that would spring from them[2] (E. Gatti Pertegato, 1994a,b; E. Gatti Pertegato & G. O. Pertegato, 1995). In turn, this changed the direction of her professional interests, as Burrow's writings were of such importance, from both the historical point of view and their theoretical–technical content, that her projects connected with them progressively increased.

The subsequent research revealed an extraordinary unpublished paper dealing with the outline of the "Eight propositions of group analysis", that is, with the systematisation of the theoretical structure of group analysis (Burrow, 1928; E. Gatti Pertegato, 2005), which can be found here and there in his previous essays, where, in a relatively explicit way, they act as the basis of Burrow's researches.

Along the way, the involvement of Giorgio O. Pertegato was required, first as a translator of the essays of this volume into Italian, then as a collaborator on some papers, and, finally, as co-editor of the present work.

Furthermore, we have to highlight the role played by the review *Psicoterapia e Scienze Umane*, which, under the banner of "Classics of psychoanalytic research", published Burrow's paper (1927b, trans. 1994) on the basic method of group analysis.

Another significant contribution to the digging up of Burrow's work has been made by Paolo Migone (1995) who, in the historical magazine *Rivista Sperimentale di Freniatria*, encompassing a multidisciplinary vision, traced a historical outline of group analysis from its origins, revealing the influence of some innovative ideas of Burrow on social psychiatry, on Sullivan's interpersonal theory, on the psychology of organisations, and on the studies of countertransference. But, as we shall see, all this happened in an almost clandestine way.

In a wider context, we should mention our papers on Burrow's thoughts that we submitted to the IAGP International Congresses (E. Gatti Pertegato & G. O. Pertegato, Buenos Aires, 1995, London, 1998, Jerusalem, 2000), to the XII Symposium of Group Analytic Society (Bologna, 2002), and to the Lifwynn Conference (New York, 2006a, 2010),[3] as well as a paper published by the journal *Group Analysis* in a special section dedicated to Burrow (E. Gatti Pertegato, 1999), an introduction to his work which describes, through mostly unpublished correspondence, the frustrating relationship with Freud, along with the ostracism from the Vienna Group.

This collection of Burrow's essays, thus, is not going to be set in an empty place. On the contrary, owing to the series of papers mentioned above, it is introduced in the context of historical knowledge about the vicissitudes that marked Burrow's relationships with psychoanalytic thought and institutions, about the origin and development of group analysis, as well as the comparison of Burrow's concepts with those of S. H. Foulkes. The aim of this volume, which reconsiders the evolution from psychoanalysis to group analysis, is, then, the prosecution of the unearthing of Burrow's original endowment of studies and research, which led Ackerman (1964), without any hesitation, to refer to him as a "giant figure".

As a matter of fact, in the USA, besides the valuable contribution by Max Rosenbaum (1986, 1992; Rosenbaum & Berger, 1963) and by Nathan Ackerman (1964), the Lifwynn Foundation is systematically bringing to light Burrow's work. It has been doing this for many years and achieving considerable results in the field of human sciences in general and in that of group psychotherapy, working to overcome the deep silence from psychoanalysis and the lack of a significant response from group analysis. In Europe, the attempts to rediscover and reconsider Burrow's concepts by Juan Campos (1990) in Spain and Claude Pigott (1990) in France received some modest resonance. The same response was given to Burrow's writing, in which—in advance of the times—he had recourse to instrumental investigations, forestalling the present neuro-scientific research; such work was published in Italian by the review *Archivio Generale di Neurologia, Psichiatria e Psicoanalisi* (Burrow, 1933, translated in 1934).

This resistance to acknowledging Burrow's work provided further impetus to the publication of his original writings.

Topicality and relevance of Burrow's thought

Another question might arise: what sense is there in presenting to today's students and professionals essays written in the first decades of the last century?

First of all, it is a duty to rescue them from oblivion, if only to fill a gap in the historical–epistemological point of view. Indeed, it is a work destined to revolutionise our knowledge about the evolution of psychoanalysis, the origin and contents of the group analytic perspective, and to provide a systematic viewpoint on various aspects of human relationships, their conflicts and distortions. Burrow was the first to have highlighted the social nature of the individual and his interaction with the environment about him (family, cultural, social), in contrast to the deterministic and individualistic vision that prevailed in Freud's thought.

Through this theoretical position, Burrow transformed the psychoanalytic paradigm based on the vicissitudes of the drives into a historical–relational one, becoming the *precursor of the relational approach in psychoanalysis* and anticipating by around half a century the leading figures of the English School of Object Relations (Balint,

Fairbairn, Winnicott, and Guntrip). Furthermore, he was the first to apply psychoanalytic principles to group therapy (Oberndorf, 1953). It is noteworthy that his thinking evolved from psychoanalysis to group analysis not on the basis of mere theoretical presuppositions, but through group empirical experimentations, using what he called the "laboratory consensual method", or "group analysis", invented and developed by Burrow himself and his collaborators, which gradually resulted in the formulation of its theoretic–methodological structure, as we will clearly see from his writings published here.

Another interesting contemporary aspect—although ignored by psychoanalysis and mostly unknown to the group analytic field—is that Burrow's "laboratory method", or group analysis, besides being a therapeutic tool, is primarily a perspective on the social nature of human behaviour and an effort to supply, through an inclusive and interdisciplinary approach and through connecting its findings to biological foundations, a scientific basis to the conflict affecting individuals and society (Burrow, 1937a). One could state that Burrow surpassed Freud (1913j) in the aim to find a contact with biology as a bedrock not only for the psychic field, but also for the social one, overcoming the mind–body, nature–nurture dichotomies, in favour of *man's organism as a whole* in interaction with the social context. Already, in 1927, Burrow wrote his first group analytic book, with the significant title *The Social Basis of Consciousness,* which points to the "totality of personality" as "biologically tenable" and to the social implication of human pathology *vs.* Freud's "limitation of the conception of the neurosis within the bounds of individual consciousness" (p. 109). Furthermore, from the 1930s onward, there took place a significant evolution in group analysis, whose research was increasingly integrated by recourse to psychophysiological experiments and also through instrumental recordings (1935, 1937b, 1941, 1943, 1945). Although, at that time, Burrow could not rely on today's sophisticated technology as a means of investigation, his findings of instrumental evidence of man's primary biological norm of behaviour and of his deviations from it, which correlated with the earlier group analytic researches (Burrow, 1950), are substantiated by neuroscientific studies, which increasingly demonstrate that "the mind develops at the interface of neurophysiological processes and interpersonal relationships" (Siegel, 1999, p. 21).

Almost fifty years ago, Ackerman (1964) affirmed: "Evidence accumulates in the field of biology and the science of human relations to support the importance of a basic current of interdependence and cooperation throughout animal forms. Burrow's theory rests on firm biological ground" (pp. xv–xvi).

From the following essays, we will get a wide and significant overview of Burrow's contribution to psychoanalysis and of the basis of group analysis, as he envisaged it.

The psychoanalytic period, which ranges from 1909 to 1918, shows, as early as 1913, the evolution of the "principle of primary identification" along with its clinical application, and, in 1914, Burrow draws attention to "the social aspect of neurotic disorders—unrecognized disintegrative forces existing quite generally in socially accepted behaviour" (Syz, 1957, p. 147). Although his intellectual freedom caused him to take into consideration the role played by social factors, thus theoretically differing from Freud, as far as psychoanalytic procedure is concerned, apart from his adoption of a flexible attitude to the setting, essentially he followed the Freudian method of individual psychoanalysis.

From 1918 to 1924, there was a hiatus, during which he interrupted either the writing of essays or his psychoanalytic practice. What happened? During a psychoanalytic session, he was suddenly confronted by his analysand, Clarence Shields, with a contradiction between theory and practice and, consequently, with the inadequacy of classical psychoanalysis to meet the problems of the individual as a totality (Burrow, 1926a; E. Gatti Pertegato & G. O. Pertegato, 2010). From that moment on, he set aside the psychoanalytic procedure and, after attempts at first reversing roles, with Shields as analyst, and then mutual analysis, Burrow wholly dedicated himself to experimentation with the social principles, already included in his first psychoanalytic formulations, through group research (see "The group analytic period: the group processes as a person's structure", p. lxiv).

The development of group analysis proceeded step by step, through trial and error, solely based on the "consensual observation" and analytical evaluation of what was happening "here and now", that is, of the group interchange during the sessions, which emerged as representative of the "there and then", that is, of the individual's relationships with the original environment about him, as well as his community at large (Syz, 1961).

At last, in 1924, Burrow had much to communicate about his six years of research dedicated to the application of psychoanalysis to groups. Consequently, he broke this long silence and began to write one essay after the other, on both psychoanalysis and group analysis. This new cycle started with two quite theoretical writings "Social images versus reality" (1924), and "A relative concept of consciousness" (1925a), where he presented the new principles that he believed should be at the basis of group analysis. It is noteworthy that Burrow explained and re-explained his thesis, reprised and developed his ideas several times, as if he, fully conscious of his completely new and demanding conception, was afraid of possible misunderstandings.

In the other essays included in this second group, Burrow resumed and rethought, according to this new perspective of group analysis, some theoretical–technical psychoanalytic subjects, such as the transference, the resistance, the psychoanalyst's attitude, etc. It must be emphasised that he considered group analysis to be a *development* of Freudian psychoanalysis, through "an interpretation based upon a social conception of consciousness" (Burrow, 1927a), and certainly not as a separate discipline or in opposition to it, even if Freud thought otherwise. Anyway, at that point, theory and practice were no longer contradictory, but being enriched by feeding into and reflecting each other.

To approximately the same period, from 1924 to 1930, belongs the third group of papers, in which Burrow established the theoretical and methodological basis of group analysis. Our criterion of selection regarding these essays was to privilege what we call the first group analytic period, where one can follow the origin and evolution of group analysis and its fundamentals through the concepts of social images, social unconscious, social neurosis, transgenerational and transpersonal processes, along with the handling of technique and of therapeutic factors.

More particularly, these essays are of undeniable topicality and relevance, because of the richness and originality of the themes developed, in both the psychoanalytic field and in the group analytic one, which are still open as an object of study, within which we can mention:

- in the "preconscious phase", the *principle of primary identification* during prenatal life and the early months of life, a concept that

Burrow has connected with the theoretical–clinical study of neurosis (1914a), of narcissism, of homosexuality (1917a), of incest (1918), and, in the group analytic phase, of social neurosis (1926c);

- a relative concept of consciousness (1925a), and the consequent abrogation of both the absolutist conception, inherent in observation as reality's mirror, and of the psychoanalyst's neutrality;
- criticism of the individualistic basis of psychiatry and psychoanalysis through the concept of the *personal equation* (1926d), owing to its deforming effects on both interpretation and therapeutic process;
- interrelatedness as fundamental to the group analytic perspective, relating both to the social conception of the human being and to the psychopathology, along with its consequent feedback on the psychotherapeutic practice, not only on the group setting, but also on the dyadic one, first of all via the relational conception of *transference* (1927c) and *resistances* (1927d);
- the concept of *social images* (1924) as raw material of the prejudice and conflict expressed at individual, interpersonal, and social level, to which is strictly connected the concept of the *social unconscious*;
- the *questioning of so called "normality"* (1930) and the formulation of the concept of *social neurosis* (1926c) as an illness unconsciously shared between individual and society.

The psychoanalytic period: from drives to relationships

Who was Trigant Burrow? How did he come to psychoanalysis? What was his pathway and the motivation that brought him from psychoanalysis to group analysis?

Contemporaneous with Freud and Jung, Trigant Burrow (1875–1950) was among those psychoanalysts that, in 1911, together with Ernest Jones and others, founded the American Psychoanalytical Association (APA),[4] where he held important positions and became its president in the year 1925–1926. With his numerous works, he actively contributed to the introduction and spread of psychoanalysis in America, by means of journals issued by the American Psychological Association and the American Psychopathological Association (of which he was a member) and those on medicine, psychiatry, and human sciences in general.

His encounter with psychoanalysis was quite unusual. Burrow was working at the New York State Psychiatric Institute as a collaborator of A. Meyer—the pioneer of American psychiatry—with whom, in September 1909, he attended a performance at Hammerstein's Roof Gardens, with illustrious guests passing through New York, such as Freud, who, with Jung and Ferenczi, by invitation of Stanley Hall, had come to America for the first time in order to give the famous "Five lectures on psychoanalysis" at the Worchester Clark University. According to Cesare Musatti (1977) "such an event did mark the beginning of the international diffusion of psychoanalysis" (p. xi). During the intermission, Burrow and Meyer were introduced by A. A. Brill to Freud and to the other two guests. Burrow had a sudden inspiration, so that, at the end of the performance, he had already decided on his training in psychoanalysis and arranged his analysis with Jung, at that time Freud's favourite disciple, his designated heir.

That is why, in September 1909, Burrow, at thirty-four years old, together with his family (his wife and two children), left New York for Zurich, where they stayed for one year, paying for it through selling some assets he inherited from his father. He returned from Europe in the autumn of 1910 (Burrow, 1958).

Burrow as a psychoanalyst

It is worthwhile to say a few words on Burrow's psychoanalytic training and attitude as a psychoanalyst in order to try to dispel suspicions, insinuations, and misinterpretations with regard to these issues.

Taking as an apt example the incorrect conclusions Richard Crocket (1999) drew about the duration and the validity of the analysis Burrow underwent with Jung, one finds a plain contradiction to them in several of Burrow's letters to his mother (Burrow, 1958), in which he furnishes details about it and gives precise information on the procedure of his psychoanalytic training and education as a whole.

Besides his attendance with Jung and other colleagues at occasional medical meetings, Burrow was engaged, together with the American psychiatrist August Hoch and two other disciples, in an intensive study of psychoanalysis: "Much of time, of course is actually spent with Jung, and then there is an enormous amount of reading to be done—all in German—and so I seem quite cramped for time" (letter of 21 November 1909, p. 27).

The reading was interspersed by Jung's interesting and winning lectures, by which Burrow was entranced:

> I sat spell-bound during the entire conference held in his esthetic study overlooking the beautiful Zürich Lake. Our next meeting was called for this afternoon at 5:00. . . . On our arrival Dr. Jung suggested that we take our talk out on the water. We were quick to agree to the suggestion and a moment later found us sailing across the lake while Jung descanted upon the psychology of various psychoses. It was very interesting listening to this wonderful man relating with its characteristic ardor his theories and discoveries in the realm of his interest. . . . *I believe it is to be the year of my life.* (Burrow, 1958, p. 24, our italics; letter of 8 October 1909)

We can also see Jung's appreciation of Burrow as a disciple:

> Jung . . . also said a thing that delighted and encouraged me very much—that he had early recognized in me a readiness to grasp his psychology, that my questions showed my aptitude for this method and teaching." (Burrow, 1958, p. 26; letter of 27 October 1909)

It was during his stay in Zurich that he wrote his first article on psychoanalysis, "Freud's psychology in its relation to the neuroses" (Burrow, 1911), in which he gave "some account of Freud's and Jung's psychoanalytic method" and which he read to Jung who was "much pleased with it" (Burrow, 1958, pp. 30, 34).

About the project of his own analysis, which, in Jung's words, "would be the greatest assistance to me in handling others", it was a depressive reaction Burrow felt "out of all proportion to the *exciting* cause" that induced him to initiate it. But it is noteworthy to specify that, although with Jung many aspects of the setting evolved with respect to the early days of psychoanalysis, there exists no doubt about its rigour and adherence to the basic analytic criteria, as Burrow himself had communicated to his mother:

> I resolved to go to Jung and he said immediately that the trouble lay deeper and that he agreed with me and recommended treatment. *So I*

> *am going to his office an hour each day*, and hope to be greatly benefitted after his analysis and psychotherapy. (Burrow, 1958, p. 26, our italics; letter of 27 October 1909)

In this connection, Juan Campos (1992), who also studied Burrow in depth, placed a high value on Burrow's psychoanalytic training by underlining that

> Trigant Burrow was the first native American psychoanalyst to practice psychoanalysis in America and to be able to do so, the first one also to subject himself to a didactic analysis—five times a week with Jung in Zurich between 1909–1910. (p. 3)

Furthermore, according to Burrow's own descriptions of his year in Zurich, another singular aspect about Jung's behaviour style calls for our attention: although rigorous in his teachings, as a training analyst he appears to be far from both the rigidity of the setting and the analytic neutrality prescribed by the Freudian technique, being very empathic, both outside the context of sessions and in his formal teaching: "Dr. Jung this afternoon introduced me to his wife who also speaks English and he has invited us to call" (Burrow, 1958, p. 24). And it seemed that Burrow met with Jung independently of his role as a training analyst, just for leisure: "This afternoon Dr. Jung and I went to a café together as we often do. We all went for a sail" (p. 27).

Therefore, Crocket's (1999, p. 287) under-evaluation of Burrow's psychoanalytic training, according to which his "Jungian 'analysis' . . . amounted to a 3–4-month visit to Zurich in 1909 or 1910" and was limited to "long walks with Jung" in order to discuss "ideas current at that time", is quite misleading. Moreover, Crocket's supposition that Burrow "gave up his membership" of the American Psychoanalytic Association is groundless, since Burrow was expelled in 1932 because of his social conception of the human being. And, given that the "first group analytic period" should be distinguished by the second one, which constitutes a development, contrary to Crocket, we maintain that people "in group analytic practice" ought to be interested in Burrow's ideas not "only in an academic or historical context", but also and above all in his writings of the 1920s, where he laid the foundations of group analysis, either in its theoretical structure or its methodology. Curiously enough, most of them are very similar to

Foulkes's, even if the latter's are without Burrow's rigour. Through the knowledge they disseminate, one may realise that Burrow still has much to say to us about today's complex problems, as is evident in his psychoanalytic and group analytic essays published here.

In the face of such frequent misunderstandings, we are inclined to think that perhaps Crocket, like many other group analysts, lacks much information due to the difficulty of finding all Burrow's original writings. However, he has the merit of picking up Burrow from Foulkes's very scant references and of recognising being influenced by "his systematisations" (p. 287).

And what about Burrow as a psychoanalyst? Besides being one of the first American psychoanalysts to undergo his training in Europe, no less with Jung himself, before introducing group analysis, during the 1910s and the early 1920s, he practised psychoanalysis for many years either in private practice or in the Phipps Psychiatry Clinic School of Medicine directed by Adolf Meyer. Between 1911 and 1927, he made a remarkable contribution to psychoanalysis through his twenty-four psychoanalytic papers on various subjects, both theory and technique; some of them were sent to Freud, who categorically rejected Burrow's thesis (see "Censorship and ostracism of the psychoanalytic orthdoxy", below). And yet, notwithstanding the orthodoxy's obstructionism, there were some American psychoanalysts who were sympathetic to Burrow's views. For example, MacCurdy (1922), an APA founder member, dedicated a chapter of his book *Problems in Dynamic Psychology* to a basic concept of Burrow's by titling it "The primary subjective phase of Burrow", and Oberndorf (1927), in his outline of American psychoanalytic history, emphasised Burrow's distinguished and fundamental contribution to the principle of "the primary identification of the infant with the mother".

Moreover, as shown in his book of selected letters (Burrow, 1958), it was Burrow's lifelong professional habit to contribute to enriching exchanges of writings and to correspond with outstanding students belonging to various scientific disciplines, including, to name a few, W. B. Cannon, G. E. Coghill, J. Dewey, L. K. Frank, K. Goldstein, C. J. Herrick, A. Korzybsky, C. R. Rogers, L. Von Bertanlanffy, and G. B. Watson. Furthermore, in *Science and Man's Behavior*, Burrow (1953) interlaced a debate on human behaviour with twenty-nine eminent scientists in the fields of psychology, philosophy, physics, physiology, psychiatry, neurology, medical sciences, anthropology, and sociology, feeling that "the exchange of views contributed much toward the fuller formulation of his position" (W. E. Galt, 1953, p. 2).

In the light of the data mentioned above, we cannot deny that Burrow's credentials as a psychoanalyst were exceptional. In fact, we are faced with a "giant figure", as Ackerman (1964) stated.

In short, from the letters to his mother, Burrow's enthusiasm for what he called "the new psychology" emerges clearly, particularly the high esteem he held for Jung, whom he considered a "brilliant psychologist" and a "most picturesque personality" (Burrow, 1958, p. 24).

Back in America, Burrow devoted himself with the utmost care and trust to psychoanalytic practice, but the question about the efficacy of Freudian instinct theory became more and more insistent. What spurred his shift from an enthusiastic attitude for Freud's theory to such growing disappointment? It is Burrow himself who shows us its evolution:

> Yet, this factor of denied desire, of repressed libido, however hospitable a latitude was given it in Freud's interpretation, did not appear to me the whole account of things. Though it seemed to explain much that had long been puzzling in the behavior of the neurotic personality, it seemed also to leave out of reckoning much that was equally significant. The situation was not at first clear to me. (Burrow, 1964, p. 2)

What was overlooked in the Freudian approach that Burrow thought was "significant"? In his own writings, years later, he gave the clear-cut explanation that, in his psychoanalytic practice, he was soon led to pay attention to social factors with which the individual interacts through the following unequivocal assertion: "*almost from the outset of my work in psychoanalysis I became interested in what seemed to me the social implications of the neurosis*" (Burrow, 1958, p. 559, our italics. Letter to W. L. Phillips, 4 March, par. 8)

Ackerman (1964) commented that Burrow, from early on in his psychoanalytic practice, "was convinced that something was wrong, something was missing" in assigning the neurotic and mental disorders to the isolated individual; thus, he arrived at the conclusion that "the neurosis of society is primary" while "the neurosis of the individual is secondary". Such a concept is firmly linked to the statement that "normality must be distinguished from health" (p. viii). Ackerman, who, with Max Rosenbaum, is one of the few who has thoroughly studied Burrow's work, emphasised, "He was a prime founder of the culture-personality school of thought. In his original distinction between normality and health, he opened a vast area of investigation of the relation between human values and mental health" (p. x).

Burrow's cultural and professional matrix

What were the reasons that led Burrow, from the beginning of his psychoanalytic practice, to assign a fundamental role in the individual's development to the environment? What was his cultural and professional background before moving towards psychoanalysis?

In this connection, we should turn to the history of human sciences. Pines (1991) provides a valuable historical perspective of the European context of thought that prepared the ground for the matrix of group analysis. However, it seems that such a cultural context did not prove sufficiently meaningful to Foulkes to induce him to experiment earlier with those ideas, as it seems that it was only in the 1940s, in Exeter, that he took such a decision.

Further, as we shall see later, since he had read some of Burrow's papers in the 1920s, we might ask why he waited for over two decades (Foulkes, 1948) before putting them into practice (E. Gatti Pertegato & G. O. Pertegato, 1995).

We should consider, too, that at the time of Pines' analysis, Burrow was still mostly in the shadows, especially in Europe. Furthermore, owing to Foulkes's very vague statements about the relation of his work to that of Burrow, on the one hand, and to the fact that he would not miss any opportunity to underline that group analysis was first introduced by himself (1948, 1964, 1975) on the other hand, one was rather prevented from knowing whether a few elements of doubt crossed his mind or from knowing more about such vicissitudes through investigating them.

However, notwithstanding the rather diffused belief facing Burrow's group analytic writings, one cannot deny the reality that the matrix of group analysis sprang from the USA and that Foulkes introduced it in the UK, but omitted to clearly quote its founder. As Abse (1990) wrote, "Burrow's views stimulated Foulkes to consider the possibility of group analysis as a means of treatment, so that *the inception of group analysis in the U.S.A. found in him a transatlantic response*" (p. 10, our italics).

Regarding the USA's cultural context, despite appearances, American people's attention to the environment is deep-rooted in its history. Max Rosenbaum and Milton Berger (1963) report:

> Philosophical tradition in the United States stresses the ethic of individual responsibility, with, historically, little emphasis on the group and its relationship to the individual. Nevertheless, the country is in fact group oriented. (p. 1)

It is well known that although the pioneers did extol the rights of the individual, the realisation of their ambitious projects was asking for "group functioning". Furthermore, owing to the subsequent impact of industrialisation and new waves of immigration, "the individualistic forms of living were supplanted by highly organised forms of group living". It follows that the students of human behaviour were compelled to study the individual in his own group or community. For example, an eminent figure was John Dewey (1859–1952), philosopher, pedagogue, and social theorist, who, in the course of time, exchanged letters with Burrow (1958). His "philosophy of experience" brought him to elaborate a deep reflection on the essentially social nature of human behaviour, based on the "dynamic relationship between environment and human organism". Such a concept sounds as though it was affected by pragmatism, brought in by C. S. Peirce and developed by William James, who spread it at a worldwide level, so that it became one of the main currents of thought in the first years of the twentieth century (Enciclopedia Europea, 1976).

According to Rosenbaum and Berger (1963, p. 2), group psychotherapy is supposed to be a consequence of the pragmatism of American psychiatry, which appeared willing to explore any new and possibly helpful technique. Even though Burrow might be in some way influenced by it, his primary motivation towards group analysis was not caused by merely technical and applicative issues, as we shall see. Instead, it was due to his break with the individualistic imprint of psychoanalytic theory and practice, owing to his feeling of failure (1926b) and the resulting urge to conduct research aimed at gaining a comprehensive knowledge of man's nature, that is, of his relationships with the environment, conflict, and behaviour disorders.

Burrow himself did not hesitate (1930) to reveal the presuppositions that were the origin of his thinking and to acknowledge the great influence on him of Adolf Meyer, with whom he had collaborated at Phipps Psychiatric Clinic, and who had trained generations of psychiatrists to strictly follow, in their clinical practice, the observation of the individual as inseparable from his own environment. The school of thought based upon Meyer's theoretical orientation "stressed the integration mechanisms of the biological, the psychological and the social experiences" (Reber, 1985).

This is also confirmed by Burrow's writings included in this book:

> In my very first acquaintance with the teaching of Adolf Meyer some twenty years ago, what impressed me was the fact that here was the application of definite principles of biology to mental and social disharmonies. In Meyer's study of the individual patient, *it was not the individual alone that he saw before him, but a socially integrated situation that related the individual to the community as a whole*. The entire impetus of the school of psychiatry that originated with Meyer . . . lies precisely in the generic and inclusive inferences derived from the specific data under observation. . . .
>
> When, under the stimulus of Meyer, I undertook the study and the application of psychoanalysis to the problems of individual adjustment, it was inevitable that I should apply to the analytic field, with its latent manifestations of man's consciousness, the same underlying principles I had learned from Meyer. (Burrow, 1930, pp. 113–114, our italics)

However, he then went *beyond* the teachings of his masters, Meyer and Freud, through their development by means of the *application of psychoanalytic principles to the group*, and this marks his *passage from psychoanalysis to group analysis*:

> With my associates I came to realize the necessity of applying under conditions of actual laboratory or group analysis the methods which Freud had developed in the treatment of individuals. The outcome of our work has been the gradual recognition of the necessity to base the processes of our observation upon methods involving a social or consensual technique that is as definite of that of the laboratories of objective biology. (Burrow, 1926a, p. 347)

It took several years of experimentation with a variety of groups to get to the theoretical elaboration of group analysis, which was considered both as a social conception of the human being, of the conflict, of the psychopathology, and as a therapeutic and research tool. He himself clarified that

> for several years I have, in association with others, been daily occupied with the practical observation of these interreactions as they are found to occur under the experimental conditions of actual group setting. (Burrow, 1928b, p. 198, note)

In short, it clearly emerges that, following his encounter with psychoanalysis, Burrow's innovative contribution consists, first, in having applied "those factors of integration which Dr Meyer has for so long emphasized" to the psychoanalytic procedure and, successively, in having been driven to test them in the group setting, developing them on the basis of the relativity of observation as well, borrowed from Einstein's theory of relativity (Burrow, 1925a). Thus, we can deduce that, moved by his own cultural and professional matrix, integrated with the Freudian one, Burrow began to consider, in a dissimilar way to Freud, the data arising from his psychoanalytic practice, coming then, over the years, to the formulation of the *social basis of human consciousness as an original datum* (Burrow, 1927a; E. Gatti Pertegato, 2001a).

Therefore, the importance Burrow attached to the role of environmental factors for the individual's development and its distortions is rooted in the cultural excitements of his time and in his training and psychiatric experience, when he was working closely with Meyer, the "father of the American psychiatry". Nothing can be born from nothing. How fitting is Goethe's maxim that one gets everything from his own fathers should be developed creatively. In fact, it reflects exactly Burrow's attitude towards his own "fathers", first Meyer, and then Freud, by building on the basis of what he inherited from them.

But, as happens in the parent–child relationship, so in the cultural, professional, and institutional fields; the "fathers" do not always accept the necessary separation and foster the consequent self-creativity of their disciples or collaborators, instead inducing them to conformism, to the reproduction of their "word", otherwise the punishment is expulsion, as Burrow himself experienced. The opposite could also happen, that is, the sons could refuse more or less categorically what is passed on by their fathers, rather than based upon their own subjective and creative potentialities, in a virtual transgenerational chain, thus transforming it and contributing to the growth and evolution of knowledge and culture. These dynamics are emblematic of the history of psychoanalysis and also of group analysis.

At the beginning there was . . . the relationship

Burrow's theoretical–technical thinking marks a crucial turning point in psychoanalysis, owing to the emphasis put on the significant role of the environment, starting from the primary one—represented not only by the mother, but also by the father and the professional and educational figures moving around the unborn and the newborn child.

Already, in 1913, in "Psychoanalysis and life", an unpublished paper included in this book, Burrow shows that he had a unitary idea of the human being, as opposed to any dualisms, such as mind–body, nature–culture. As we shall see, he postulates in the pre-natal life the existence of a "preconscious subjective phase" which constitutes the matrix of consciousness.

The term "matrix" was used first by Burrow (1913) very shortly after the beginning of his activity as a psychoanalyst, to focus on—in both pre-natal and very early postnatal life—a primary *subjective* phase he called the *preconscious mode,* since not only does it precede the formation of consciousness, but it also becomes its integral part. In such a phase, the *preconscious mode* is characterised by the *primary identification of the infant with the mother,* which is developed from the physiological continuity of the vital processes between mother and child, along with the feelings and reactions that the unborn child and the infant are experiencing.

It is glaringly obvious that, through such an innovative formulation, Burrow anticipated the concept of the "proto-mental system" posited by Bion (1961)—even if it conveys a somewhat different meaning—and of "psyche–soma", a theory of Winnicott's (1954) which is very similar to that of Burrow. Oberndorf (1953), historian of American psychoanalysis, in referring to the psychoanalysts who made an outstanding American contribution before 1920, mentioned "Trigant Burrow's emphasis of a 'primary *subjective* phase' in the infant chronologically preceding the Oedipus situation" (pp. 132–133), which, in Freud's theory, takes place in the objective phase of consciousness.

Such a primary affective phase—*not conflictual and pre-sexual*—is considered crucial in that it constitutes the "biological matrix" of subsequent development. In fact, here is set "the preconscious basis of the human experience" (Burrow, 1964), which represents the prototype of relationships with the world, both in the direction of a subjective, creative approach and of its encroachment, when, because of the environmental pressures, the "social image" substitutes for the individual's "reality". In this case, the result can only be the dissociation and the subsequent development of a "false identity", which Burrow named "I-Persona",[5] which causes the individual to imitate the induced relational modes, so that

> the judgment of the individual is not, as we suppose, the natural expression of a spontaneous idea, but it is the reflection of the social systematization about him that he has unconsciously come to embody. Thus the individual is not sponsor of the idea for which he is spokesman, but rather he is unconsciously sponsored by it. Instead of actuating his ideas, he is actuated by them. And not only the individual but the collective personality is rendered equally servile to such unconscious systematizations. (Burrow, 1926c, p. 306)

As a consequence, "a profound cleavage develops both within the organism and between the organism and the physical and social environment" (Gilden, 1999, p. 258).

It is impressive how Burrow (1928a) described in detail the genesis, phases, and modalities of the *process of dissociation*, along with its repercussions, as a consequence of the transmission of social images from the mother environment to the baby, starting from his early development.

> The child is about to reach out with all his feeling, all his interest toward the object, . . . the wholly *spontaneous gesture* toward the object is suddenly checked in the child and it is conveyed to him . . . that this is naughty, this is taboo. He must not. Gradually the objects of the child's universe, gradually every impulse of the child's life comes to be measured in the light of this implied code. (p. 11, our italics)

Thus, in such a superimposition of the environment, there is the origin of compliance, as it will "win love or approval", and the concomitant loss of the individual's spontaneous behaviour. Burrow's comment is incisive: this *"is not a healthy gesture"* because it happens *"under restriction,* [it is] *dominated by fear,* [it is] *subject to a division"* (Burrow, 1928a, p. 12; E. Gatti Pertegato & G. O. Pertegato, 2006b, our italics).

Winnicott—in whom several conceptual affinities seem to accord closely with Burrow (E. Gatti Pertegato, 2009a)—would say that *"the mind dominates the psyche-soma"*, so that the "true-self" remains split off from the living experience and there develops a "false-self" that deprives the individual of both spontaneity and creative potentiality (E. Gatti Pertegato, 1987[1994]; Winnicott, 1954, 1960, our italics).

Diego Napolitani (1987), inspired by such theories, identified the two fundamental poles of the individual's identity, based upon the interaction with his environment, whose pathogenic outcome is the individual's *subjugation* to environmental models, instead of being the *author* of his own development, thus losing, partially or completely, his conceptive–creative attitude towards the world. *Burrow would say that social images substitute for individual's authentic reality.*

It follows that, according to Burrow's perspective, the conflict shows an interrelational connotation and it is secondary to the environmental pressures that induce a distorted development. In such an eventuality, the individual can only be a *"potential artist"* (Burrow, 1913, our italics) because, in his initial relationships with the world, he was unable to express his original creative impulse, that is, his *spontaneous gesture,* remaining more or less conditioned. Above all, in the earlier phases, the quality of individual–environment interactions is a determining factor in allowing or blocking the capacity to establish a subjective, constructive relationship with the world. But also, in the intercourse of subsequent life, it could interfere with the individual's ability to cope with the imposition of serious life adversities. Such a concept is completely different from the Freudian individualistic formulation concerned with instincts, according to which the conflict has intrapsychic origins, being the result of their vicissitudes.

Antithetical to that vision (that ended by prevailing over the relational intuitions, yet present here and there within Freudian work, from the so-called theory of sexual trauma to *Group Psychology and the Analysis of the Ego* (Freud, 1921c)) in Burrow's work, we are faced with a *historical relational perspective*: where the individual is a social being interacting from the beginning with his significant environment that, if it is not *respectful* of his own subjectivity and initiative—that is, the "spontaneous gesture"—mortifies its intrinsic tendency to opening to the world in his own personal way, hence interfering with the emerging of his own authentic potentialities, paving the way to conflict and distorted relational modes, neurosis and psychosis included.

We can also consider an incontrovertible confirmation of the strict interdependency between biological–psychological and social processes, more and more substantiated by the neurosciences, among them the important researches by Edelman (2006) and Kandell (2005), who heartily wish for a dialogue with the human sciences in general and psychoanalysis in particular.

The "scientifically grounded synthesis" of the vast neuroscientific researches presented by the psychiatrist Daniel Siegel (1999), emphasised that the biologic determinism, that is, "a view of psychiatric disorders as a result of biochemical processes, most of which are genetically determined and little influenced by experience", was no longer corroborated, in that

> the recent findings of neural science in fact point to just the opposite: Interactions with the environment, especially, with other people directly shape the development of the brain's structure and functions. . . . Although it is important to be aware of the significant and very real contributions of genetic and constitutional factors to the outcome of the development, it is equally crucial that we examine what in fact is known, how experience shapes development. (Siegel, 1999, pp. x–xi)

In short, the keyword seems to be *interaction* between brain, mind, and experience, so that Siegel (1999) speaks of "social brain" (p. xiv). The complexity of the human mind, then, requires an approach based upon an interdisciplinary comparison and the overcoming of the rigid contrapositions of mind *vs.* body, nature *vs.* culture, and of the consequent dichotomous conceptions either in biology or psychology.

Relationship, sexuality, and sex

At this point, if the individual is constitutively a social being, what is the meaning of the sexuality that, in Freudian theory, has a basic role? In this respect, Burrow (1926b) himself in the end came to state that his altered conception entailed "a distinct departure from the accepted psychoanalytic position" (p. 211). And to what cause, then, can the neurosis be traced?

As emerges from the early essay, "Notes with reference to Freud, Jung and Adler", included in this volume, Burrow (1917b) reports some interesting details on either the motive for his disagreement about sexual repression as a basic agent in the conflict and psychopathology, or his view on this topic emerging from his clinical practice. He was in agreement with Jung on the existence of a "primary presexual mode", that is, "a phase of consciousness which precedes the desire or the sexual phase", but he did not share the "non-continuity with the sexual mode" expressed in Jung's concept of "vital energy", in contrast with Freudian theory. On the contrary, Burrow considered his "conception of a presexual mode being not only not incompatible with Freud, but . . . a requisite correlate of his teaching"; as such it was seen as "a distinction that is based solely on a developmental difference" in respect to Freud's fundamental findings.

Yet, in spite of the fact that the psychoanalytic establishment was far from sharing Burrow's views, he firmly held his position and continued his researches, the outcome of which was "entirely at variance" with the prevailing psychoanalytic conception that "nervous disorders are the substitutive manifestation of a repressed sexual life" (Burrow, 1926b).

Actually, from the beginning, Burrow (1964) realised the weakness of such a perspective:

> The psychoanalytic conception of repressed libido as the sole element in neurotic disturbances failed, it seemed to me, to take account of evidences of another trend, that was revealed in the analysis of various types of patients. (p. 2).

Burrow considered Freud's observation about "sex as a content underlying the symbolic disguises of unconscious" to be correct, but stated that it "fails to include all the elements composing the human personality" (p. 3). Ackerman (1964), in referring to Burrow's position, expressed his conviction that Freud "by-passed a significant problem", illustrating it by a vivid metaphor:

> It seems to me he got derailed in his evaluation of some aspects of the sexual drive. Just as all is not gold that glitters, so, too, everything that looks like sex is not sex. I believe that Freud failed to read correctly

those kinds of human behaviors, in which sex is just a disguise of other motives. (p. xii)

Burrow's (1926b) objection concerned the relation of the two factors of the replacement and sexuality, as he clearly specified:

> I do not regard this replacement *primarily* a replacement for sexuality as we now know it. On the contrary sexuality . . . as manifested to-day amid the sophistications of civilization, is itself a replacement for the organic unit of personality arising naturally from the harmony functions that pertain biologically to the primary infant psyche. This original preconscious mode I regard as the matrix of personality. (p. 210, original italic)

Thus, Burrow, coming to the conclusion that "the repression is not the outcome of sex", but on the contrary "the sex is the result of the repression", reversed Freud's viewpoint. What drew him to make such a statement? Quite in agreement with Jung "that there is contained in dreams, as in life, a non-sexual clause", he writes,

> I think there is in life a factor that is preclusive of sex. I do not mean the repressive factor, exhibited in the censorship of social inhibition. This is a quite secondary, artificial proscription, reacting in response to an external agency. But I mean a primary and inherent non-sexual tendency, the biology of which is traceable to the *embryonic matrix of consciousness* represented by the *preconscious mode*." (Burrow 1917b, p.7, our italics)

Clearly showing that he would not be diverted by preconstituted theoretical restrictions, and rigorously following the data emerging from his own clinical experience instead, Burrow came to reckon that

> a patient *study of life*, such as it is given the psychoanalyst to pursue, *brings to light yet deeper-lying factors*, beside which the intense craving for self-satisfaction expressed in sex, notwithstanding its insatiate affirmation, is revealed as an anomalous exaggeration—a sporadic miscarriage of affectivity representing *the distortion of an originally harmonious principle of life*. (Burrow, 1917b, p. 7, our italics)

In Burrow's perspective (1964), then, we meet with this explicit and seemingly paradoxical formulation: "According to my thesis, man is primarily, genetically non-sexual", where, however, the word "sexual" should be interpreted in the accepted meaning of "an inherent urge toward the satisfaction of physical sensations for their own sake" (p. 40), consequently disjoined from relatedness and to the detriment of what he called the "originally harmonious principle of life" (Burrow, 1917b, p. 7), that is, of his own creativity and inherent social nature.

> The sexual repression which Freud has so rightly emphasized in individual neurotics is, I am convinced, quite secondary to this more general mood-interdiction within the *social* instinct of man. The pathological effect of this arbitrary social mood in repressing man's natural societal instinct is traceable throughout our social institutions everywhere. It is the position of group-analysis that the concurrence between this wide-spread social repression and the general social increase of insanity points to a definite causal relationship. (Burrow, 1928c, p. 15, original italics)

Therefore, the pathology takes root when the person's wholeness is undermined and deprived of the "social instinct" that allows the subjective development of his intrinsic potentialities through the interaction with the environment *vs.* all the more or less masked forms of hindrance, possessiveness, or dominance. This represents a watershed to Freud's position, since he assigned to sexuality a central function in the neuroses.

Further, it should be clarified that Burrow (1926b) made a clear-cut *distinction between sex and sexuality.* On what basis did he come to such a contraposition? By relying, as usual, on his psychoanalytic practice first and the group analytic one second, he could observe that

> the modern substitutions existing under the name of sexuality, whether repressed or indulged, are but a symptom of this organic denial of the inherent life of man. Sexuality is not only utterly unrelated to sex but it is intrinsically exclusive of sex. Sex is life. It is life in its deepest inherency. Sex is the spontaneous expression of a natural hunger. In the instinct of sex there is felt a yearning from the depth of man's soul for mateship and reproduction, while sexuality is the personal coveting of momentary satisfaction in mere superficial sensation. By sexuality then I mean something very different from sex. I mean the restless, obsessive, overstimulated quest for temporary self-gratification that everywhere masquerades as sex. (pp. 210–211)

And, coherently, in no uncertain terms, he asserted that the whole meaning of sexuality "is substitution, compensation, repression" (1926b, pp. 210–211).

Yet, since his early psychoanalytic writings, it has emerged that, more important than "sex or its vicarious palliations" that have become for the individual "the affirmation of existence", Burrow (1917b) thought that "*there is something deeper still, more native to man, than all this*". He referred to "the primacy of relatedness" springing out of the preconscious mode, that is, the "non-conflicting" subjective phase of the primary consciousness, which, through its creative and progressive interaction with the objective world, is expressed in the bond between the human beings, in the solidarity, in the urge to search and strive for "the pursuit of common good" (p. 8, our italics).

> It is this quality of harmoniousness and unity inherent in the social aims of man that is, it seems to me, the strongest principle of man's consciousness. *This it is that men have called love.* This, it seems to me, is *the true affirmation of life* and its prototype is the harmonious principle of the preconscious. (p. 8, our italics)

Indeed, Burrow's conception of the preconscious mode—being the matrix of the affectivity and subjectivity preceding consciousness but always interacting with it—was the cornerstone of his psychoanalytic and group analytic researches, according to which it could not be ousted by the mind or be overwhelmed by sexuality with impunity for the human being.

Furthermore, besides questioning the importance assigned by classical psychoanalysis to sexuality in the individual's development, from Burrow's work it emerges that aggression—the other instinct identified by Freud as the basis of his drive theory—is secondary to environment pressures.

Also with reference to aggression, it is evident that Burrow anticipated Winnicott (1950), who considered it a reaction to impingement on the part of the environment.

But Burrow (1914b) goes beyond that by singling out the conflict even in what is called "normality" and, as mentioned before, he does not deem it a criterion of health, because, compared to the neurotic,

> society is hysterical too. Society has its elaborate system of defence-mechanisms, its equivocations and metonymies. The difference is that

> society's counterfeits possesses the advantage of universal currency, and so the record of its frailties is set down under the name of *custom* rather than *pathology*. (p. 6, our italics)

That was a crucial point he would return to and develop in 1930 in "The so-called 'normal' social relationships expressed in the individual and in the group, and their bearing on the problems of neurotic disharmonies" (herein included) and that he faces constantly in his writings, being, along with conflict, the focus of his psychoanalytical and group analytical research. We find a significant confirmation in a letter that appeared in his posthumously published book, *Science and Man's Behavior* (1953), which Burrow addressed in 1948 to a group of eminent students belonging to various fields of science, in order to instigate with them a debate on his theses just before they became the subject of his book *The Neurosis of Man* (1950). In his "invitation to scientists", he emphasised:

> For years my analytic quarry has been the state of mind fallaciously yet universally known as 'normality'—the social reaction-average of an artificially conditioned species. For our medical investigations showed that abnormal processes motivate also the so-called 'normal' behaviour of man. They indicated the extent to which a 'social neurosis' now dominates human motives and institutions. (p. 15)

In short, we are faced with a revolutionary theory that postulates a *well defined shift from drive to relationship* that is not ineluctably weighed down with conflict. In fact, Burrow (1926a, p. 349) assumes the existence of a "common substrate of feelings and reactions" that ties together human beings; therefore, co-operation *is primary compared to conflict and division*, even if the "social reaction-average, arbitrarily called *normality* tends to obscure it".

Ackerman (1964), in his remarkable analysis presented in his foreword to Burrow's posthumously published book, *The Preconscious Foundations of Human Experience* (1964), points out,

> Steadily, the evidence mounts in biology, ethology, social psychology, anthropology, and psychiatry to substantiate Burrow's main theses of a primary biosocial union, a fundamental principle of cooperation in human relations. Burrow was correct in alleging that, in the evolution of society, this principle has somewhere been pathogenically aborted and derailed. (pp. xi–xii)

The writer Thomas Merton (1955), greatly emphasised man's interconnectedness *vs.* isolation. In his most famous book *No Man Is an Island*, he expressed his deep conviction that nobody can exist on his own by commenting on and echoing a famous passage by the poet John Donne in *Meditations*, from which Merton's book's title is drawn:

> Only when we see ourselves in our true human context, as members of a race which is intended to be one organism and "one body", will we begin to understand the positive importance not only of the successes but of the failures and accident in our lives.
>
> Every other man is a piece of myself, for I am a part and a member of mankind. . . . (p. xii)
>
> Nothing at all makes sense, unless we admit, with John Donne, that: "No man is an island, entire in itself; every man is a piece of a continent, a part of the main" (p. xxiii).

The social underlying thread connecting Burrow, Binswanger, and Fabrizio Napolitani

At first sight, it might be seen as hazardous to relate Burrow's group analytic perspective to Ludwig Binswanger's (1955) anthropological–phenomenological one, so different are the respective initial theoretical references, the ambit of their clinical experiences and therapeutic methods, but we will see that, in some aspects, this is to judge only by appearances. And what has Fabrizio Napolitani got to do with either of them? Well, he is undoubtedly connected to them, having introduced a pioneering group therapeutic method in Binswanger's psychiatric clinic.

Considering that delving into the correlations between Burrow's and Binswanger's research is not the aim of our work, nevertheless, some general characteristics should be taken into account: in fact, what is common is their strong interest in psychoanalysis, and also their striving after an end that could impart rigorous foundations to human sciences, where the individual should not be considered as a separate unit from his own world, but in strict interaction with it.

But how might they be reciprocally connected? Burrow at first, and Binswanger later on, although attracted by psychoanalysis, were, however, unsatisfied with both its theoretical formulation and its method, focused as it was upon an objectifying and individualistic basis. Thus, they dedicated themselves to a passionate and painstaking search for the social foundations of human consciousness, not with the aim of opposing psychoanalysis or of building up a school of their own, but only with the aim of contributing to its development through a *constructive critique* that would set free both psychoanalysis and psychiatry from the dualistic conception of the physical sciences based upon the split of mind *vs.* body, subject *vs.* object, individual *vs.* his own environment.

Thanks to the introduction of some changes connected to the relational conception of the psychotherapeutic situation, Burrow practised psychoanalysis for several years until 1918. Binswanger (1956) courageously brought it into his psychiatric clinic—The Sanatorium Bellevue at Kreutzlingen (Switzerland)—raising hostile reactions on the part of German psychiatrists, who branded his decision a "death sentence" for the Institute (p. 37, translated for this edition). This did not happen at all, but, as Binswanger himself wrote, "it took ten years of hard work and disappointments" to realise the limits of psychoanalysis, which induced him to adopt—for a few patients only—what he called "a psychotherapy led according to a psychoanalytic point of view", resolutely sticking to his idea of psychoanalysis as "a branch of psychiatry" (Binswanger, 1956, p. 30, translated for this edition). Although following different routes, the respective theoretical–methodological elaborations do then show several points of contact. Burrow, through his study of the phenomenology of the psychoanalytic setting at first, and subsequently by years of group experimentation, or "laboratory method" (1926a), will arrive at the formulation of "man's instinctive group principle" as the social basis of consciousness and the foundation of group analysis, according to which the individual cannot be dissociated from his own environment.

Binswanger, with one interested, yet critical, eye toward psychoanalysis and the other toward Husserl's phenomenological philosophy (descriptive at first and transcendental later on), and to Heidegger's existential one, although the influence of either one or the other prevailed at different stages, tested and reworked them in a dialectical mode through his psychiatric practice (Borgna, 1990). So, he laid down the basis of anthropo-analysis, according to which "psychology never deals with a person deprived of his own world" (Binswanger, 1955, p. 95, translated for this edition), coming to state, in a powerful and significant metaphor, that the split between subject and object, introduced by Descartes and adopted until recent years by science, is "the cancer of every psychology" (1946, 1973, p. 22, translated for this edition).

As for Burrow (1913), he qualified as a "potential artist" the individual who, in consequence of environmental impingements, was unable to express, in his relationships with the world, his subjectiveness, instead assimilating inauthentic, alienated relational modes, the source of ailment and pathology.

As far as Binswanger (1944) is concerned, in *The Case of Ellen West*, who had problems with food all her life, he traced the origin of such a disorder to the fact that "since the beginning, the construction of her own world had been realised in sharp contraposition to the world of coexistence", that is, "to those persons who tried to be opposed to Ellen's singularity" (pp. 60–61, translated for this edition). In *Delirium* (1965), Binswanger's last work, he stated that in schizophrenia the patient's "being-in-the-world" is expressed by "his/her *being at the mercy of or enslaved*" to others; consequently he/she "cannot any more realise himself/herself authentically as a Self" (pp. 13–15, original italics, translated for this edition). In this failure, he identifies "a defect of transcendence" representing the unique mode of a possible existence.

As Borgna specified (1994), psychotic experiences are nothing other than "*distorted* modes of 'being-in-the-world'", or "disorders of communication" in which there can be traced their "meaning's concatenations", certainly not the "anarchic aggregations of symptomatology" (p. 13).

On the basis of such few but significant remarks, it seems apt to deduce that Burrow's group analytic perspective, considered in its underlying philosophic presuppositions, foresees, albeit with different modulations and language, the anthropologic–phenomenological approach that was later introduced into the psychiatric ambit by Binswanger's (1955) existential or anthropo-analysis. Both of them were dedicated passionately to the investigation and understanding of the pathologic "being in the world" in favour of an authentic one, distinct and yet connected by interpersonal relations. William Galt (1964), one of Burrow's closest collaborators, in referring to the "preconscious mode" as a matrix of the social consciousness and mentioning Binswanger, provides an authoritative confirmation of such relation: "His emphasis on this deeply positive and constructive element in man's consciousness and behavior anticipated the conceptions presented more recently by some exponent of existential psychiatry (Binswanger)" (Galt, 1964, p. xvii).

Last, but not least, there is something more to say in connection with this. We cannot fail to mention the important meeting between Ludwig Binswanger and Fabrizio Napolitani, at the end of 1957 in Kreuzlingen, Switzerland, whose purpose—contrary to what Valeria Babini (2009a,b) wrote in her historical works—was not about his training, which he had undergone in Brazil, but about his collaboration with Binswanger, based both on group techniques, to which he had had recourse in Claudio De Araujo Lima's Psychiatric Clinic, and on his knowledge of Binswanger's thought, which strongly appealed to him (Cuomo, 1996).

At that time, as F. Napolitani (1985–1986) himself reports, he could rely on ten years of experience regarding "intense, although diversified, professional experiences" ranging from "the management of group situations in traditional, closed psychiatric departments to those made by patients and operators of therapeutic communities" and "from the conduction of therapeutic groups in psychiatric outpatient departments, to those constituted by groups of patients in the private practice" (p. 135).

That meeting would act as a further, albeit indirect, link with Burrow's group perspective, since it would prove decisive for the introduction of innovative community and group techniques in the therapy of psychotic patients.

In fact, as reported by Cuomo (1996), who was his closest collaborator and at present is still continuing and developing his thinking and methodology (2009), Binswanger immediately accepted F. Napolitani's project, which took shape in 1958 as a result of his appointment as head of the Villa Landegg department of Binswanger's Psychiatric Clinic, directed by himself. Within a few months, Napolitani (1961) transformed the department into a "psychiatric therapeutic community self-administered by patients", who were called "guest-members". The isolation from the city context was eliminated, and, if permitted by their conditions, they could enjoy the liberty of going out by being "entrusted with the key to the house". It should be stressed that such a measure, as well as similar ones, was only applied after it had been discussed with the patients in group meetings.

Thanks to a flexibility respectful of each person's exigencies, in addition to group analytic sessions, there was the possibility of individual integrative psychotherapeutic interviews; moreover, all decisions were commonly agreed and taken during regularly scheduled community meetings. As a witness to the vitality and creativity of that unusual management, as well as the "committee for entertainment and cultural programmes", there was the so-called *Merle Curieux* (The Curious Blackbird), the house newspaper produced by those same guest-members, in which they could "freely express their opinions and criticisms of everything and everyone, including *their physicians*" (F. Napolitani, 1961, p. 108, original italics).

We would like to highlight the feature of total self-administration by patients, achieved by what F. Napolitani (1961) described as a "*special* therapeutic community", in that the psychiatrists stayed with patients, sharing a good part of their lives and eating with them, "with the absence of all other personnel whatsoever", in the hypothesis that this "might make possible an advance in the therapeutic effectiveness of such a community" (p. 108). In particular:

> Thus, in this unit *all* the tasks normally performed by the usual house and nursing personnel have been completely taken over by the patients and are performed only by themselves. . . . It might be important to mention that the patients are paid for their work at the end of each month. It is understandable that such a concrete economic recognition has the purpose of emphasising the importance and value of the patients' activities in the community. (p. 108, original italics)

It is also worthwhile reporting what F. Napolitani (1985–1986) himself pointed out about the prerequisites of *complete self-administration by patients*:

> Such innovation had been possible not only thanks to a systematic and composite socio-therapeutic program, but above all *thanks to the fact that the patients had their daily sessions of analytic group-psychotherapy and the psychiatric staff underwent special training groups.*[6] (p. 135, original italics)

It was the first experiment of that kind in a psychiatric institution, so that in a short time it became the longed for destination of psychiatrists, both from Italy and other countries, some of whom were allowed to stay there for a certain time, on approval of the patients' meeting, in order to learn from their own direct experience of the community and group psychotherapy techniques (Cuomo, 1996). Subsequently, Binswanger assigned to Napolitani the direction of another department, Villa Roberta. The high esteem in which he held F. Napolitani is shown also from the dedication written on his photograph in 1960: "To the great maestro Fabrizio, Ludwig Binswanger" (Cuomo, 2010)

Upon his return to Italy in 1963, Fabrizio Napolitani, on the basis of the same therapeutic criterion of "self-government" he had made use of in Villa Landegg, founded the Therapeutic Community of Rome, "a hospital whose therapeutic methods are based on the modern principles of Social Psychiatry and Psychoanalysis". It is noteworthy that, in Italy, it represented a *dynamic training centre in group analysis* for the various operators in the psychiatric and psychoanalytic field. The brochure of such a community[7] is indeed an extraordinary document, showing in detail its objectives, the range of the sociotherapeutic activities[8] and specific therapies, besides assistance to the patients' relatives and the "post-therapy outpatient's consultation".

It clearly emerges that the *humanisation* of the relationship of doctor–patient–institution is connected to the rigour of treatments: by psycho-pharmacological methods when required, although "reduced to the minimum necessary" by group analytic sessions and individual consultations, were they needed, potentiated by the community context that socialises patients and helps them to become self-responsible. Most of all, it was an approach to the person in its entirety, aiming at considering the mentally disturbed patients not as objects identified with their disease, but as subjects with the right to keep up their relationships with the outside world and their affective bonds.

From a historical point of view, it preceded the experimentation conducted in Italy by Franco Basaglia, who, in his capacity as director of the Gorizia Psychiatric Hospital, initiated in the autumn of 1964, based upon Maxwell Jones' model, "the constitution of the first 'therapeutic community' in a long-term patients' department"; in 1965–1966, the experiment was extended to the "major part of the department sub-systems" (Slavich, 1968). Nevertheless, no one was free to leave the hospital area (Corbellini & Jervis, 2008). Moreover, as Basaglia (1968) himself stated, his approach excluded "whichever group psychotherapy" and the experience of the therapeutic community that was "revealed ambiguous", so that, in the end, it resulted in "the first steps towards a *denial* of the mental hospital reality" which, starting from 1971, would be realised in Trieste, at the San Giovanni Psychiatric Hospital (Parmegiani & Zanetti, 2007).

F. Napolitani's innovative methodology of "self-administration by patients" attracted the keen interest of Maxwell Jones and Tom Main, who paid a visit to him in Rome in order to see personally the further developments of the therapeutic community (Cuomo, 2010) of which they were the pioneers and which "constitutes still nowadays a required point of reference for those who deal with therapeutic communities, family-houses, therapeutic daily centres" (Cuomo, 2006, p. 159) and, in any case, is a precious source from which one can get ideas and hints about the psychiatric patients' treatment in Mental Health Departments.

The social conception of consciousness and Binswanger's overture to group and community therapies in his clinic through F. Napolitani, represents a sort of underground social link connecting both of them to Burrow, a pioneer of group analysis and of an experimental community, the Lifwynn Foundation for Laboratory Research in Analytic and Social Psychiatry, which he established in 1927 with the aim of "carrying on the study of man as an integral part of man's community life" (Burrow, 1958, p. 172).

Moreover, a comparative study might fruitfully demonstrate integrations between Burrow's research on the primary phase of consciousness and its development, and that part of Binswanger's work that the deep analysis by Mario Galzigna (1994, pp. 49–50) indicates as "intrinsically incomplete", being historically the "daughter of the mental hospital institution". It follows that "the defective ways of the presence are described and known in their very least details" while the description of the passing from the "extended social network" to the "restricted social network" specifically "about the patient's relational style before the pathological process" is inadequate. Binswanger (cited in M. Galzigna, 1994) also acknowledged that "the psychiatric clinic is able to examine only some single segment of the route of the being-in-the-world".

The group analytic period: the group processes as a person's structure

According to Burrow's assumption, then, the human being should be only conceived in relation to his environment, and, thus, his psychoanalytical practice was marked by the consideration of patients' interpersonal relationships, of their exigencies, and of reality data, which he did not retain, as it was subject to rigid rules. Nevertheless, it is noteworthy that the adoption of such a relational theoretic view and flexible attitude to setting do not appear, *per se*, to be sufficiently strong reasons to lead him to conceive group analysis.

The birth of group analysis

What, then, induced Burrow to move towards group analysis? The determining factor cannot be traced to a rational elaboration, but is likely that it stemmed from his analysand, Clarence Shield, protesting against the discrepancy between theoretical statements and his attitude as a psychoanalyst. This provoked the questioning of the psychoanalytic setting, which was then given a more social connotation with the attribution of fundamental importance to the analyst–patient relationship. Thus, it implied the abrogation of the authoritarian and detached position of the psychoanalyst in favour of his involvement: it is the coming of countertransference, of a circular, emotional interchange which upset the established view of the psychoanalyst's role as a mirror.

The new approach, in which we can distinguish three stages, began with the acceptance, albeit very painful, of the challenge issued by Shields to exchange roles between analyst and analysand. In the course of a short time, this modality revealed its problems, in that it resulted in, to use Modell's terms (1984), a "one-personal" conception of the psychoanalytic situation, instead of a "bipersonal context" (E. Gatti Pertegato, 2001b): the analysand, in his new capacity as a psychoanalyst, reproduced the self-same authoritarian attitude. This awareness led to the relinquishment of the exchange of roles, which in turn evolved into the common decision to experiment with mutual analysis, preceding Ferenczi, who adopted it in 1932 but subsequently abandoned it. Burrow, differing from Ferenczi with regard to various aspects (E. Gatti Pertegato, 1999), would continue with it tenaciously by involving other people.

It was from these very fruitful group experiments, notwithstanding many difficulties that emerged due to the absence of any precedents, and through a painstaking elaboration of what was resulting from the group interaction, that Burrow originated group analysis by establishing its group method and principles. It required several years of studies and intensive researches with groups of various types, numbers, and duration (E. Gatti Pertegato, 2009a). In "The group method of analysis", as well as in other papers, Burrow (1927b) highlighted the means by which he established of his procedure:

> I have stated what seems to me the inadequate basis of the private method of analysis. In various writings I have made as clear as I can the altered position to which I have been brought through the *researches of my students and myself* during recent years. (p. 273, our italics)

And in "The problem of the transference", he stressed that group analysis is not traceable to deductions from a preconceived theory or from a position as a detached observer:

> The reader is here reminded that this position is not a mere expression of my view. It should be understood that all I am saying is the *report of a laboratory or group finding* with respect to *my own processes and those of other individuals who have submitted themselves to the group analysis.* (1927c, p. 201, our italics)

In connection with this, we can derive another significant hint from one of Burrow's unpublished papers (1928a), in which, in order to give "an understanding of the principle and method and the purpose of group-analysis", he systematises group analytic principles already present in his previous papers by establishing eight "basic propositions". But he warns that they

> have been empirically determined as a *result of an experimental procedure* in which individuals and groups of individuals have sought to observe with accuracy and with the absence of bias the supposedly unbiased and too often inaccurate reactions and interreactions of these self-same individuals and these self-same groups. (Burrow, 1928a, p. 1, our italics; E. Gatti Pertegato & G. O. Pertegato, 2006b)

Moreover, in reporting the "very definite results" there had been in group analysis, although not demonstrable in objective terms "like an experiment in chemistry", as some people would expect, he points out that "the course and development of man's life is a process", it is not a "static, fixed condition" and warns us

> that the spirit of the mere onlooker at processes common to all of us as social beings is very far removed from that of the direct investigator of those processes as they may be witnessed within oneself, and that 'results' must of necessity have a different connotation according as they are perceived from within or without. (1927b, pp. 273–274)

Some years after the inception of group analysis, referring to the fact that his analysand, in the role of the analyst, reproduced his detached attitude, Burrow (1927a) spoke of a "crucial revelation" which marked the direction of his group analytic research.

But what is meant by *group analysis*? First of all, given the still widespread tendency to give it the reductive meaning of a group treatment, it might be opportune to clarify that, in Burrow's view, the term "group analysis" designates primarily a social conception of the human being, as well as describing a research method for human behaviour and treatment of people's disorders.

Therefore, the word "group" that precedes such a designation connotes the *group principle as constitutive of the individual*, so that the dichotomy individual–group is overcome in favour of the continuity of the individual with the group about him and with the human species in general, starting from the physiological continuity of the child with the mother (E. Gatti Pertegato, 1994b).

In this connection, also in Burrow's time, the term group analysis was subject to erroneous interpretation on the part of colleagues who, in "adopting what they have supposed to be the group method of analysis, have assumed the role of analyst to a group of people", so that Burrow felt the urge to clear up such misunderstanding:

> Contrary to a frequent misinterpretation, *group analysis is not my analysis of the group but it is the group's analysis of me or of any other individual of the group*. 'Group' does not mean a collection of individuals. It means a phyletic principle of observation. This phyletic principle of observation as applied to the individual and to the aggregate is the whole significance of the group analysis. (Burrow, 1927c, p. 201, original italics)

However, in order to confound the confusions and misinterpretations which such locutions continued to perpetuate, starting from the 1930s, Burrow was compelled to return to the matter of the true meaning of group analysis, explaining it by unequivocal statements and eventually deciding to substitute it with the term "phyloanalysis".

> I should especially like to make clear at the outset, however, that the method of group-analysis is not so named because the procedure is carried on by groups of people. This circumstance is really wholly accidental and subsidiary. 'Group' merely means the integral or inclusive method characteristic of the laboratory as it relates the function of the individual organism to the community or species as a whole. . . . The meaning of 'group' in the collective sense should be carefully distinguished from 'group' in its integral or inclusive meaning. The former applies to the imitative automatisms of our secondary, psychological adaptations, the latter to the spontaneous, physiological reactions of the organism as a whole such as are the basis of man's conscious, creative individuality. (1930, pp. 104–105)

It might be worthwhile to specify that group analysis is but a synonym for phyloanalysis, as is seen repeatedly in Burrow's writings, where he speaks of "group or phylum", of "group analysis or phyloanalysis". Thus, "group analysis" was never totally discarded, as Foulkes (1948, 1964) states, but sometimes it was used interchangeably with phyloanalysis to refer to the same group principle and procedure. Still, today, at the Lifwynn Foundation, there is a preference for the term group analysis (Gilden, 1999), from which the specific technique "social self-enquiry" has been developed.

It should be emphasised that an innovative peculiarity is that the group method of analysis, introduced by Burrow, is conceived as the "analysis of the group *by* the group" and, therefore, must be differentiated from the analysis of a group of individuals on the part of a therapist, whether *in* group or *of* the group.

Further, given that "the social medium is represented quite as completely in the single individual as in a group of individuals", and that specific to group analysis is the *group principle of observation*, it follows that group analysis as a therapeutic tool is applicable not only to the group setting, but also to the dual one. In "The autonomy of the 'I' from the standpoint of group analysis", Burrow (1928c) reasserted this basic concept. "In my private analysis, I do not cease to adhere to a *group principle of analysis* because there is only one individual to be analyzed" (p. 6, our italics).

According to Burrow, then, in view of the social nature of human being, the individual analysis should be carried on the basis of the group analytic perspective, where the object of analysis is the interpersonal vicissitudes and the reproductions in actuality of models of distorted internalised relations, either in the psychotherapeutic setting or in life.

In this light, even the contemporary forms of relational psychoanalysis, which Burrow undoubtedly anticipated by many decades, present remarkable convergences with group analysis as applied to individual patients in a dual setting.

This reflects Pines' (2011) thought, where, in his recent interview with Tubert-Oklander and Hernández-Tubert (2011), he states with conviction that "*psychoanalysis is slowly moving to where it should be*, which is *group analysis*" and that "through relational psychology and self psychology, it's moving in that direction" (p. 10, our italics).

In this respect, in facing the group analysts' prevalent adherence to the view of group analysis as a group treatment, Nitsun (2001) raised the opportunity of promoting "a valid and distinctive group-analytic approach to individual therapy", which he considers important "not only for theoretical reasons", but also, in referring to the debate inside the Institute of Group Analysis, in order to "develop its own individual training" (p. 474). More particularly, he suggested that "the time has come, it seems, to consider whether it would not be more appropriate for the IGA to provide an individual training, one that reflects more clearly the group analytic philosophy and value system" (p. 474).

Diego Napolitani (1987), who critically rethought Freud's and Foulkes's work, arrived at a historical–relational perspective which presents points of confluence with Burrow's approach, particularly on this topic, where he states that the prefix "group" should not be intended reductively as an application of psychoanalysis to groups, but "designates a collective, transpersonal basis of the individual identity" (1994, p. 3).

Consequently, from the beginning, the Italian Group Analytic Society (SGAI), in adherence to the principle of man's social nature, reworked group analysis both as a dual and a group treatment.

We cannot but say that in this connection, too, Burrow stands as a true forerunner.

Social images and the pathology of "normality"

What does Burrow mean by the concept of "social images"? The need to distinguish the word "group" in the connotation of group analysis has its parallel in the notion of "social image", where the word "social" is not intended "in the customary acceptation of the term, either scientific or popular", but as interiorised relational modes, that is, values, modes of thinking, of feeling and of acting induced by environmental contexts—familial, cultural, social, institutional—considered "normal", but that do not reflect the true reality of individual and community (Burrow, 1924). This is in strict accordance with group analysis's cardinal concept of *internal groups* (D. Napolitani, 1987), based upon identification models that have marked the relationships of the individual with his environment, starting from the original relationship.

And what are the social images' implications for the individual and society? *Social images* are the raw material of the unconscious, which cannot but have a social connotation; hence, Burrow speaks of *social unconscious* either in the individual or in the group. In contrast with the individual's and community's reality, social images induce conflict and division until dissociation both in the individual and society, so much so that Burrow formulated the concepts of "I-persona" and of pseudo-normality, respectively.

In fact, Burrow's findings led him to question the so-called "normality" and his statement "Normality too, then, may be neurotic" (1926b, p. 212) should command our attention, since today's society is more and more dominated by distorted social images unconsciously accepted as normal.

With regard to this topic of the questioning of "normality", it is evident that Burrow is the undisputed forerunner of authors "from many different theoretical traditions" who, as reported by Mitchell (1993), a few decades ago became "interested in the problem of pseudonormality as, perhaps, the central clinical issue of our time", so that some were led to coin new diagnostic tags: the "normopath" (McDougall, 1985, p. 156) and the "normatic personality" (Bollas, 1987, p. 137). But other authors had caught such a phenomenon. Fromm (1990, 1991) denounced the "pathology of normality", while Gruen (1992) published a book emblematically entitled *The Insanity of Normality*. Before the sociologist Lawrence K. Frank (1948) wrote the book *Society as the Patient*, which is on the same wave-length as Burrow's concept of ill society, he was acquainted with Burrow, had exchanges of correspondence and writings with him, had met him at least once, enjoyed their talk very much, and felt that they should meet again in order to deepen their discussions of such a fundamental subject.

Moreover, in the epigraph we chose for this book, Kahlil Gibran, in the dialogue of the visitor with the "madman", who, albeit with shyness and reluctance, outlines the picture of his historical truth, represents so effectively the transgenerational nature of human experience and the insanity of the world of the "normal" people:

> My father would make of me the reproduction of himself; so also would my uncle. My mother would have the image of her illustrious father. . . . And my teachers also . . . and each would have me but a reflection of his own face in a mirror.
>
> Therefore I came to this place. I find it more sane here. At least I can be myself.

And when the visitor was asked whether he was also "driven to this place by education and good counsel" and gave his clear-cut answer: "No, I am a visitor", strikingly, the madman burst out, "*Oh, you are one of those who live in the madhouse on the other side of the wall*".

Is there a more convincing confirmation of Burrow's concept of "ill society" or of "social neurosis", of normality as a "shared illness"? In this respect, we cannot avoid a disquieting question and may ask with Ackerman (1964, p. xv), "And who is sick?—the individual, the family, society? What do we mean when we exclaim with horror that our world is going mad? We must rethink this whole question".

Considering that "Burrow saw the conflict enacted not only in the individual's repressive and defensive devices, but also in the accepted codes and conventions of normal social living" (Syz, 1961, p. 149), he consistently *rejects the concept of adaptation*. If the goal of group analysis is the adaptation to so-called "normality", then it would collude with the family, the social group, the institutions, and society in general in keeping the patient subjected to "social images". As Ackerman (1964) synthesises: "Normality must be distinguished from health. Normal behaviour is a brand of shared sickness" (p. viii).

In fact, the outcome of "the group basis of observation" is that "the discrimination between the neurotic and the normal becomes an artificial one". But let Burrow speak for himself:

> Perhaps the most interesting feature of group-analysis is its tendency to break down certain demarcations in the field of mental pathology,

> particularly the differentiation between normal and neurotic reactions. As far as our group observations have progressed, it would seem that from the basis of the group inquiry *there is no difference whatever between the social images of the neurotic and social images as they occur in normal individuals.* The origin and mechanism of their development would seem to be identical in both. . . . Not only is the normal as completely a prey to the images comprising his latent social content, but he is quite inaccessible to a rational attitude toward these private images occurring in himself as the neurotic is inaccessible to a rational view of these images as they occur in him. (1928b, p. 202, our italics)

Consequently, the object of group analysis is not the isolated individual, but the individual in interaction with the environment of which he is an integral part; it is not only the individual considered neurotic or mentally disturbed, but also the individuals, social groups, and institutions which, though apparently seen as representative of "normality" but in reality just like neurotic or psychotic subjects, equally unconsciously base their interactions with others and with society in general upon "social images", alienating themselves and their interpersonal, group, and institutional relationships.

It must, however, be emphasised that, from Burrow's perspective, a circularity is established where if the neurosis of the individual is secondary to that of society, in turn the individual concurs with the social neurosis.

> The reason is, as I see it, that the individual with all his personal subordination to the social system about him is at the same time an integral and necessarily contributory part of this same unconscious social organism. *At one and the same time the individual is both victim and aggressor. He is at once both the aggrieved and the offender.* (Burrow, 1926a, p. 354; our italics)

In these dynamics the *transgenerational, transpersonal, and mirroring processes* come into play, through which social images are transmitted "from individual to individual and from generation to generation", giving rise to a "social collusion of universal extent". Social images are originally reflected socially from the parents (thus involving the father more and more in the child's nurture from early infancy), who unconsciously induce in the child distorted relational modes that, in turn, they themselves might have experienced in relation to their own original familial and past and present social environment. This is specifically addressed in the unpublished paper "The element of group analysis" (Burrow, 1928a; E. Gatti Pertegato, & G. O. Pertegato 2006b), which presents a systematic theory of group analysis, and also in "Social images versus reality" (Burrow, 1924), included in this volume.

The aim of group analysis, then, is to break this perverse drive chain and "to challenge the neurosis in its individual as well as in its social intrenchments" [*sic*] by the *analysis of the social unconscious*, both at the individual and social level (1924, p. 235). Burrow felt that, "without including a consideration of the social neurosis, understanding and treatment of the individual's disorder must remain inadequate" (Syz, 1957, p. 151).

The concepts of "social image" and of "social unconscious" mark out the evolution from psychoanalysis to group analysis, and account for the individual's intrinsic social structure. *Without social interaction, there would be no individual.* As far as group analytic practice is concerned, the group is considered representative of society at large, and, like the biologic laboratory, constitutes a laboratory *in vivo*, not only with therapeutic aims, but also of research for the study of interpersonal and social relations, both normal and pathological. The group analytic procedure, initially connoted as a "laboratory method" in psychoanalysis and then as "laboratory of group analysis", does not consist in the analysis of the individual by another individual or individuals, but in the *analysis of the group by the group*—including the group analyst—of those feelings, thoughts, and motivations which are expressed in the here-and-now of the group setting, and which are nothing other than the reproduction in the group reality of fictitious social images. In fact, "group analysis occupies itself with social images or with images shared among people generally, regardless of whether they are designated as neurotic or normal" (Burrow, 1928b, p. 204). While reminiscences and private ruminations are disregarded, emphasis is placed on "the latent social content of consciousness, revealed beneath the manifest material represented in the habitual opinions and discussions of social interchange", which becomes the sole material of analysis (p. 205)

Burrow (1928b) clearly states,

> Whatever manifestation a member may present, in no circumstance is he made answerable for it as though it were a reaction particular to him. Whatever it may be, the manifestation is viewed as the

> expression of a latent content that is common to the group as a whole. Under no circumstance is the reaction of anyone regarded as isolated or separated. Nor does the group as a whole mean any particular group as differentiated from another group, but by 'group' is meant the social constellation generally with its ramifications throughout the community at large, the immediate group being but a constituent of this larger unit. (p. 202)

Through different intensities and technical modalities in the dual situation with respect to that of the group, there are specific therapeutic factors at work, the most relevant being free communication, exchange, mirroring, and resonance. Regarding some important aspects, above all the technical ones, *it seems to be Foulkes speaking*. Thus, we might ask ourselves why these concepts introduced by Burrow have been divulged under the name of Foulkes, resulting in the oblivion of Burrow, a topic which was developed in a specific paper to which readers are referred (E. Gatti Pertegato & G. O. Pertegato, 1995). However, we believe it would be opportune in the future to explore the question further through a comparative study of Burrow and Foulkes, with the aim of defining not only the debt of the latter to his predecessor, but also his own real personal contribution to group analysis.

Censorship and ostracism of the psychoanalytic orthodoxy

The considerable and wholly original contribution given by Burrow to psychoanalysis is borne out by his vast output of writing, which, together with the group analytic work, includes seven books and about seventy papers. As shown by his work, his attendance at IPA congresses, and his correspondence with Freud and with the circle of his European followers, such as Radó, Federn, Eitingon, and Jones, Burrow was a highly active and well-known member of the circle of international psychoanalysis, although troublesome particularly for the group gravitating around Freud, representing the heart of orthodoxy. We might ask, then, how is it that his work has remained almost unknown, both in the field of psychoanalysis and of group analysis?

The social and professional ostracism of this eminent psychoanalyst who had a passion for research is, at the least, perplexing, and throws dark shadows upon the methods and institutional relations inside psychoanalysis, as well as upon the world of group analysis, and the questions that this raises are disquieting. Why was Burrow censored so extensively? How is it that still today one either does not find, or finds so difficult to obtain, traces of his thinking? Why has he been so long ignored even by group analysis? Who has not allowed his thinking to come to light, and why?

On the basis of the above-mentioned reports, it is evident that the underlying motive that caused Burrow's name and work to be object of censorship, or, in the best hypothesis, undervalued for so long, should be researched on the basis of the fact that—as deduced from correspondence—Freud and his followers were disturbed by Burrow's theoretical perspective, the focus of which consisted in the importance attributed to social–relational factors in the genesis of neurosis, seeing in it a deviation from Freud's classical psychoanalysis, instead of a development of it, as it was viewed by Burrow.

One can imagine the kind of welcome he received when, before the international psychoanalytic community at the 1925 Bad Homburg IPA Congress, Burrow, in his capacity as President of the American Psychoanalytical Association, presented for the first time to such an august audience the outcomes of his group analytic research, centred around its main thesis that "*man is not an individual. His mentation is not individualistic. He is part of a societal continuum* . . ." (1926a, p. 349, our italics).

Given that such a statement unequivocally denotes the *social structure* of the human being, the reciprocal interaction between individual and society, and the transgenerational nature of human experience, it must have sounded *subversive* to the psychoanalytic orthodoxy. Burrow himself euphemistically reported that the reception of his presentation, mitigated by his office of president, had been rather cool: Jones "made what effort he could to discredit my position with our German colleagues", he stated, even if some of them showed interest in reading his paper (Letter to Hans Syz of September 5, 1925c; in Burrow, 1958, pp. 110–111). In fact, the consequences were swift in coming: censorship and ostracism were actuated at once through the rejection of his papers from the official psychoanalytic journals and the loss of his university ties, and his isolation went on until 1932, when he "was in effect evicted from the American Psychoanalytic Association of which he had been a founder and one-time President" (Burnshaw, 1984, p. xi). And his paper "The laboratory method in psychoanalysis. Its inception and development", which he had read at Bad Homburg, was rejected when submitted for publication. That is what led Ackerman (1964) to express his quite eloquent disconcertment:

> But how was I to understand this piece of history: Burrow dismissed from his university appointment, excommunicated from the American Psychoanalytic Association, and then a virtual taboo placed on his name? Burrow, a dedicated researcher in human behaviour, tossed into scientific exile! (p. vii)

However, if we consider more closely his relation with Freud, as disclosed in his correspondence with him and by his writings, *Burrow sharply draws away from both the dissenting disciples and from the complacent ones.* His divergence was not meant as a contraposition to Freudian theory aimed at breaking off with it; rather, expressed in an explicit and closely argued style, it was without acrimony and marked by a *constructive* critique of psychoanalysis, so much so that he considered his thinking as "a position" *inside* psychoanalysis aiming at its development. In fact, both in his writings and in his correspondence with Freud, to whom he used to send some of his papers in the hope of receiving his approval and words of encouragement, we find several statements that *his group approach was but an extension of Freud's discoveries in the individual analysis in the direction of a social perspective.* In particular, these letters clearly showed that Burrow never missed an opportunity to express the continuity of his thinking with that of his Master and to recognise in him his own matrix, even when he defended, in a passionate yet reasonably argued way, his ideas about what he maintained to be unfounded in Freud's arbitrary objections.

Nevertheless, he was met constantly by Freud's inflexible opposition. Sometimes, his attitude was marked by crushing criticisms, other times by sharp sarcasm. And, as also reported by Behr (2004), "Freud's criticism of Burrow is breathtaking in its harshness" (p. 334). But, in the case of the paper "Social images versus reality", faced with Burrow's (1925b) accurate confutation, which confronts him with his macroscopic misinterpretation, Freud (3 May 1925), in his letter of response, is compelled to self-criticism: "I am satisfied I was mistaken in my judgement of your second article and I am ready to correct my judgement", and also recognised: "I was prejudiced".

From correspondence with the editors and leading figures of the psychoanalytic journals, behind which was supposedly Freud's *longa manus*, the vicissitudes which Burrow's psychoanalytic papers encountered when submitted for publication, in the *International Journal of Psychoanalysis*, *Imago*, and *Internationale Zeitschrift für Psycanalise*, come to the surface and one is confronted by a chain of somewhat masked refusals. His last paper published in a psychoanalytic review dates back to 1927 (E. Gatti Pertegato, 1999).

It is well known that Freud was always well disposed to revising his own concepts, but it seems that he was not at all so inclined when proposals for modifications came from others. Eugen Bleuler, for instance, was attracted by psychoanalysis and had recourse to it in order to develop "an interpretative model of schizophrenia", thus founding a dynamic conception of psychiatry; but, on the other hand, he kept himself at "due distance" from it, declaring openly his opposition to its dogmatism (Rossi Monti, 2006). According to what was reported by Weiss (1970, p. 28), "Bleuler . . . had been a member of the Swiss Psychoanalytic Society, but he had then left it because, in his opinion, Freud was too much intolerant of the conceptual modifications or additions introduced by others" (p. 28).

Again, it is well known in the psychoanalytic movement that such an attitude was the rule with Freud, which had mown down many illustrious victims. The first outstanding breakings off due to conceptual divergences were carried out by Freud's closest followers: Adler in 1911 and Jung in 1913.

This was the atmosphere that hovered above Freud's Viennese circle and the other European psychoanalysts in which Burrow's story is set. Although there was an ocean between Europe and the USA, and a major liberation in the American Psychoanalytic Association in questioning some theoretical concepts and technical modalities (Oberndorf, 1927), they joined together in the IPA, falling, in some measure, under Freud's and his most faithful followers' control, a control which was exercised in all its rigidity through the firm defence of orthodoxy and the consequent ostracism of Burrow's writings.

Thus, it is reasonable to assume that the refusal of Burrow's ideas might have been influenced by Freud's intolerant attitude, probably accentuated by the preconceived distrust that, as reported by Jones (1955, 1959), Oberndorf (1953), and Ruitenbeck (1966), Freud nourished toward the American people. In addition, there is Rosenbaum's

(1992) interesting hypothesis, according to which Burrow's analysis with Jung might have entailed from Freud a negative influence "related to the disastrous outcome of his relationship with Jung", so that "hostility from this may have spilled over onto Burrow" (p. 11).

Such censorship, transmitted by Freud to his disciples and then from generation to generation, still persists nowadays, especially in the official psychoanalytical ranks. We ourselves have also experienced its effect in our attempts to publish the Italian edition of Burrow's writings: accepted by the publisher, it was rejected by two series editors belonging to the Italian Psychoanalytic Society (SPI); thus, we strongly rejected the publisher's offer to insert it in a generic series. Such an effect has even been experienced by Professor Leonardo Ancona (1996), at the time director of the Psychiatric Clinic of the Catholic University of Rome, a group analyst, and a psychoanalyst of the SPI, whose paper—which dealt with a confrontation between psychoanalysis and group analysis, aimed at establishing "convergences and possibilities of exchange rather than their merits and contrasted positions"—was rejected by the *Rivista di Psicoanalisi* (the official journal of the SPI), as recently testified by Ancona (2007), whose paper was published soon afterwards in *Gli Argonauti*, an independent psychoanalytic journal.

In short, a thick fog, as we shall see, was intermittently dispersing, allowing us a glimpse of Burrow's patrimony of studies and research, which has been misappropriated, alongside which is an impenetrable silence that envelops Burrow's work in darkness. Campos (1990) defined such a reaction with the meaningful phrase, "conspiracy of silence".

Although being eclipsed in the world of psychoanalysis, Burrow did not deflect at all from his objectives and, with his group of co-workers, carried on with his research, as well as continuing as usual to keep in touch with the world of human, physical, and biological sciences, so that his writings became more and more wide-ranging and will continue to be published in the journals of psychiatry, psychopathology, biology, psychology, sociology, and psychotherapy. Burrow read before the APA fifteen papers in which he developed his new formulations in the psychoanalytic field, the first in 1912 and the last in 1927, when censorship reached its zenith after he had presented his first paper on group analysis at the 1925 Bad Homburg Psychoanalytic Congress, and continued to be a contributing member of the

American Psychopathological Association, before which he delivered his twenty-four papers that spanned the years 1913 to 1944.

The elusive and distorted elaboration of historiography

What is yet more striking is that the axe of censorship also fell on the historiography of psychoanalysis, where, except with Oberndorf (1927, 1953) and Ruitenbeck (1966), Burrow's name does not appear at all or, if mentioned, it is swiftly dismissed, underestimated, or disparaged.

Jones (1955), in his book *Sigmund Freud: Life and Work,* mentions him twice, hastily, and in circumstances in which he cannot avoid doing so: the first when he refers to Jung in Zurich, where, among others present, there was a certain Trigant Burrow from Baltimore; the second when he draws up the list of the founder members of the American Psychoanalytic Association (APA). There is not a hint about his writings, or even scattered notes of the tasks he was charged with inside the Association. And yet, Burrow was a most active member, either "in organizing and extending psychoanalysis in America", or by "serving as one of its first councilors, and later as a president" (Burrow, 1958, p. 38). Even subsequently, when, in his book *Free Associations: Memories of a Psychoanalyst,* Jones (1959) reports on his frequent visits from Canada to the USA, particularly to Baltimore, in order to introduce psychoanalysis in the Phipps Psychiatric Clinic of the Johns Hopkins University, directed by Meyer, he totally ignores Burrow, who worked there as a close collaborator of Meyer, and, still in this circumstance, he limits himself to naming him among the founder members of APA.

We can get further confirmation of the censorship of Burrow from MacCurdy (1922, pp. 38–39), another founder member of APA, who was sympathetic to his research and dedicated a chapter of his own book to Burrow's new concept of "primary subjective phase", considering particularly significant that "the most original contribution to psychoanalysis of recent years received no attention from Freud and his strict followers". In this connection, MacCurdy stated,

> *Burrow must be given credit for adding to our psychological schemes two most fundamental principles—that of the primary subjective state and that of*

> *primary identification*, together with the corollary that they occur together. ... The principle of identification is practically, therapeutically of vast application. Its meaning we are only beginning to grasp. (p. 199; our italics)

Nevertheless, censorship continued.

More recently, Pigott (1990) too, in drawing attention to the importance of its utilisation in a theoretical–clinical conceptualisation, states, "Strangely the primary identification is not mentioned at all in Strachey's Index of the *Standard Edition*" (p. 65).

Most strangely, Burrow is ignored even by Paul Roazen (1975), who dedicated his interesting volume *Freud and his Followers* to the more or less troubled events of Freud's disciples "who broke away to found their own movements and of the loyalist" ones. Also, subsequently, in his critical analysis "of the works of the 'official' historiography of psychoanalysis", he does not hesitate to define them as "highly filtered products, which leak out only the version welcome to the conservatives of the Freudian orthodoxy" (1995, p. 76), but there is no trace of Burrow and of the blatant censorship to which his work was subjected.

And, surprisingly, neither is there any reference to Burrow in the volume edited by Alexander, Eisenstein, and Grotjahn (1966), *Psychoanalytic Pioneers*, which outlines a comprehensive history of psychoanalysis as seen through the lives and the works of its more eminent teachers, thinkers, and clinicians. Instead, Gay (1988), in his book *Freud: A Life for Our Time*, in referring to the discord aroused in some American analysts by Rank's "quite heady disorienting experience" in his first visit to America, owing to his theory of the birth trauma and to "his propaganda for short analyses", mentions in a deprecating reference "the psychiatrist Trigant Burrow", who informed Freud on these issues, by qualifying him as "a curious amalgam of physician and crank and an inconstant supporter of psychoanalysis", to the point that "Freud thought of him a 'muddled babbler'" (p. 476).

As far as Italy is concerned, Burrow is ignored in the classic "Treatise of Psychoanalysis", by Cesare L. Musatti (1977), remains entirely absent even in the historical volume by Silvia Vegetti Finzi (1990) "History of Psychoanalysis", while in the "Treatise of Psychoanalysis: Theory and Technique" by Antonio A. Semi (1989), he is censored as a psychoanalyst, but mentioned by Silvia Corbella as "the first who tried to utilise in groups the technique and the concepts of psychoanalysis" (1988, p. 771). However, the author does not attribute to him the space and relevance his work would deserve, which is instead reserved for the later authors, such as W. R. Bion and S. H. Foulkes. But, at the time, Burrow was almost an "illustrious unknown man", and after the series of papers which brought him to light (E. Gatti Pertegato, 1994a,b; E. Gatti Pertegato & G. O. Pertegato, 1995), in her subsequent works, Corbella (2004, 2006) quotes a very significant passage on the unavoidable relation "individual–group", which begins with an apparently paradoxical statement: "Man is not an individual . . ." (Burrow, 1926a; E. Gatti Pertegato, 1994a).

Also in the group analytic historiography, we meet an analogous censorship in the form of heavy undervaluation and distortion, traceable above all to James Anthony, even if its underlying motivations seem different in respect to the psychoanalytic work, which was due to Burrow's social approach.

It is astounding that even Anthony (1971), Foulkes's close collaborator and historian of group analysis, excludes Burrow from the history of group psychotherapy, where he maintains:

> Although he had a background of psychoanalytic knowledge and working in groups, *he did not strongly affect the field of current group psychotherapy. Essentially, he does not belong to the history of group psychotherapy*" (p. 10, our italics).

In the face of such a macroscopic misconception as Anthony's historical estimate of Burrow's work, which is, after all, in contrast with the irrefutable reality of Burrow's writings and with other evaluations by those who studied Burrow's thinking in depth, we ask: is this misinterpretation imputable to a scant knowledge of Burrow's work and/or perhaps to an exorbitantly subjective component connected—as will be shown later on—to the issue of the paternity of group analysis on the part of Foulkes?

And, as far as the field of dynamic group psychotherapy is concerned, what about Scheidlinger's (1980, p. 4) historical account, which puts himself in a similar position to that of Anthony by stamping on Burrow's work in favour of Redl's "Group emotion and leadership" (1980), arguing that, although published over twenty years after Freud's *Group Psychology and the Analysis of the Ego*, Redl "picks up where Freud left off"? It is noteworthy that, curiously enough, Scheidlinger (1980, p. ix) heavily criticised Irvin Yalom's (1975) "otherwise excellent book" as an example of "biased" literature, in that, among other things, he "totally ignored the relevant contributions of Freud and of Redl", while he himself quite overlooked Burrow, who not only developed Freud's theory into a relational orientation, but also first conceived group analysis by experimenting with the application of psychoanalytic principles to groups.

However, how is it, for example, that Tuttman (1986) can write in terms totally opposed to Anthony and Scheidlinger, clearly attributing to Burrow the founding of group analysis?

> The pioneering works of Burrow (1927), Schilder (1939), Slavson (1943, 1964), and Moreno (1946) *are particularly important from the viewpoint of psychoanalytic group therapy*. . . .
>
> Because he believed the psychoanalytic focus upon the individual excluded social factors, *the American psychiatrist and psychoanalyst Trigant Burrow* (1927) *developed a method he called "group analysis"* as a means of conducting research in social psychiatry. For him, *the group was a milieu for the study of human behaviour as well as a treatment mode.* (p. 500, our italics)

And, again, how is it that van Schoor (2000) is in line with Tuttman and sharply in contrast with Anthony's and Scheidlinger's positions?

> In the psychoanalytic arena, Burrow was breaking new ground. The individual was envisioned as an interactive part of the larger sociobiological whole . . . Burrow's investigation of an individual's neurotic deviation within the context of the interrelational structure of groups may be seen to have been *the only forerunner of analytic group psychotherapy at that time.* (p. 443, our italics)

How to understand such historiographical distortions? History is complex *per se* and, over the years, other factors might have further contributed to their interlacing with one another. Documented facts, whenever possible, are of great help in broaching the thorny subject of the origin of these distortions.

Undoubtedly, these ungrounded historical accounts by two such prominent figures as Anthony and Scheidlinger might have had considerable weight in misrepresenting Burrow's work and in marginalising him or, in the worst case, in throwing him out of the history of group analysis. Scheidlinger's (1987) commentary to an appreciative article on Burrow's pioneering work by Rosenbaum (1986) presents his quite negative evaluation, which he calls "a more parsimonious, historical perspective" (p. 74), and in which he extrapolates from the context of Burrow's letters and writings a series of passages that he misinterprets and heavily distorts, thus betraying their original true meaning. He even charged Burrow with being "the unwitting cause of Freud's dropping forever the theme of group psychology", in that he "over many years kept besieging Freud with reprints and letters with extravagant claims for his group methods" (p. 76). In truth, in Burrow's letters there is no trace of "besieging" or "claims". Burrow was a very polite person. Rather, he never missed any occasion to express to Freud his indebtedness, and respectfully objected to his misunderstandings and endeavoured to show him how his own group research was but a development of Freud's findings in the individual field as applied to man's social sphere. But Burrow's hope of getting Freud's approval met with disappointment. However, although Freud and his strict followers acted with a heavy hand, Burrow was not discouraged from carrying on with his group researches.

Regarding Scheidlinger's allegation that Burrow might have "alienated Freud from the idea of groups as a therapeutic medium", Behr (2004) firmly objected by arguing, with a note of sarcasm,

> This was a hard trip to lay on Burrow. It set him up to be marginalized within the psychotherapeutic community and probably made it difficult for those psychoanalysts who were sympathetic to the idea of group therapy to openly acknowledge their indebtedness to his ideas. Freud's excursion into group psychology carries no kernel of an idea that the group might become a potential forum for the practice of psychoanalytic psychotherapy. (p. 335)

Further, Behr draws one's attention to the fact that, by his remarks in a letter to Burrow, Freud (1926) proves "to be adamant in his view that groups are potentially dangerous places and therefore unsuitable for therapeutic purposes" (p. 335).

Moreover, what about the diffused ignoring of Burrow's name and work specifically on the part of many of Foulkes's epigones? Besides the generic and very elusive accounts of Burrow by Foulkes himself (see "Appreciation and ransacking", below), it seems that a significant role in this more or less unconscious prejudice might have been played by Anthony's (1971) misleading historical rendition of group analysis. In turn, such a prejudice, in the absence or difficulty of a confrontation with the original sources, might have nourished the successive historical accounts which, thus, were based on second-hand groundless sources, so that it has been transmitted from generation to generation. It is striking how it is often taken as gospel truth and persists even when the most rigorous evidence is provided.

But, on the other hand, objectively one should not ignore that the little, or lack of, attention paid to Burrow's work might also be traceable both to the oblivion caused by the psychoanalytic censorship, first, and then by the general ransacking to which it was subjected. Even Ackerman (1964) himself was unaware of it and reported that his enquiry to his psychiatric colleagues around the 1960s met with either the confirmation of disinformation about Burrow or with a "vague recollection" of his writings, which were discarded because they had been somehow felt too advanced, as if he would be off the common track. Here is how Ackerman puts it:

> Who was this man, and by what odd fate were his early discoveries buried? Only a few years back I had not so much as heard his name. Could this have been simply my personal ignorance? Stirred to curiosity, I made an inquiry among my colleagues in psychiatry. They were mainly as uninformed as I. It is true, some had a vague recollection of his writings, but they seemed to dismiss him quickly as one who had gone off the path. This seemed very odd. (p. vi)

It is noteworthy that these evaluations reflect those by Mullan and Rosenbaum (1971), who point out:

> In the history of psychotherapy there has been little attention given to Burrow—a great and original thinker of the early years of psychoanalysis who has been oddly neglected in surveys of contemporary psychotherapy. His pioneer group analytic studies were largely ignored and only currently is he receiving some recognition. (p. 5)

It is curious that, while Burrow enjoyed the high appreciation of outstanding novelists and poets (see "Writers' captivation by

Burrow's thought") and eminent scientists, inside the field of the psychoanalytic and group analytic establishment, in Behr's words, which are in line with those of Ackerman, as well as Mullan and Rosenbaum, "Burrow's works gathered dust". In fact, "Burrow remained largely unquoted and unacknowledged" (2004, p. 334) and he finds this very puzzling, given that, alluding to writers, Burrow has been

> highly regarded by prominent figures outside the world of psychotherapy, who saw in his visionary outlook a blueprint for society. . . . His under-acknowledgement remains something of a mystery, since he influenced several schools of psychotherapy, including [as reported by Ettin (1992)] those developed by Harry Stack Sullivan, Karen Horney and Irvin Yalom. (Behr, 2004, pp. 335–336)

Similarly, it was just as incomprehensible to the writer Herbert Read (1949) that Burrow "has not received the recognition due to one of the greatest psychologists of our time" (p. 115). And Ackerman (1964), referring to the reaction to Burrow's "startling discoveries", speaks of "a strange and mysterious tale" (see "Appreciation and ransacking", below).

Yes, it is indeed difficult to understand such generalised lack of acknowledgement, particularly as, we should point out, Burrow's papers and books, although banned by the psychoanalytic orthodoxy, were available overseas, since they were issued by both English journals and publishers, even if today they might be unlikely to be easily accessible. We should also remind readers that, in the past decades, from time to time, in *Group Analysis* itself significant articles appeared by both Abse (1979[1990]) on "the inauguration of group analysis in the U.S.A." and by Rosenbaum (1986) on the "pioneer" Burrow; later, in 1999, a "Special Section" of the journal was dedicated to "Trigant Burrow's Group Analysis".

Thus, for many different reasons, most of them due to the "conspiracy of silence" (Campos, 1990), some preconceived, some justified as a consequence of the misinformation, some others induced by misappropriation, Burrow's work was the object of every sort of oversight. To limit ourselves to a few coming from outstanding group analysts: from Brown and Zinkin (1994), who indicate that Foulkes was the "founder" of group analysis, to Winship (2003), who iterated

Foulkes's statement that "Karl Mannheim was the first to use the term 'group analysis'" (p. 37), followed by Verdecchia's (2004) confutation, which drew attention to the fact that "group analysis" had been coined by Burrow (E. Gatti Pertegato, 1999; Gilden, 1999); from a recent book (Hopper & Weinberg, 2011), dealing with the concept of the social unconscious in its various articulations, and, previously, to some articles as a part of a wide debate on such a concept, which took place in *Group Analysis*, without Burrow being mentioned (Brown, 2001; Dalal, 2001; Hopper, 2001), and so on. Beyond the merit of that debate and without going into the heart of the matter, we want to emphasise that the social unconscious was introduced by Burrow as early as 1924, in "Social images versus reality", here published, where one can obtain knowledge of his original formulation of this basic group analytic concept. So it is for the introduction of the term group analysis, regarded either as a theory of personality or a psychotherapeutic tool.

Anyway, whatever are the complex reasons for Burrow's oblivion, we do hope that at long last this book, containing Burrow's original writings, might fill the gap left by the many previous omissions and distortions and serve the cause of the historical truth.

As far as Italy is concerned, although Burrow's work is better known among professionals, since the publication of the series of introductory papers on the history of group analysis, on Burrow's thinking, and on the censorship to which it was subject can be traced to over fifteen years ago (E. Gatti Pertegato, 1994a,b; E. Gatti Pertegato & G. O. Pertegato, 1995; Migone, 1995), Burrow is not taken into consideration in the historical accounts in recent books on group analysis, except for the volume by Rocco Pisani (2000). At most, one can find brief generic or misleading hints, even without quoting the source of them. And yet, since the mid-1970s, Burrow has made sporadic appearances on the scene of Italian group analysis (Ancona, 1983; Borgogno & Calorio, 1976; Campos, 1990; Pauletta d'Anna, 1990), though sometimes in an imprecise form, without arousing interest or exciting curiosity in the experts or insiders. This sounds more surprising as, in the title of Borgogno and Calorio's abovementioned paper, there is an explicit reference to the "foundation of group analysis" and, in the subtitle, to Burrow's work. Most recently, besides the Italian edition of the present book with Burrow's original writings, other papers were issued on the history and theory of group analysis (E. Gatti Pertegato, 2009a,b; E. Gatti Pertegato & G. O. Pertegato, 2006b, 2009).

Nevertheless, in a recent text, which is presented as a foundations' group analysis handbook (Di Maria, & Formica, 2009), such references are totally ignored and Burrow himself is not only misinterpreted, but also mentioned in a generic way as if he did not practise group analysis—*which he founded!*—but, rather, just another nameless and mysterious form of group psychotherapy.

Historical recurrences, one would say! This short outline raises disquieting questions and throws dark shadows upon the rigour and the reliability of the sources which are utilised in the drawing up of both psychoanalytic and group analytic history.

As group analysts, it is essential to pay the utmost attention to the history at every level, in order to avoid its repetition and to understand the present and project the future. Burrow (1934) firmly objected to the writer Leo Stein, who had questioned the importance of history in the study of neuroses,

> You are quite mistaken in thinking I am interested in the paleontology of the neurosis. A history of consciousness or of tendencies of reaction possesses interest for me only as it throws light upon the reaction in the immediate moment. How could you of all people so far have missed my meaning! . . . Maybe a paper I read two weeks ago at the 'Psychopathological' will help make clearer to you my position in its immediate, practical implications. . . . I don't wonder you are not sympathetic to what you have conceived to be a sort of Neanderthaloid psychology! (Letter of June 18, 1934, in Burrow, 1958, p. 281)

In short, to use Behr's felicitous expression, our primary task is "to bring the past alive" (2011, p. 456) by attaching due importance to history, not only in our group analytic theory and practice, but also in the personal, interpersonal, community, and institutional plane, our institutions included.

From censorship to misappropriation and to re-emergence of Burrow's work

We remain steadfast in examining more closely the range of the vicissitudes Burrow's work met with concomitant with psychoanalytic aversion to his views, first, and the censorship, second. These range from dense oblivion to deprecation and ostracism, from appreciation to misappropriation and ransacking, but also from rediscovery to reappraisal and recognition by the world of dynamic group psychotherapy.

Further, what is most amazing is the fact that, despite overwhelming psychoanalytic rejection, Burrow's social conceptions met with some eminent writers' high estimation, which acted as a sounding chamber within the literary field and, through the writers' works, within their readers, among whom it seems there were outstanding psychoanalytic figures, such as Fromm and Horney.

Appreciation and ransacking

After a few decades, in some circles, the "virtual taboo" placed on Burrow's name (Ackerman, 1964) seemed to dissolve, and his work met with a remarkable enhancement of appreciation, which, nevertheless, happens mostly in a furtive form. In fact, a contradictory phenomenon takes place: if, on the one hand, Burrow's work continued to lie persistently under the iron censorship of the psychoanalytic orthodoxy, on the other hand, it began to become the object of great interest, but through *a copious* ransacking, so that his concepts ended up giving rise to, or nourishing, various relational, interpersonal, group approaches. In this respect, Foulkes stands out, since he had constantly presented group analysis as his own original creation, limiting himself to mentioning some quite summary and generic historical accounts of Burrow's work, even contradicting between them, without which there might be a *reference to the paternity of whatever concept* (E. Gatti Pertegato & G. O. Pertegato, 1995)

From some viewpoints, it is possible to deduce how this might have happened. Burrow's writings, which, before censorship, had been published in psychoanalytic journals or books that also circulated in the Anglo-Saxon world, notwithstanding the fact that, at an official level, a gravestone had fallen on them, must have been the object of careful reading by some authors of the succeeding generation. Among them were some exponents of the psychoanalytic and group analytic field, who could derive selectively from his concepts but present them as their own original discoveries, thus founding schools of thought of relational, interpersonal, and group orientation. *A curious aspect is that this selective appreciation took place after Freud's death.*

Except for Schilder (1936) and Wender (1936), who, supporting one another and inspired by the group dynamics and the therapeutic factors discovered by Burrow, though avoiding giving him credit, made use of group psychotherapy, each in his own way, by applying for the first time in a psychiatric institution the psychoanalytic principles to a group situation, that is, to psychotic inpatients and outpatients. Owing to the brevity of the treatment, imposed by the patients' time-limited stay in hospital, they could be considered *the forerunner of short term group psychotherapy in the public institutions* (E. Gatti Pertegato, 2001c; E. Gatti Pertegato & G. O. Pertegato, 2003). In particular, Schilder, who served as Clinical Director of the Psychiatric Division at New York Bellevue Hospital, as reported by Wolberg and Aronson (1979), used to grasp the opportunity to work with group dynamics arising from patients' free discussion even during the hospital rounds, so that the department itself was transformed into a group situation with therapeutic potentialities. As Bender (1979) stated, "he was fully aware of both the scope and the limitations of classical analysis as a therapeutic tool" (p. 8), and in the end, just like Burrow, Schilder was expelled from the American Psychoanalytic Association, although he was from Vienna and, before extending the psychoanalytic principles to groups, he enjoyed Freud's appreciation.

Regarding the persistent exclusion of Burrow's name and work from the group analytic field, the principal actor appears to be Foulkes, who, like some exponents of other schools, with the advantage of the blanket of silence cast over them, derived some basic theoretical–technical concepts from Burrow's work, privileging its methodology (E. Gatti Pertegato & G. O. Pertegato, 1995).

Such an active and diffused form of reintroducing Burrow's concepts, which took place with the denial and removal of their authorship, aroused indignation in Ackerman, who, having through the Lifwynn Foundation discovered and studied Burrow's thought, in the foreword of his posthumously published book, *The Preconscious Foundation of Human Experience* (1964), puts the following disquieting questions:

> As far back as the 1920's and 1930's, *Burrow made some startling discoveries. . . . The reaction* to Burrow and his studies in mental health *is a strange and mysterious tale.* His writings were provocative, piercing, even shocking; *they were shelved. Presently, some thirty years later, the*

> *same ideas, one by one, are being rediscovered*. They represent now, in essence, the vanguard of a new social–psychiatric approach to mental health, the core of an advancing science of human behaviour. Why, for the major part of a half century, were Burrow's theories bypassed? ... How could this *giant figure* have remained so obscure, and for so many years? (p. vi, our italics)

Here are the answers he tries to give to such questions.

> A generation ago, Burrow's theories were far in advance of his time. They were too radical, too threatening to conventional systems of thought. ... his discoveries concerning the pathology of normality—his ideas must have been felt to be a danger to the then-popular concepts of psychiatry and psychoanalysis. Even more important, his approach challenged the established self-identity of investigator and therapist and the implications of his theories for a revolution in established social forms were possibly such to impel what amounted to a mass avoidance, an unconscious complicity in protest and denial. (pp. vii–viii)

Ackerman does not hesitate to qualify such behaviour as "surely one of the strangest episodes in the history of psychiatry", and, we can add, of psychoanalysis and group analysis. Furthermore, in view of the subsequent growing interest in Burrow's work, he does not make a mystery of the underhanded form in which such a change was taking place:

> Now, the truth will out. Now comes a curious and paradoxical shift. *One by one, Burrow's concepts begin to re-emerge in the current literature, but, oddly enough, not as coming from him*. Piecemeal, they reappear and gain strength in the writing of contemporary scholars in the field of mental health. (p. viii, our italics)

Then, in outspoken terms, Ackerman clearly corroborates the thesis of a *generalised plagiarism* based on the statement that a large number of authors derived concepts from Burrow's work without giving him due credit.

In the psychoanalytic field, there are some surprising examples of this in the case of some outstanding exponents of the Interpersonal School. In *Personal Psychop;athology*, written between 1929 and 1933 but published posthumously some forty years later, Harry Stack

Sullivan (1972) does not acknowledge any indebtedness to Burrow, though clearly reflecting his thinking. Given that Sullivan and Burrow became acquainted in Baltimore at the Phipps Psychiatric Clinic of the Johns Hopkins Medical School directed by Meyer, it is interesting to discover that Sullivan certainly had knowledge of Burrow's writings, which were regularly sent to him by none other than Burrow himself (1949a), as is unequivocally confirmed in the following:

> I have not myself read either Fromm or Horney, but a good many people have spoken of what they felt was *the tendency of these authors to borrow rather freely from my thesis. Harry Stack Sullivan helped himself lavishly to my material. I knew him at Hopkins and he received through the years all of my reprints*. (Letter to Thomas Sancton of September 28, 1949; in Burrow, 1958, p. 584, our italics).

This is further confirmed in a letter by Alfreda Galt (1974), at the time secretary of the Lifwynn Foundation:

> Burrow and Sullivan were acquainted with each other and I have been reviewing the correspondence between them which consists of about fifteen letters and notes between October 1924 and January 1927. It is cordial for the most part and the last letter from *Dr. Sullivan requested that Dr Burrow continue to send reprints*. But . . . later Dr. Burrow felt that Dr. Sullivan had based some of his theories on Burrow's reports without acknowledgement. (Letter to Dr. Ralph Crowley of December 9, 1974; our italics).

Moreover, according to the historical account by Ettin (1992), a good example of historical fidelity, Burrow's work "certainly represents an early experiment in interpersonal psychotherapeutics", and, as reported also by Behr, "it in fact influenced the later practices of the interpersonal school of psychiatry as represented by Harry Stack Sullivan, Karen Horney, and Irwin Yalom". Ettin also let us know that "Samuel Slavson Archives, housed at the headquarters of the American Group Psychotherapy Association, contains many reprints of Burrow's writings". And he emphasises, "Though underacknowledged, *Trigant Burrow's work represented an innovation in the treatment of the individuals as social beings*" (p. 69; our italics)

What is more, through Swick Perry (1971) and Levenson (1983), one discovers also that it was Sullivan's habit to draw from other authors' basic concepts, in a variety of ways, sometimes even changing their names. Swick Perry relates that, in a 1970 talk with Kempf about his relationship with Sullivan, she "became aware of the extent to which Dr. Kempf's vocabulary and ideas were reminiscent of the vocabulary and conceptions of Sullivan" (p. xvi). Thus, once she was able to locate Kempf's *Psychopathology* (1921), dealing with the "new dynamic psychiatry on psychotic patients", she found confirmation that, in comparing Sullivan's thought "to even a part of Kempf's long study, one is immediately struck by many similarities" (p. xvi). Just as, we can add, remarkable similarities exist between Burrow's basic concepts and those of Sullivan.

Swick Perry argues that "he [Sullivan] had an extraordinary ability to take the cream off the thought in his own generation and to early recognize a seminal thinker" and that "Sullivan never recognized clearly his basic indebtedness to Kempf" (p. xix).

We also know that Ferenczi's work met the same fate as that of Kempf and Burrow. As Sabourin (1985) reports, Cremerius made a list of important authors who "have reinvented what Ferenczi had written long before them, but without quoting him" (E. Gatti Pertegato, 2009a).

Getting back to the group analytic field, something similar took place with Foulkes in respect to Burrow. It becomes evident throughout various statements that Foulkes aspired to propose himself as the founder of group analysis, as one may notice, starting from his paper "On group analysis" (1946), in which he presented his work with groups for the first time to his psychoanalytic colleagues , to his subsequent books (Foulkes, 1948, 1964), up to his last one, where he opens its first chapter by insisting on drawing one's attention to the fact that group analysis was "initiated" by himself , that it "grew out of" and was "inspired by" his "experiences as a psychoanalyst" (1975, p. 3). Furthermore, we thoroughly examined the contradictions in his references to how many Burrow's papers he had read—one "communication", "one or two papers", or more?—and the omission of the titles of the papers which "stimulated" him about group analysis. Thus, one meets with generic assertions and just as many generic and belated recognitions. In any case, it emerges that, when Foulkes took the decision to experiment for the first time with the psychoanalytic approach to groups at Exeter, it was "more than twenty years ago" that he "came across" Burrow's thinking (Foulkes, 1948, p. 37). In this regard, Behr (2004) points out, with a touch of irony,

> Having paid scant acknowledgement to Burrow's contributions in the 1940s, Foulkes went on later to state that the idea of group analysis as a form of treatment was put in his mind by a paper of Burrow's he had read in the mid-1920s. (p. 337).

But why did he not make any specific reference to any of Burrow's concepts or papers? Why did he privilege the method, mostly overlooking the theory? Furthermore, why did he never write a book on theory if, as reported by Rosenbaum (1975), Foulkes himself informed him that "he always aimed to build up the foundations of a comprehensive and really adequate and specific theory for group analysis" (p. xii)? In this respect, besides Foulkes' meaningful sentence after his first group session, "I remembered Trigant Burrow – nobody else did at the time " (1964), besides his rather evident aim to obtain primacy in the founding of group analysis, other motives might have played a role that linked with the previous ones. In the Milan SGAI group research, it turned out the hypothesis that his bond connected to his position as a training analyst of the British Psychoanalytic Society might have prevented him from mentioning Burrow, that is, an unnameable "heretic" (E. Gatti Pertegato & G. O. Pertegato, 1995). His loyalty to Freudian perspective might have made him incapable of reproducing integrally either Burrow's concepts or re-elaborating a coherent group theory, being in contrast to the psychoanalytic theory he was teaching: in adopting the so-called "bifocal registry" between the individual and the collective mind, psychoanalysis and group analysis, his thought ends with the negative result "to keep those dichotomies he declares to want to overcome" (D. Napolitani, 1981, 1987). As a consequence, group analysis, besides being lacking on the theoretical plane, presents various ambiguities, even if, in one of his last writings, Foulkes (1973) opts for "the multipersonal hypothesis of mind" (p. 280).

The critical analysis of Foulkes's work by Napolitani (1987) was followed ten years later by that of Farhad Dalal (1998), who points out its "confusions and contradictions", which result in paradoxical consequences: "In the *practice of group analysis* almost all of Foulkes interpretations are couched in individualistic terms, and often in Freudian language. Even group specific concepts like scapegoating are given an individualistic basis" (p. 12, original italic).

So, Dalal speaks of the existence of "two Foulkes, a radical one and a more orthodox one. The two Foulkes set out two sorts of theories", and Dalal's exploration traces these to the fact that "Foulkes is constantly torn between Freud and Elias" (p. 13). May we add that, as far as the theory of group analysis is concerned, Foulkes was also "torn" between Freud and Burrow's thinking—whom Dalal does not mention at all—and to which may be traceable what he calls the "radical Foulkes"? Thus, far from undervaluing the influence of Elias's social views, given that Foulkes, though in a surreptitious form, drew plenty from Burrow's method, ultimately, we are inclined to attribute such ambiguities, theoretical deficiencies, and contradictions mostly to the *mutilated form* in which, owing to the various reasons mentioned above, Foulkes's group analytic theory was borrowed from Burrow's (E. Gatti Pertegato, 2009b).

In Burrow, instead, there is no confusion, in that he does not strive to keep simultaneously in the same field the contradictory aspects present in Freud between individual psychology and social psychology (D. Napolitani, 1987). His perspective, although conceived as a social extension of Freud's psychoanalysis, implies a radical reversal of Freud's prevailing individualistic anthropology, and, thus, he made "a choice of field also on the epistemological level": psychology cannot avoid having a social basis (E. Gatti Pertegato, 1994b, p. 28).

In Italy, too, despite the growing interest in Burrow's group analytic thought, up to now there persists a certain ideological defensive position, refractory even to the most rigorous historical documented facts. We are faced with a hard core of orthodox group analysis to whom the fidelity to Foulkes seems to exclude, *a priori*, every objective approach aimed at deepening the relation of his work with that of his predecessor.

However, some historical accounts, based on the examination of Burrow's group analytic writings on the part of exponents of the dynamic group psychotherapy in general (Ackerman, 1964; Berne, 1963; Ettin, 1992; Mullan & Rosenbaum, 1971; Rosenbaum & Berger, 1963; Tuttman, 1986), definitively contradict Anthony's evaluation, and consider Burrow the originator of the application of psychoanalytic principles to the group setting some 15–20 years in advance of subsequent authors. Indeed, Burrow's work paved the way for entire generations, as significantly emphasised by Burnham (1946–1950):

> Only later did many modes in which Burrow's thought appear of great importance—the significance of nonverbal behaviour, analysis of

> a holistic group, the pathogenic potential of the person's concept of self, interdisciplinary approaches to neurosis, the psychophysiological study of eye movements, breathing and EEG. Much of its importance lay, therefore beyond his own day, in the way in which his writings gave courage to a later generation of pioneers in a number of different areas in psychological–psychiatric research. His example at first encouraged a number of workers to try a group setting for individual psychotherapy, and much later his writings were an inspiration to organic group analysts, particularly in the family analysis movement of the 1960's. (p. 131)

Rediscovery and reappraisal from the world of dynamic group psychotherapy

The world of group psychotherapy, then, for some decades, has begun to rediscover Burrow's work, giving him the recognition that was denied him by the major part of group analysis. And this is yet more incomprehensible if we consider that, in the early 1970s De Maré (1972), an outstanding exponent of the Group Analytic Society, in his book *Perspectives of Group Psychotherapy. A Theoretical Background*—which even has a foreword by Foulkes—refers to Burrow by describing extensively his thought and, although with some imprecisions, he acknowledges that "the one-time psychoanalyst Trigant Burrow recognized the significance of the interactive matrix of society for individual growth, 'phylic' [or group] cohesion" and "saw clearly the individual as a 'socius', as part of the larger sociological structure" (p. 21). It is noteworthy that of the "psychoanalysts who played a crucial role in the development of an actual technique of group analysis", and that "deserve a special mention", De Maré underlines that

> *it was the psychoanalyst Burrow who first coined the expression 'group analysis'* and in whose praise under the title of "A new theory of neurosis", D. H. Lawrence reviewed Burrow's book, *The Social Basis of Consciousness*, in a 1927 issue of the *The Bookman*. The importance of Burrow's work for group therapists can easily be underestimated, partly because his style of writing is difficult, partly because it is extremely advanced; indeed *we may still have much to learn from his writings*. (p. 62, our italics)

And Malcolm Pines himself (1981) refers to Trigant Burrow as "the first to show" how the group "is a powerful social situation with its own dynamics" (p. 277), and, in a paper emblematically entitled "Forgotten pioneers", he dedicates a conspicuous part of the paragraph "Forgotten pioneers in group psychotherapy" to Burrow's work, where he starts off as follows.

> I shall begin in America, where Trigant Burrow in the 1920s and the 1930s explored the dynamics of small and large groups under what he called 'laboratory conditions'. Neglected and opposed for much of his life by his former fellow psychoanalysts, *he significantly influenced Foulkes who had read his papers in German in the 1920s.* (1999, p. 21, our italics)

In examining the origin and "the distorted role of fictitious social images", Pines continues by mentioning the enormous influence exercised by Burrow:

> Not only was this exploration remarkable, anticipating developments that took place 20 or 30 years later by Schilder in America, by Foulkes in England, Lacan in France, after World War II by the Encounter Movement, but he early realized that these social deceptions are not the property of any one individual but of the group as a whole as a microcosm of the wider society. (1999, p. 26)

Last, but not least, "Burrow's earlier psychoanalytic papers written from 1914 onwards, are novel and anticipate the work of Kohut and the School of Self Psychology when he writes of the 'preconscious' experience of the infant which remains part of our psyche throughout life" and "anticipates the work of Mahler on separation–individuation" (1999, pp. 28–29).

Despite the persistence of some still deep-rooted misinterpretations of Burrow's research, such as that of Hinshelwood (2004), who, besides some imprecision and erroneous dates, ignores the first group analytic period in which the foundations of group analysis were laid, confusing it with the second period, and quite bypasses the role of social images, either in the individual or society, for some years now more and more signs of a favourable change have been emerging from the Anglo-Saxon group analytic world, as reported by Behr (2004):

> At last there seems to be a resurgence of interest in Burrow, thanks largely to a dedicated group of colleagues across the world and to

> those who worked with him at Lifwynn . . . [so that] *Burrow's star may be in the ascendant.* (p. 336, our italics)
>
> . . . Burrow in particular, I believe, is slowly being restored to his rightful place as an *innovator and profound thinker in the field of group analysis.* (p. 338, our italics)

And subsequently, in their book *Group-Analytic Psychotherapy. A Meeting of Minds*, Behr and Hearst (2005), in the historical account of Burrow's contribution, stressed that "his views on the social nature of man are germane to modern group analysis and there is a current renewal of interest in his writings" (p. 17).

Moreover, in the Italian group-analytic ranks, in the wake of incontestable historical sources, an opening to Burrow's work has been taking place in various contexts over the past decade, which is not only progressively eroding the prejudicial attitude of denial, but also arousing the interest of those who were entirely in the dark or had only a partial knowledge of it. An example is the value that discovering Burrow's thought assumed for Leonardo Ancona (2007), a historical figure of group analysis, which he came to through Fabrizio Napolitani, the "master" who captivated him with his "therapeutic and didactic seriousness", and who transmitted to him his "praxis and scientific experience" (Montesarchio, 1993). In the early 1970s, through an innovative initiative with F. Napolitani, Ancona introduced group analysis in the university, marking the beginning of a productive collaboration. Despite being an academic, he held the role of "his first observer in training" in the conduction of therapeutic groups in the outpatient clinic department, a role in which he involved, in a second group conducted by F. Napolitani, the then scholarship holder Corrado Pontalti (2008). It must be said that group analysis was taking its first steps in Italy. Notwithstanding his long and substantial association with the Foulkesian approach, after the reading of the paper on the first theoretical structure of group analysis outlined in the "Eight propositions" (E. Gatti Pertegato & G. O. Pertegato, 2006b), in referring to Foulkes's selective plundering of Burrow's work, Ancona, with an extraordinary intellectual freedom and an open-minded attitude to the new, did not hesitate to revise his own position, which he expressed in an eloquent comment:

> Foulkes has overlooked the most important part . . . Burrow has aroused enthusiasm in me! It's the first time I have become

> enthusiastic about reading something . . . *He really opened the horizon for me!* So much so that I see Burrow's concept of social images is applicable to individual psychoanalysis too, because it goes into much depth. When we have to deal with the attachment level, which is the early phase of relation with the world, there we meet with transgenerational and interpersonal transmissions, whose origin, as you will remember, is in Burrow. (2007, our italics)

And we may add that recently Burrow has also opened up the horizon to the newly graduated Francesca Mazzotta (2009a). It is significant that the name and the studies of an author, then unknown to her, but of whom "there hypothesised as a precursor and pioneer of the work with groups", had captured her imagination to such an extent that she involved herself in demanding and passionate research into his life and work for her degree with the aim "to enhance and to introduce Trigant Burrow, a pioneer of analytic work with groups, who, in the early twentieth century, made important contributions through his main concepts of social image, transpersonal process, and transgenerational process". Such concepts give evidence of "a multipersonal approach of the mind". Here is a significant proclamation she made, in an excerpt from her thesis:

> The research was interesting and stimulated my desire to deepen the study of the analytic work with groups and allowed me to enrich my store of knowledge . . . What aroused strong emotions in me was Burrow's conviction in considering the individual an integral unity, part of a primary *continuum*; that in considering the individual he assigned importance to all his fund of induced and acquired feeling and behaviour. . . . Moreover, his conception of conflict, which is social, on normality, which is a shared illness that represses the innate creativity of each of us through the adoption of false social images. I like to imagine a man who really believed in what he continuously experimented with and tried to make emerge—the creativity which is inherent in every individual. Just as he himself theorised, he was the victim of a social mechanism based on the adherence to rooted social images.

Such a study was rewarding also for the members of the Committee. The thesis discussion, introduced by Professor Maurizio Gasseau, who underlined the historical importance of Burrow and the reappraisal of his studies, anticipating the current ones by many decades, aroused in the Committee Members "interest", "curiosity" about the similarity of Burrow's thought with that of Foulkes, and "astonishment because Burrow is so little known, though he was the first to experiment with the social dimension of the individual" (Mazzotta, 2009b).

Finally, we cannot avoid mentioning the significant, even if isolated, acknowledgement of Burrow's group activity emanating from the American psychoanalytic field through the historian Oberndorf's unequivocal statements (1953):

> Trigant Burrow, one of the earlier American analysts, made use of the reactions of individuals within a group setting for psychoanalytic interpretations and therapy as early as 1920 . . . [and] first applied psychoanalytic concepts in group therapy. (pp. 237, 256).

Writers' captivation by Burrow's thought

We cannot omit to mention the strong attraction that Burrow's thought exercised for some famous American and English writers. It is surprising that, despite the majority of his psychoanalytic colleagues' steadfast rejection of it, Burrow's work was read and greatly appreciated by some outstanding writers, who saw in its emphasis on the "social implications of the neurosis" a great innovation in respect to Freud's psychoanalysis, so that its social approach influenced their works. Let us briefly mention some significant witnesses by those writers whose deep interest in his thought led them to seek a close relationship with him.

Sherwood Anderson, whose interest in Burrow's ideas was of long standing, fostered also through a captivating correspondence with him—there are twenty-one of Anderson's letters written between 1919 and 1937 (Burrow, 1958)—became acquainted with Burrow through his wife, Tennessee, who had spoken enthusiastically of him. It is Burrow himself that lets us know some details about their encounter: "When I first knew Anderson many years ago, Freud's ideas were just beginning to reach this country. Yet Anderson was already acknowledged an outstanding novelist" (Letter to F. J. Hoffman, October 2, 1942, in Burrow, 1958, p. 442)

They met for the first time in 1915 at a camp on Lake Chateaugay, as guests of a common friend, where they used to take the midday meal. But it was the following summer of 1916, at Burrow's Lifwynn Camp, that there was more frequent contact and, in the course of long walks, they used to discuss, animatedly and frankly, psychoanalysis in relation to human existence. In particular, they discussed Anderson's pessimism about the capacity of the psychoanalytic tool to meet the individual's needs and also to enable him to delve into his own malaise, which had resulted in neuroses, *vs.* Burrow's belief in it. It is noteworthy that one of these talks with Burrow on the aim and efficacy of psychoanalysis, taking place after a long walk in the woods, turned into a significant experience which affected both of them so deeply that it became the creative stimulus for writing about it. Let Burrow speak for himself:

> Sherwood and I set out on a two and a half mile jaunt to Rocky Brook. We sat there beside the brook and talked the lifelong day, and our talk was entirely along psychoanalytic lines. It was a delightful midsummer day, and I have thought back upon it many times. Of course, there were other days and other talks during this and as well as the previous summer, but the talk that especially stands out in my memory is the day long discussion we had beside the brook. (Letter to W. L. Phillips, March 4, 1949; in Burrow, 1958, p. 559)

Well, that heated and unusually long discussion on psychoanalysis versus life in 1916 imprinted itself so strongly on their memory that, even after some years, it led Anderson (1921) to dramatise it in *Seeds*, where, as confirmed subsequently in a letter from Burrow (1942) to a student, he is "the analyst to whom Anderson referred in this story" (p. 442). And, ten years later, some vivid excerpts from those talks were reported by Burrow (1926d) in his paper "Psychoanalytic improvisations and the personal equation".

It is clear that Burrow's social conception of the human being and of the role of social factors in his wellbeing or uneasiness had a strong hold on Anderson. In *Winesburg, Ohio* (1919), a masterpiece which brought him fame, Anderson analysed the frustrations, the solitude, and the repressed desires of a small city and, in his subsequent novels he re-proposed analogous themes of the individual's maladjustment and bewilderment in a more and more mechanised society. He had a relevant influence on some contemporaneous writers; in particular, he constituted a model for Ernest Hemingway (Enciclopedia Europea, 1976, Vol. I).

Burrow tends to minimise his influence on Anderson's writings, preferring to stress an enriching reciprocity. Through the re-reading of all of Anderson's letters to him in order to answer a student's queries for his dissertation on Anderson's *Winesburg, Ohio*, Burrow (1949b) was able to reconstruct the dates of his relationship with him, withdrawing what he had mistakenly written before:

> I think now that there is no question but that my acquaintance with Sherwood antedated certain of his writings which, at the time I wrote Hoffman, I thought were written before I knew Anderson. So that it would now appear that Anderson was not uninfluenced by my talks with him on psychoanalysis. I should mention, however, that almost from the outset of my work in psychoanalysis I became interested in what seemed to me the social implications of the neurosis and it was this aspect of our talk that took strong hold with Anderson. I do want to emphasize, moreover, that Sherwood Anderson was an original psychologist in his own right and, if he profited by any insights of mine, I also profited in no small measure by the exceptional insights of this literary genius. (Letter to W. L. Phillips, March, 4 1949, in Burrow 1958, p. 559).

Again in response to the above-mentioned student, Burrow (1949) stated that he "did not analyze Anderson" and "at no time did Anderson take part" in his "researches in group- or phylo-analysis", which were a much later development of his work, and specified that, simply, their "relationship rested upon a quite unusual sympathy and understanding of one another that was spontaneous, immediate" (p. 560).

D. H. Lawrence never met Burrow, even if both of them longed to do so. At the time of their correspondence, Lawrence was in Florence. Notwithstanding, as soon as he had the opportunity to read some of Burrow's early psychoanalytic papers, he became a great admirer of his thinking. But how could the English Lawrence get closely in touch with an American psychoanalyst and feel so in synchrony with his writings, given that he essentially lived in Europe, the land where psychoanalysis had its birth and was first disseminated and which looked with suspicion at the American Psychoanalytic Association? It is Burrow himself who, in response to a letter enquiring how he came to make the acquaintance of Lawrence, gives us a hint about the circumstance which gave rise to their deep mutual understanding and fellowship:

> A student of mine, interested him in some of my earlier writings and through them he was prompted to put out the little volume he called *Psychoanalysis and the Unconscious*. Lawrence was very sympathetic to my trend at that time and showed an uncommon insight into it. (Letter to F. J. Hoffman, October 2, 1942; in Burrow, 1958, p. 443).

On 3 August 1927, Lawrence expressed his deep sharing about Burrow's book *The Social Basis of Consciousness* (1927). In this letter, as in others, it emerges that "cut-offness" seems to be have been Lawrence's deep distress and main concern. He longed for a meeting with Burrow and aspired to undergo group analysis, but this project was destined to fail because of Lawrence's health problems. However, they kept in touch through correspondence:

> Your book came three days ago, and I have now read it. I found it extremely good. Your findings about sex and sexuality seems to me exactly it: that's how it is: and your criticism of psychoanalysis as practised is to the quick. I believe as you do—one must use words like believe—that it is our being cut off that is our ailment, and out of this ailment everything bad arises. I wish I saw a little clearer how you get over the cut-offness. I must come and be present at your group-analysis work one day, if I may. Myself, I suffer badly from being so cut off. But what is one to do? One can't link up with the social unconscious. At times, one is *forced* to be essentially an hermit. . . . One has no real human relations—that is so devastating. (Lawrence, 1927a, in A. Huxley, 1956, p. 687)

In a previous letter, dated 13 July 1927, Lawrence had written to Burrow:

> What ails me is the absolute frustration of my primeval societal instinct. . . . *I think societal instinct much deeper than sex instinct—and societal repression much more devastating.* There is no repression of the sexual individual comparable to the repression of the societal man in me, by the individual ego, my own and everybody elses's. (Lawrence, 1927b; in A. Huxley, 1956, p. 685, our italics)

Burrow's (1927g) long response dealt with the many questions Lawrence raised about man's "cut-offness" and the role of "social images", life in general, and their own personal life, religion, and love, psychoanalysis and group analysis, physical and psychological ailment and health. The tone of the following excerpts show how friendly and sympathetic was the relationship existing between them:

> My dear Lawrence,
>
> you have been very much in my thought. Your letter was so heartening and so very kind. I want to say to you first, though, how sorry I am that you have been ill . . . It is so good of you to have in mind the thought of possibly writing a review of my book. It would mean much to me to have your very understanding comment on it. And I, too, hope very earnestly that we shall meet. . . . I do hope you will be well soon and that you will keep in mind how much I enjoy having your good letters. (Letter to D. H. Lawrence, Florence, Italy; September 9, 1927, pp. 184–187)

In particular, Lawrence greatly contributed to expanding Burrow's new social views, first through his book *Psychoanalysis and the Unconscious* (1921), as soon as he had read Burrow's early psychoanalytic writings. Subsequently, it was Lawrence's (1927c) enthusiastic review of Burrow's first book, *The Social Basis of Consciousness* (1927a) in *The Bookman*, whose appealing title was "A new theory of neurosis", that, beyond expectations, *was very well received generally outside the psychoanalytic field*, especially between writers, who became deeply interested in Burrow's social conceptions which, in turn, converged with their own works. According to Herbert Read (1943), "Lawrence was much influenced by Trigant Burrow, and in this way some of Dr. Burrow's ideas have been diffused among people who had never heard his name" (p. 198). Rosenbaum and Berger (1963) echo Read's words and suggested that Fromm and Horney became acquainted with Burrow's thinking through Lawrence's novels, of which they were fond readers: "It has been conjectured that Burrow's impact upon D. H. Lawrence, who admired Burrow, indirectly came through to Fromm and Horney, who were familiar with Lawrence's writings" (p. 6).

With respect to this, we should like to underline that among "Lawrence's writings", there were also the two important ones of 1921 and 1927, mentioned above, dealing specifically with Burrow's work. In addition, in contrast to the criticisms of *The Social Basis of Consciousness*, which "in so far as they were antagonistic, mainly by the Freudians" (Read, 1943, p. 198), it stands out that Lawrence's review of it introduced Burrow with the utmost consideration, and he stated how "far-reaching, and vital" his outcomes were in comparison to Freud's view:

> Dr. Trigant Burrow is well known as an independent psychoanalyst through the essays and addresses he has published in pamphlet form from time to time. These have invariably shown the spark of original thought and discovery. The gist of all these essays now fuses into this important book. . . . He set out years ago as an enthusiastic psychoanalyst and follower of Freud, working according the Freudian method, in America. And gradually the sense that something was wrong, both in theory and in practice of psychoanalysis, invaded him. Like any truly honest man, he turned and asked himself what it was that was wrong, with himself, with his methods and with the theory according to which he was working?
>
> This book is the answer, a book for every man interested in the human consciousness to read carefully. Because Dr. Burrow's conclusions, sincere, almost naïve in their startled emotion, are far-reaching, and vital. (1927c, pp. 162–163)

Lawrence continued with a thorough description of Burrow's basic concepts, such as the social nature of man, the questioning of normality, and the role of the picture which dominates man's life, even sex, of which we report some significant statements.

> The real trouble lies in the sense of 'separateness' which dominates every man. . . . What man really wants, according to Dr. Burrow, is a sense of togetherness with his fellow men, which shall balance the secret but overmastering sense of separateness and aloneness which now dominates him. And therefore, instead of the Freudian method of personal analysis, in which the personality of the patient is pitted against the personality of the analyst in the old struggle for dominancy, Dr. Burrow would substitute a method of group analysis, wherein the reactions were distributed over a group of people, and the intensely personal element eliminated as far as possible. (1927c, pp. 163–164)

In his reply to Lawrence's review, Burrow (1927f) expressed his deep gratitude and appreciation, together with the unexpected news that *The Social Basis of Consciousness* was gaining a wide recognition "among readers generally".

> I am ashamed of myself I have not written you before this to tell you how deeply I appreciated the very kind and sympathetic review of my book that you sent to *The Bookman*. It was such a generous recognition on your part and has, I am sure, *stimulated no little recognition among readers generally*. It was very good of you and I have appreciated deeply your thoughtfulness in this. You will be glad to know, and perhaps as surprised as I am, that the book is really being read and finding not a few favourable reviews. . . . (Letter to D. H. Lawrence of December 21, 1927, Florence, Italy; in Burrow, 1958, pp. 195–196, our italics)

Among the writers who, through Lawrence's review, became sympathetic to Burrow was Leo Stein, whose review of the same book by Burrow was emblematically entitled "Psychoanalysis psychoanalyzed" (1927). Burrow (1927h) expressed his deep appreciation to Stein for his support, pointing out at the same time how his research was at its inception:

> Your review of *The Social Basis* that appeared in *The New Republic* two weeks ago reads most delightfully. It is finely cut and will do much to bring my thesis to the notice of those who may venture along its way. I am most grateful for your sponsorship of an endeavor which I realize, and which I know you realize also, is yet far too limited and incomplete. (Letter to L. Stein, December 29, 1927; in Burrow, 1958, p. 196)

There were exchanges of their respective writings and profound and demanding correspondence with Leo Stein, and, in response to his enquiries or objections, Burrow explained how the meaning of his research led him to be "primarily interested in the health of man as a biological organism, individual and social", rather than in the "analysis of the 'I' by the 'I'", which "simply has no longer any place with me". He goes on by emphasising:

> It just does not have any longer a part in the domain of my processes of feeling and thinking as a social organism or as a student attempting to explain to himself the social organism that he himself, along with others, constantly embodies. (Letter to L. Stein, June 18, 1934, in Burrow, 1958, p. 281)

Particularly fascinated by Burrow's writings was Sir Herbert Read, an eminent English poet and writer on art, whose theoretical–critical essays were integrated by a very up to date and extensive psychological documentation. It is amazing that the art magazine *The Tiger's Eye*[9] published a long review of Burrow's last book, *The Neurosis of Man* (1949), in which six artists each articulated their opinions of the work.[10] The review was introduced by an Editorial, which began:

> The provocative book by Dr. Burrow which appeared recently is of especial interest to the TIGER'S EYE, for many of the points emphasized in this study of human behavior are parallel to the aesthetic tenets held by the magazine. . . . What is important is his meticulous uncovering of human behavior and his recording the research so that it will be recognized seriously today. For those of us who are not scientists it is curious to remember that his proposal of a group analysis has been the natural method of most novelists. (Stephan, 1949, p. 114)

Read's review comes first and relates the way in which he was led to Burrow's thinking:

> Somewhere and somehow, round about 1927, D. H. Lawrence communicated to me his enthusiasm for a new psychologist, Trigant Burrow. . . . From that time, more than twenty years ago, I have been a devoted student of everything Dr. Burrow has written, and I have never been able to understand why, in his own country, he has not received the recognition due to *one of the greatest psychologists of our time*. . . . What distinguishes Burrow's psychology from the rest, and makes it so important? It is undoubtedly his insistence on the primary importance of the problem of consciousness—a consciousness that is phylic (one has to avoid the misleading word racial) and socially unified, and the consciousness that is self-regarding and isolating—the self over against other selves. (Read, 1949, p. 115, our italics)

Subsequently, in his foreword to *A Search of Man's Sanity* (1958), a posthumously published volume of Burrow's selected letters, which, "by revealing the man, explains his work" (p. viii), a "book very moving", Read wanted to relate the precise circumstance of his encountering Burrow's writings:

> It was D. H. Lawrence's review of *The Social Basis of Consciousness* in *The Bookman* in 1927 which first drew my attention to Dr. Burrow's name and work, and from that time *I was an attentive reader of all he published*. By a happy coincidence, ten years later after this hearing his

> name I was to become a director of the firm that was publishing his works in England, and from that time onward *I was in personal contact with a man for whom I had conceived an unlimited admiration.* (Read, 1958, p. vii, our italics)

What, in particular, aroused in him such admiration?

> . . . It is because I believe that Dr. Burrow has, more clearly than any other living psychologist explained the secret of cultural vitality that I personally find such a source of inspiration in his work. Others have contributed to the definition of this problem—Nietzsche, Burckhardt, Lawrence, Whitehead, Jung, Buber—but only Trigant Burrow suggested a method, even a technique, by means of which our social aberrations can be corrected. My own feeling is that the "therapy" of group-analysis must be widened to include the whole process of upbringing. . . . But essentially *what Dr. Burrow is proposing is not a psychological experiment, but new foundations for the next phase in human evolution.* (Read, 1949, p. 117, our italics)

In considering Freud's negative attitude toward "Burrow's extension of psychoanalysis to the social sphere", Read argues,

> This indifference, no doubt influenced the attitude of the scientific world in general. One word of approval or encouragement from Freud would have made an immense difference to the general acceptance and diffusion of Trigant Burrow's main thesis. This thesis . . . points to the anciently recognized truth that *man is not a detached particle of life, pursuing a separate orbit, but that we are part of one another.* From that fact it follows that *the analysis of the individual can never be completed without a consideration of the group of which he is an organic part.* (1958, p. ix, our italics)

Furthermore, Stanley Burnshaw, in his acute and meaningful introduction to Burrow's *Toward Social Sanity and Human Survival* (1984), a selection of his concepts, recounts that it was just four decades before that, through H. J. Muller's book *Science and Criticism* (1943), he first "encountered" what Muller called a "*revolutionary social theory*", that is, "*the theory detonated by Trigant Burrow*" based on the concept of the *organism as a whole*, in whose implications "*biology approaches sociology*" (p. viii, our italics). In Burnshaw's words: "Hence, when I read his opening page on 'Social Biology', I knew I had touched something crucial" (p. viii). At the time, Burnshaw "was striving to master the final version of what, in a drastically different form, would much later (1970) appear as *The Seamless Web*" (p. vii), where with eager attention he could "draw heavily" from Burrow's *Preconscious Foundation of Human Experience* (1964), by trying to express in it his "sense of its supreme significance for the story of man on earth and the 'science' of man" (p. xii). On the cover of *The Seamless Web* one can read: "A new challenging exploration of the arts as the expression of the creator's total organism."

We have to say that the meaning of Burrow's basic concept of the *organism as a whole* was clearly grasped by writers and had such a strong hold over them that they embraced divulging and deepening it, either through their own works or through reviewing Burrow's books. It is a stark confirmation of Freud's statement that novelists, poets, and artists in general are more inclined to catch by intuition the deep meaning of human nature than the experts, such as the psychoanalysts, by often preceding them. In the case of Burrow, we are faced with a creative interchange with the literary and artistic world in general.

Paradoxically, then, Burrow's thought was more widely known and valued outside the psychoanalytic and group analytic circles, his original families, where, until recent years, he had been substantially unknown, or censored, or ransacked, both in America and in Europe.

Indeed, Burrow met with an unenviable fate: he was a rejected son of psychoanalysis as well as a rejected father of group analysis, even though, at least in this latter field, for some years now a considerable change has been occurring in that there is a growing interest in Burrow's thought.

Finally, it should be remembered that in 1949 the American Psychoanalytic Association, in a sort of belated *mea culpa,* assigned to Burrow, as a past president of APA, a gold medal, the Abraham A. Brill Memorial Medal. He could not personally receive the medal, which is now kept, together with his writings, at the Yale University Library. It was very moving to take it from its elegant case and hold it in hand.

Conclusion

Though Burrow's work seems at first sight dated, its contribution and its meanings are of surprising topicality, and constitute a source of fruitful reflection and development, in particular to those relational orientations which have revolutionised classic psychoanalytic thought, of which Burrow was the indisputable and impassioned anticipator and advocate.

As far as group analysis is concerned, one may state that the distinctive feature of group analytic thought, introduced *ex novo* by Burrow, is identifiable in the extension of Freudian ideas centred on the individual to the study of the social factors with which the individual interacts.

Among Freud's followers, he can be considered the one who continued Freud's thought, recognising in him his own matrix, which he rethought in a reflexive and well-grounded way through a radical but constructive critique of the Freudian conception, and, progressively, he went on by developing new ideas and by making a clear and consistent choice of sides. If Freud dared to uncover the boiling pot of the *individual unconscious*, Burrow extended his enquiry to the environment, thus uncovering the boiling pot of the *social unconscious*, whether it is set in the individual's most intimate recesses, or hidden within the folds of society: that is, in the usages, customs, rules, and attitudes of the community one belongs to, of society at large, and its institutions.

It might be said that Burrow's thought triggered off a process, which, being compelled by censorship to remain underground, like the karst phenomena or the forest tree, then crops up again in a myriad of rivulets or buds: we refer to the host of authors who were inspired by Burrow, but it is a great pity that they more or less ignored the spring, or the original base. Apart from everything else, the denial of original, own roots or "matrix", be they personal, professional, or institutional, is anti group analytic: it is the equivalent of mutilating a fundamental part of one's own history, which, if necessary, must be reflexively rethought, analogously to what happens for our patients.

The examination of Burrow's work is worthwhile not only for its pertinence to the present-day situation, but also because, owing to the selective extracting of his concepts, converging in an almost furtive way as founding criteria of the various theorisations, it has been subjected to fragmentation and mutilation which compromised the unity of his thought. In fact, there are significant elaborations and intuitions of Burrow that are not adequately known or are even wholly ignored.

"Burrow, the scientist and analyst" (Behr, 2004), through his work is revealed as a "remarkable man" and a "dedicated researcher" (Pines, 1998, 2012), as a "true explorer" and as a "man of profound personal and scientific honesty" (Ackerman, 1964), as a "great observer" (Berne, 1963), as a "great and original thinker" (Mullan & Rosenbaum, 1971) of psychoanalysis and group analysis and, in general, of the study of human relations and its distortions. Read (1949) qualified him as "one of the greatest psychologists of our time", and, as D. H. Lawrence (1927) stated, "his finding is surely much deeper and more vital, and also, less spectacular than Freud's".

Just like a true pioneer, braving hostile surroundings on unknown and uneven terrain, he was able to *dare* and to go *ahead*, eventually throwing open the door to a world unexplored until then. His thought constitutes a deep well from which we can draw in order to deepen our knowledge of the individual's complex interrelatedness with the social context of which he is an integral part. And it might help us to understand something more about the many problems and conflicts which nowadays, more than ever, afflict both individual and society, its organisations, and institutions—in fact, the entire world. In conclusion, Trigant Burrow's thought, represented in these essays, is of historical, epistemological, theoretical–clinical, and socially relevant value.

Its reappraisal in some ways follows the same path as Ferenczi's thought, rediscovered in these latter years after decades of censorship and now of great topicality, besides being the object of appreciation and an essential point of reference. After all, the analogy between these two great men of psychoanalysis, beyond their suffering personal vicissitudes in their relationship with Freud and their experiences with reciprocal analysis, may be traced to the urge to question those aspects of the theories and technical modalities which, instead of being in attunement with life, are the antithesis to it, or restrain it, or mortify it.

Notes

1. The Lifwynn Foundation for Laboratory Research in Analytic and Social Psychiatry is the first group analytic society, founded by Burrow and his co-operators in 1927.

2. I will be always grateful to the research group members: Sergio Audenino, Roberto Carnevali, the late Claudio Mattioli, Claudio Migliavacca, Paola Pazzagli, Valeria Plateo, and Paola Ronchetti for their valued contribution during our debates, and especially to Diego Napolitani whose encouragement to write and critical support were essential.
3. Papers presented by E. Gatti Pertegato and G. O. Pertegato at the following IAGP Congresses: "Trigant Burrow's conception of prejudice as the underlying cause of individual and social conflict", Buenos Aires, 1995; "Language and conflict in both individual and groups in Trigant Burrow's conception", London, 1998; "Trigant Burrow's eight propositions of group analysis from conflict to cooperation", Jerusalem, 2000. "12th Symposium in Group Analysis", Group Analytic Society, London, Istituto di Gruppo Analisi, Bologna, "Trigant Burrow, a pioneer of *relational goods* through psychoanalysis to group analysis and to dialogue with scientists", Bologna, 2002. Lifwynn Conference, "Burrow's concept of wholeness versus divisiveness: in the individual, in society and scientific world", New York University, July 25–27, 2006; Lifwynn Conference and C. G. Jung Foundation, "The role of social images in conflict and pathology of 'normality'", New York University, October 29–31, 2010.
4. The other APA founders were: Ralph C. Hamill, August Hoch, Ernest Jones, John T. MacCurdy, Adolf Meyer, J. J. Putnam, G. Lane Taneyhill, and G. Alexander Young.
5. Regarding the concept of I-Persona, it should be clarified that "I" is not linked to the concept of the structural theory by Freud (1923b), but is simply the personal pronoun; "Persona" comes from the Etrurian language *phersu* and from the Latin word *per-sonare* (to resound through) and it is associated to the rugged-featured "masks" the ancient Greek and Roman actors put over their own faces, so that the (face) expression and the voice could be well seen and heard by the audience. From that moment on, it has been common to use the word "persona" to indicate the character shown on stage (Pianigiani, 1990). Therefore, as in a scene in both ancient and modern theatre, the individual represents a part, plays a role.
6. Such pioneer experience was presented by F. Napolitani (1961) in plenary session at the Third World Psychiatry Congress in Montreal, Canada. One year later, the progression of the experiment was the object of another report presented by F. Napolitani (1962) at the Fifth International Psychotherapy Congress in Vienna, Austria.
7. Many thanks to Dr Giusy Cuomo, who provided us with the original booklet of the "Therapeutic Community of Rome –Founder and Medical

Supervisor: Dr. F. Napolitani – Affiliated Organisation of the World Federation of Mental Health – Institute of Socio-Therapy and Group-Analysis", Rome, 1963.

8. The "guest-members" were keeping as much as possible in touch with the external world; through "sociotherapeutic assistance", some of them "continued studies or new courses or working activities outside the TC".
9. *The Tiger's Eye* was a magazine of art and literature published in nine quarterly issues from 1947 to 1949.
10. The reviewers were: Herbert Read, the poet and writer on art, and S. I. Hayakawa, the semantic scholar and editor of *ETC*, both of whom were familiar with Burrow's studies; the poets Jean Garrigue and Richard Eberhart, the novelist Seymour Krim, and the painter–writer Barnett B. Newman also added their opinions.

Editors' note

Carrying forward the conception and the realisation of this book has been stimulating and greatly interesting, but so onerous that it has taken several years to complete. In fact, the vicissitudes we met with were so great that they jeopardised our objective: to bring to light Burrow's thinking.

The selection of essays comprising this book offers a panorama of the evolution from Burrow's particular psychoanalytic perspective to the founding of group analysis. However, we have to say that making such a selection also created problems for us, in that it entailed the exclusion of many other papers, including the group analytic studies of the 1930s and 1940s concerning the instrumental body of research on the physiological concomitants of both conflict and authentic integration.

Another aspect we want to stress is the peculiarity of Burrow's language in connection with the introduction of new concepts and the distinctive use of some terms, sometimes resulting in a rather difficult style of writing. No less a figure than D. H. Lawrence, who held Burrow in high esteem, while appreciating and disseminating the article "Psychoanalysis in theory and in life", complained about his style, and Burrow (1927e) readily recognised that this criticism was "terribly true". He did his best to ameliorate it, forwarding to Lawrence another paper, "The reabsorbed affect and its elimination", accompanied by the plea, "See if my language is not improving in this essay I am sending you today" (p. 163). Again, it sounds as if he wanted to reassure Lawrence when he wrote, "In the last weeks I have been trying to make amends for the obscurities and difficulties in *The Social Basis of Consciousness* by putting together material from more recent notes" (1927f, p. 195).

In truth, what was considered Burrow's "involved style" could be attributed to the complexity of the quite new field he was studying and to the lack of existing terms to describe it. For example, as A. Galt (1984, p. 2) pointed out, "there were no words that carried the connotation of humanity as an organism": thus, he borrowed from Ancient Greek the word *phylum* and combined it with other words, among them *phyloorganism*, signifying "the human species as a vast interlinked whole", and *phyloanalysis*, meaning group analysis, and so on.

Doubts about our interpretations were confronted through a number of visits to America, during which we consulted original sources (Burrow's unpublished papers, his correspondence with Freud and his followers) that the Lifwynn Foundation had transferred to Yale University in New Haven. We also kept in constant touch with Alfreda Sill Galt, the then president of the Lifwynn Foundation, and later with Lloyd Gilden, her successor, both of whom were immeasurably helpful.

The editing, applied to only a few essays, has been kept to a minimum (indicated by ellipses), and relates to some unnecessary repetitions or prolixity, and some news of the time that added nothing to the author's thinking.

In the "Introdutory essay", we approached our task from the point of view of accuracy and fideltity to the text, with the clear objective of rendering Burrow's work as clear as possible to present-day readers, without simplifying it. We very much hope that we have been successful in achieving this aim.

PART I

PSYCHOANALYTIC ESSAYS PRIOR TO GROUP ANALYTIC RESEARCHES

Editors' note

From the very beginning of his psychoanalytic practice, Burrow was dissatisfied with the emphasis psychoanalysis put on the individual, to the exclusion of social factors, and began to question it. The psychoanalytic essays, covering a span of time from 1909 to 1918, are extraordinarily far in advance of his time, focusing attention on the early phases of the unborn and newborn child's primary consciousness as the matrix of the subsequent development, showing the social origin of the neuroses, the evolution of the "principle of primary identification", and its application to the comprehension of neurosis, homosexuality, and incest.

CHAPTER ONE

Psychoanalysis and life*

"Not in entire forgetfulness,
And not in utter nakedness"

(Wordsworth, Ode: Intimations of
Immortality from Recollections of
Early Childhood)

The rudiments of the mental life lie in the organic reactions of the unborn child. At first merely vegetative, later physiological, or functional, as we say, there finally occurs in the developing embryo a gradual unification of the scattered elements within the organism, representing a synthesis of function which we might call the primary, organic, mental life. It is organic because the psychic life of an organism, which is nothing more than a register of sensations that inhere within itself, being purely passive, receptive, and afferent, belongs upon a very low evolutionary plane. It is primary because the state of consciousness in this embryonic stage of development is

* Read before the New York Academy of Medicine, 14 October 1913.

simple, elemental, and homogeneous, the mental life in this early organic mode representing the primary matrix of consciousness. Here, then, in this mode which I shall call the "preconscious", is presented a phase of development in which the psychic organism is at one with its surrounding medium. Here, consciousness is in a state of perfect poise—of stable equilibrium. Here, at its biological source within the maternal envelope, this organic consciousness is so harmoniously adapted to its environment as to constitute a perfect continuum with it.

Such is the complete all-sufficing organic unity in the experiential life of the infant *in utero*, but, in due course, this pleasant epoch of dreamless plenitude is rudely interrupted. Through the shock of birth the organism's wishless peace is abruptly terminated, and with the infant's forcible extradition from his paradise of harmony and plenty, he enters into a totally different world of experience.[1]

Into this original, simple, unitary, homogeneous matrix of organic consciousness there now begin those gradual depositions of extraneous experiences, caused by the organism's enforced adaptation to the external world, and these experiences constitute the nuclei of adult social consciousness.

From now forward, life is permanently altered.[2] The fluid, current continuity and fulfilment, which characterised the life of the organism during the months of its repose within the protecting membranes of the maternal womb, no longer exist. The child has now entered a world of stubborn solidarity, and can maintain life in consistent comfort and security only upon a basis of relative adaptation to outer circumstance. Where formerly the psyche was in complete harmony with its enveloping medium, necessities of adjustment now arise that demand concession and sacrifice. The infant *in utero* wants nothing. His world is complete. But with birth, the situation changes. There are wants that are not satisfied, demands that pass unfulfilled. Indeed, it is only when the infant nourishes at the mother's bosom that he experiences a semblance of his original organic unity, completion, and satisfaction.

It is with the entrance of this altered condition that there arises within the organism the disunity which constituted the beginning of the secondary and ultimate phase of mental life, that is, the experiential or conscious phase. From now forward the psychic life is experimental, that is, mental development proceeds upon a basis of trial and error, and as experience or consciousness varies in proportion to obstacles, with the increasing demand for adjustment as life progresses, there is a steady enlarging of consciousness.

Observe the vital contrast between the two mental modes we are considering: the primary organic, preconscious, and marked by homogeneousness, simplicity, and continuity; the other secondary, extraneous, experiential, and consisting essentially of reactions to stimuli from without—that is, from stimuli which arise from a sphere which has no organic continuity with the individual. Now the first intrauterine phase of the psychic life is characterised by an inherent harmoniousness of function, whereas the second, or extra-uterine, phase is characterised by a merely *relative* harmony of function that is conditioned by the organism's acquired facility of adaptation to outer stimuli.

The mental life, therefore, is, from the moment of birth of the organism, a question of *adaptation*. The determination of the individual life is now dependent upon the manner, the degree, and the direction of its adaptation to environment. Adaptation, then, is the watch-word of consciousness. Adaptation is, thus, coterminous with the life itself—life, that is to say, considered in its subjectivity phase, viewed from the standpoint of experience; in other words, the life of thought and of feeling—life as we come to know it and to live it.

There are two central factors which compose the sum of human life; these are, broadly speaking, *love* and *work*, or, less conventionally expressed, *fancy* and *reality*, or *feeling* and *thought*.

Viewed in the light of organic psychology, or of human biology, we find that the component of experience we know as work or thought is co-extensive with the sphere of the secondary, extraneous, experiential reactions, that is, the reactions of the *conscious* ego. Work is the application of the organism to reality. Work is that element of human life which, in its psychological setting, we have recognised as conscious adaptation to outer circumstance.

Love or feeling, on the other hand, is that component of experience which embraces those aspects of life that have their biological root in the primary, inherent, organic reactions of the preconscious ego.[3] Corresponding, thus, to the sphere of the non-conscious emotions, of the primary, organic pleasure-sensations or satisfactions, love, biologically considered, is the aspect of life that embraces the whole range of affective or subjective experience. Thus, love, in general terms, is wish, temperament, imagination, interest, intuition, sentiment, and the feeling reactions generally.

The love component is, then, quite the opposite of the work component, in that the former represents primarily the organism's withdrawal from external reality, while the latter signifies the organism's adaptation to outer phenomena. As work, being adaptive, is the organism's adjustment to the external world, love, being imaginative, is the organism's disavowal of exterior circumstance. As work is the effort of consciousness toward objectivating life, love is the effort of the preconscious to maintain the ego in its primary, infantile, subjective phase.

Work and love, adaptation and sentiment, then, are the vitally opposed forces in the conflict presented in the universal drama of human biology. Now the individual who, through adequate adaptation, maintains himself in relative comfort and happiness in life, is precisely he who has secured a balanced relation between these two cardinal issues. Such a one we call the *normal individual.*

Of those accounted normal, there are two distinct types which may be classified on the basis of their relative adaptation in respect to these two fundamental factors of love and work.

There is, on the one hand, the individual in whom these factors are related, as it were, reciprocally, being balanced against one another so that the love interest occupies a place apart from the work interest. This may be illustrated by the artisan who works at his dull trade with the ulterior view of procuring thereby those things in life which, to his prosaic consciousness, seem beautiful, pleasurable, harmonious. And on the other hand, there is the individual in whom there is a tendency toward a unification, an identification of these two components. Such is the artist[4] whose labour is of itself directly beautiful, pleasurable, and harmonious, for in the life of the artist love and work must be united in a single, homogeneous current.

In other words, in the so-called normal individual, adaptation might occur in which adjustment on the basis of the secondary, adaptive phase of consciousness is dominant and, in this case, sublimations take place in exterior, objective interests such as characterise the practical, mechanical, scientific man; or there might occur an adaptation in which the adjustment entails an assimilation of the primary, original phase of consciousness, and in this case, there are sublimations in internal, subjective interest such as determine the artistic, poetic, imaginative personality.[5]

Having so far considered the underlying psychology of the normal in respect to these two dynamic issues, let us compare with this the psychology of the neurotic individual. If repeated investigation has substantiated any one principle in Freud's theory of the neuroses, it is that which assigns the chief role in the production of these disorders to the element of repression within the sphere of the patient's affective life, with a resulting introversion of the libido.

We have said that the artist is he whose adjustment is made on the basis of an assimilation of the mode of consciousness we have seen to be primary and harmonious, with resulting sublimations in internal, subjective activities. Now the neurotic is the individual who, *through repression*, fails in his attempt to assimilate in his adaptation this primary, infantile affectivity and in whom, therefore, are frustrated these sublimations which are the expression of the artist. For the neurotic, like the artist, is temperamental, imaginative, creative. The difference is, he is not successful. He has failed to objectivise his creative impulse.[6]

It may be said, then, that the neurotic is the potential artist. Now, as the artist whose activities unite work and love—a tendency which is synthetic, integrative, and makes for greater unity—represents a higher degree of mental organisation, so the neurotic, who is potentially the artist, is also potentially the more highly organised type of individual, however deplorably he has failed in his adjustment. But whether successfully sublimated, as in the artist, or obstructed or repressed, as in the neurotic patient, the essential psychological condition common to both is a super-affectivity, a super-sensitiveness.

Let us analyse this super-sensitiveness of the artistic and of the neurotic personality. Let us trace it to its ultimate source and try to discover its elementary nature.

When we consider the essential quality, the underlying motive of the artist, we find that it consists of sensitiveness to beauty, fitness, proportion, whether expressed in color, form or sound. Thus in *its essence the source of the artist's inspiration is the love of the harmonious*. As the essence of beauty is harmoniousness and as harmoniousness is the esthetic expression of that which in its moral relation is truth, the essence of what we call the artist's supersensitiveness to beauty is his innate sense of truth.[7]

Our thesis is that since this inherent harmony, which, in the artist, is sublimated through his creative genius into an expression of beauty, is an aspiration toward truth, the impulse of the artist represents a vitally *moral* trend, and that, therefore, the impulse of the neurotic, which is but the thwarted, repressed, and introverted manifestation of this same life force represents also, in its essence, a vitally *moral* impetus.[8]

As the artist's sublimation is inherently moral, in that it is nature's *successful* quest of that harmonious expression which is truth, so the neurotic's defeated sublimation is also intrinsically moral, in that it is equally nature's quest, albeit a *frustrated and unsuccessful* one, of that same organic harmony which we know as truth. As the love of beauty and of truth belongs to the affective preconscious sphere (being the derivative of the primary, unitary, harmonious phase of consciousness), it follows that, in this sense, the mental life is, in its very source, moral. It is this that I call the "*organic morality* of consciousness" (Burrow, 1914a).

I maintain, then, that the super-sensitive personality is repressed and neurotic because of his innate oneness with organic moral law, because of the vital truth within him which is shocked and outraged at the falsehood and incompatibility of conventional artifice. I maintain that the neurosis represents the struggle of the human spirit in its organic quest of truth: that the neurosis is an earnest search of the vital and invincible morality inherent in life; that the neurosis is nature's protest against civilisation's artificial suppression of the organic verities. In my interpretation, then, the suffering of the neurotic patient, whether expressed in disguised psychic equivalents or in the covert symbols of hysterical conversions, or into whatsoever disfigured and ill-shapen forms his stifled nature has been tortured, is the frantic outcry of an inherently moral organism against the outrage of artificial repression and untruth.

We have seen that *repression* consists of a limitation, a prohibition upon the life or love-component. We have seen that this component is developmentally continuous with the primary, preconscious or with the organic phase of consciousness which exists in its pure, unalloyed state in intra-uterine life and whose continuity we have traced to those affective satisfactions which the infant experiences in the intimacy and security of his dependence upon the mother, that is, in his absorbing union in the maternal love.

We know that life is the gradual process of weaning the organism from this early infantile dependence, unity, completion, and affective satisfaction, which is the vestige of his prenatal Nirvana. It is a process of receding subjectivity, of decreasing identification with the maternal interest and, correspondingly, increasing objectivisation or adaptation toward outer reality. With the so-called "normal", that is, average, individual, this process advances to a relatively successful issue.

But the neurotic, in his super-sensitiveness or super-subjectivity, tends to linger with the original model of his infant love. He is constant to the memory of the complete unity and harmony embodied in the love of the maternal image. And so, with his gradual adaptation or objectivation of experience, there is the persistence of a preconscious subjectivity whereby he ever seeks to reincarnate his cherished union with the mother. It is the repression of the sexualisation through the exaggerated persistence in the unconscious of the mother's image which psychoanalysis has revealed as the basic element in the neuroses. But it is my contention that this desire for the renewed realisation of a perfect love based upon a preconscious model of organic harmony is an aspiration toward an ideal of unity and truth, and that, therefore, as we have said, the genetic factor in the causation of neurotic disorders is an organically true moral factor.

As, in my interpretation (Burrow, 1914a), this factor of repression bespeaks in essence a morally integrative trend tending toward greater unity and synthesis of the personality, the inherent moral conflict embodied in the neurosis is biologically an economic and conservative asset of the utmost significance in ethnic evolution.

It is my position, then, that the repressed neurotic personality represents a biologically conserving and integrative tendency in the development of the race; that this neurotic diathesis is an index of a teleological tendency in mental and social evolution; and that in this tendency is again evidenced in the sphere of consciousness the biological principle of the survival of the fittest—the fittest here indicating the highest mental and *social* adaptation and being comparable to that represented in the structural sphere as the highest organic adaptation. For the stronger the preconscious assertion of this inextinguishable ideal of perfect love or organic harmony is, the greater is the tendency toward synthesis and integration in mental and social selection, that is, in the mating impulse. Repression, being discriminative and exclusive in its tendency, is a return to the principle of nature's inherent urge toward a finer, purer strain in the evolution of the species. However destructive this might be numerically, it is, on the whole, a highly constructive tendency in relation to the social survivors of this selective process, for, wisely directed, it makes for that social integration wherein lies the forward trend of the race.

From these considerations, it seems to me there is not so great a need to concern ourselves about what conventional moral standards *should* exist for society as to point to the organic moral standards that *do* exist in the evolution of conscious social beings.

Where confronted with the practical task of enlightening and training those members of society in whom there exist those thwarting introversions and distortions we know as neurotic disharmonies, there has arisen the demand for a retracing of the earliest accessible sources of the mental life, with a view to an understanding of the original springs of personality and an adjustment of life in relation to them upon a conscious, intelligent basis. In this procedure is embodied the essential function of psychoanalysis.

It seems to me only logical to believe that the indispensable regime for a really intelligent and permanent reconstruction of life is a careful psychoanalysis, or a wholesome acquaintance with oneself. I say *wholesome* acquaintance, for an attitude of wholesomeness, fearlessness, and reassurance follows inevitably from a proper contemplation of the underlying philosophy of neurotic processes as revealed through psychoanalysis.

With this ideal of psychoanalysis before us, the neurotic patient will not only learn to overcome his unconscious complexes, but he will at the same time be imbued with respect for himself, respect for inherent law, and respect for the underlying motive of his disharmony. Psychoanalysis has not come to destroy, but to build up. It is not a cynical commentary upon human records, but a devout testimony to their inherent worth. And I believe that those who come to understand psychoanalysis in its fullest biological import cannot fail to be imbued with a deeper sense of the value, the order, and the truth underlying the varying manifestations we know as life.

Notes

1. This conception of a preconscious is not a mere gratuitous inference. It is a conception that I feel follows inevitably from the empirical data of psychoanalysis. It is manifestly impossible, however, to develop here the evidence upon which it rests. As an instance of data which led to the

formulations of this thesis, the reader is referred to Ferenczi's brilliant essay concerning the unconscious influence of the prenatal and early infantile experience upon the subsequent life of the individual (Ferenczi, 1913).

2. So altered are conditions that we have accustomed ourselves to disregard entirely the life of the organism prior to birth (at least from the point of view of mental life) and to date the beginning of life from the moment of detachment of the offspring from the mother.
3. The preconscious to which I allude here, using the term synonymously with "primary consciousness" or "organic consciousness", should be carefully discriminated from "the unconscious" as specifically envisaged by psychoanalysis. Through the term "preconscious" is expressed my conception of this genetic principle of consciousness, as distinguished from the mechanistic unconscious resulting from the dynamic process of repression. The bearing of this distinction upon the interpretation of introverted mental states will be the subject of a later paper.
4. We are not here speaking of the artist as conventionally understood, that is, the producer of a work of creative genius, but of the imaginative, subjective type in general. In this sense, the artistic interest might express itself in mechanical invention, or in scientific research, or the interest might even remain wholly unproductive. Whatever the activity, though, it is essential that the element of preconscious interest or love be inseparable from it.
5. These two contrary reaction complexes probably correspond in general to the two basic mental types broadly classified by the experimental psychologist, the subjective or affective type of our grouping corresponding to the sensory type of the earlier classification, the objective or adapted type with the experimentalist's motor type. There is also indication that the type of discrimination with which we are here dealing is to be correlated psychologically with the difference of reaction type described by the writer in an earlier work [Burrow, 1909].
6. Imagination is the essence of the creative faculty. The basis of scientific discovery, research, and invention is imagination. Consider Galileo, Newton, Columbus, Darwin, Pasteur. The theory of gravitation, the theory of evolution, are the products of imaginative insight. It is only the dull, unimaginative artisan who works on with the materials of science without ever adding a single original idea to the stock with which he set out. In order that something new be created out of the old, there is need of the imaginative intellect—the inspiration of the artist, of the genius.

7. The world is surely agreed that the quality by which a work of art is adjudged great is its fidelity to the spirit of nature, its quality of truth as attested by its permanence, its capacity to withstand the test of time. As Matthew Arnold says, "To see things in their beauty is to see them in their truth".
8. "Moral" is here used in the sense of a striving toward conformity to inherent law, to organic order, and is in no sense to be allied with the morality of conventionality.

CHAPTER TWO

Character and the neuroses*

When we consider the sentiments, the interests, the general attitude of mind, the qualities of heart—in brief, the personality of the individual who, choosing to live his span of days within the cramped and gloomy walls of his self-appointed cell, has set around himself the barriers constitutive of the system of defence which we know as the neurosis, we find certain broad characterological trends that are of interest in their logical relation to that central factor which the fundamental principle of Freudian psychology assumes as basic in the production of neurotic disorders: the factor of an inherent mental conflict.

Whatever clauses of amendment students and co-workers with Freud might, in the cumulative light of investigation, deem it wise to add to the theoretical principles underlying the psychoanalytic system of psychotherapy, whether they lean to the conception of repression or regression, of infantile fixation or contemporary maladaptation, of congenital predisposition or of a primary *Inzest-Trieb*, this essential

* Read at the third annual meeting of the American Psychoanalytic Association, Washington, DC, 9 May 1913. First published in *The Psychoanalytic Review*, *I*(2): February, 1914.

factor of an inherent disquiet and inner unrest, of a mind distraught with irreconcilable dissension, will still remain the permanent and indisputable basis of the neurosis.

The terms "a nervous disorder" or "nervousness" immediately convey the idea of a state of restlessness, unhappiness, dissatisfaction, ill-adaptation, and all of these expressions contain, upon examination, the underlying idea of a mental conflict, of an inner psychic disharmony.

Psychoanalysis has shown this conflict to be traceable in every instance to the presence of primary, affective trends that are disavowed by the conventional, social ego. It has shown that this conflict consists of an inherent disaffection between organic craving and cultural aspiration; the elemental, biological impulse toward immediate erotic satisfactions meeting a rebuff from the side of the repressive, inhibitory tendency of the collective social consciousness.

Probably the chief stimulus to the evolution of consciousness, and later of self-consciousness, grew out of precisely this primary conflict, this original clash or disparity of interests between biologically related elements or individuals of a single social unit or group, as, for example, the conflict between parent and offspring within the unit presented in the primitive brood or family group.

The components of such familial aggregates had their points of contact in those common ethnic trends which are the bio-genetic or the primitive–social. Wherever, in such a biological commonwealth, a conflict of interests arose, as that already cited, for instance, between parent and offspring, naturally the demands of the stronger constituent superseded those of the weaker and, in the process of social development, the satisfactions of the child became subsidiary to those of the parent and were gradually more and more curtailed or eliminated.

It is probably by virtue of this primary social mechanism, whereby the elementary, immediate, egoistic, or autistic quests were brought into sharp conflict with the unyielding outer world of reality and of social demand, that there was quickened in the individual the primary sense of the social relation and—correlatively as it were, reflex to it—of the cognate sense of self. The conflict of the self with other and stronger selves was an uneven and futile one. The ego was at first compelled, through the exigencies of sheer physical force, to yield its demands for self-gratification to the outer, circumstantial restrictions set by the larger social demands. Later, with the further evolution of consciousness, the social prohibition became more and more rationalised; the element of fitness, of expedience, of propriety began to prevail more and more, and, thus, the child became actuated by feelings of conscience, that is, of consciousness of obligation gradually imbued through the penalties of violation, and began to yield conformity to the newly awakened, if but dimly experienced, sense of group or social suzerainty, in virtue of a suasion representing the primary moral reaction. These reactions, as we have seen, are resultant upon the friction arising between the early egoistic and the social demands. In the original social relationship, as exemplified in that of mother and offspring, the relationship is not, for the primary, infantile psyche, truly social in the sense of being objective, as it comes to be later, but there is originally an identification of the object (the mother) with the primary ego; later, as was said, a differentiation takes place through the gradual entrance of obstacles which tend to emphasise more and more the other self, or the non-ego, and the derivative self, or the secondary ego, and so is introduced the objective factor of experience, constitutive of the social relation, a relation which, thus, is not less social in respect to the self than in respect to others.

It is probable that in some such statement is to be found the biological genesis of the basic factor of repression. For, since social consciousness owes its stimulus to the discomforting contrast between the autosocial and the heterosocial demands resulting from the restrictions set upon the ego by the exactions of the group or social censor, since social consciousness is the outgrowth of the moral interaction between inner and outer, autistic and social, phantastic and actual, unconscious and conscious biological trends, it follows that the factor of repression, whereby this intrapsychic conflict is actuated, is coextensive with social consciousness.

We see, then, that the mechanism of repression is essentially a social reaction, and we have already seen that this primary social reaction comes early to be a moral reaction. For, as has been said, the moral sense is but an outgrowth of the social consciousness. *Repression, therefore, is biologically a moral reaction.*

Therefore, in dealing with the reaction of repression, we are dealing with a reaction that is moral, and this truth is brought home most forcibly to those who are concerned with the treatment of individuals whose condition is due precisely to a miscarriage of repression—that is, patients suffering from a neurosis.

Whether it is a question of the vicarious impulses and imperatives belonging to the obsessional states, or of the characteristic somatic alternatives of hysteria, or of the mitigating substitutions and replacements constitutive of paranoid mechanisms, or of the organic equivocations of the anxiety dissociations, or of the exaggerated mood reactions presented in the temperamental subterfuges of cyclothymia, or of those manifold metabolic mimicries grouped under the ample category designated by the popular misnomer of "neurasthenia", under whatever *alias* the organism might seek to elude the demand most vital to it, at the heart of the neurosis the essential situation is a *moral revulsion*.

This revulsion is directed unfailingly against the admission of primary, egoistic, organic, unconscious sexual trends. As we know, through psychoanalytic research, the different neuroses represent but varying outcomes of a fundamental effort of evasion, but the stimulus to such evasion, being essentially a reaction against prohibition, is based in every instance upon a primary, biological intuition of right and wrong. This is the tree of knowledge of good and evil of which one is commanded not to eat, as we were told long ago in the symbolic legend of Genesis. The neurosis, then, is a biologically moral integration, for it contains the assertion of the organism's innermost verity. The thesis offered here maintains, then, that the neurotic character is *an organically moral character*.

Now, we further maintain that this organic morality is an earnest of the inherent moral value of the unconscious personality. For the fact that this underlying moral trend is organic and, therefore, unconscious, blind and unreasoning, does not make it, of its essence, less moral, but, indeed, rather more moral, for being organic and unconscious it is the more native, spontaneous, and inherent. It is, of course, admitted that this unconscious repression or moral evasion is not economically wise. It is essentially nihilistic, leading to inevitable disaster. But however destructive the method may be, yet the very presence of this inherent, moral element within the organism bespeaks a characterological trend that might become an economic asset of the utmost importance for the body-social.

The essential moral situation present in the neuroses, the inherent conflict of good and ill, is, then, the dominant picture in these disorders. We have all witnessed the touchingly pathetic spectacle of a young man or woman, moving among his fellows in the grip of a great, elemental passion, against which his innermost will is staunchly, fiercely, yet ineffectively set, enduring alone, in silence and dismay, an anguish that knows no abatement. For he is, in a sense, a mere detached and helpless onlooker. Failing to understand his unremitting agony, experiencing the poignancy of his affliction, as it were, only from without, he yet vaguely senses the awful moral tragedy of the conflict within him and so, like a guilty thing, he slinks away from men, a self-distrusting, self-accusing alien, filled with the utmost sense of unworthiness and inadequacy, a prey to hideous dread and fears, alive to every suspicion of evil, dead to every hope of comfort, yet, however racked with mental woe, bearing still within his bosom the ineffaceable marks of a courage that endures.

This moral character of the struggle undergone by the neurotic patient with the innate conscientiousness that it attests and its characterological relationship to the basic principle of repression is too obvious to require insistence. But there are, besides, certain broadly characteristic traits that seem to be interestingly related to this elemental reaction and to the broader factors assumed by Freud as primarily operative in the production of the neuroses.

We are, here, disregarding entirely the relationships to be observed from the standpoint of symptomatology, as well as the definite characterological trends representing sublimations of the more specific erogenous fixations as pointed out long ago by Freud, as it is our purpose to consider, briefly, only those general social and ethical sentiments and tendencies which seem correlated with the original biologically moral and social reactions in which the neurosis has its roots.

A frequent type well illustrates these characteristics as we come to know them in the study of the neuroses. Conspicuous in the patient of this type is a certain child-like simplicity, a lack of confidence in himself combined with a readiness to exaggerate the importance of other people. Showing doubt and distrust of himself and of all that he does, he tends to overestimate the work of others. He is fearful of being misunderstood, of impressing unfavourably those about him. He is especially timorous towards persons occupying positions of authority, as he unconsciously places them in strongest contrast to himself, and best reincarnates in such persons the unconscious image of the father. The neurotic patient possesses, too, a nature that is full of gentleness. Yearning always for the pleasant security he once knew in the perfect union of the maternal love, there is in him a certain wistful tenderness and unfulfilment, in consequence of which his nature is deeply sympathetic. In his affections he is constant, for, carrying always, as he does, within his bosom the image of the complete infant love, his nature is set, as it were, to a standard of inherent loyalty. Further, because of the wound he has suffered through his early unconscious infantile renunciation, his nature is softened, mellowed, and refined.

It is here, in part, that we find the explanation of the neurotic's abiding love of beauty, especially of the sort of beauty that is, as we say, appealing in its naturalness and simplicity, such as the beauty of flowers, of little children, of a pleasant landscape. And as his love for children is called forth by their immature simplicity, so he possesses understanding and sympathy for others who, like himself, are also unconsciously detained in an early, infantile, psychic mode—the individuals whose lives are repressed, inhibited, and neurotic, like his own. This is well illustrated in the unconscious affinities which lead so frequently to marriage between neurotic persons.

As a further consequence of the introversion of the neurotic, of the folding back within itself of his interest or libido, of the mind's reversion upon itself, the individual acquires the mental habit of living within, and in relation to, himself.

On this account, the neurotic patient is pre-eminently intuitive and psychological; that is, he has a striking aptitude for putting himself in the internal situation of another. He knows without knowing why he knows. Proceeding upon the evidence of internal feeling rather than of external proof, he is actuated far more by intuitive perception than by intellectual deduction. For he is one who trusts his first impressions, knowing that they are always right.

Holding, as he does, to the unconscious phantasies of the primary ego, reality becomes the hobgoblin of the neurotic. He prefers to reside within the fluid domain of his feelings rather than to exploit the outer world of unyielding solidarity. However remote from the primary mother-complex such a characterological reaction might appear, its biological origin is unmistakably indicated in concrete instances taken from actual analysis. One patient, for example, who well illustrates the neurotic characterology, at heart a student of metaphysics and of speculative philosophy, though outwardly a hard, shrewd, matter-of-fact promoter of business enterprise, recalls how, in his very early teens, it was his especial delight to fancy to himself the philosophical condition represented by the complete cessation of flux, it being expressed by a longing to enter the quiet waters of some hidden cove—a fancy that was recalled by a dream image in which the same wish fulfilment—the return to the uterine sleep—was analogously symbolised.

The neurotic is imaginative, philosophical, artistic, interpretative, temperamental rather than literal, methodical, critical, mechanical, and deductive. If he lacks the scientific capacity of session, he compensates by a quicker philosophical insight.

It is a long theme, this of the meaning of the characterological import in the neuroses. There is much else that might be readily related to the basic circumstance of repression, which causes the blocking of the personality as we see it in neurotic disorders, but the question of most vital interest is the bearing of all this character reaction upon the practical problem of the patient's ultimate rehabilitation.

We have seen that fundamental in the neurotic character is the sense of obligation, the moral sense, or the love of truth as inculcated through the stolid organic repression of natural desire, with all the suffering it entails, out of obedience—albeit an unconscious, blind, and unreasoning obedience—to organic law as decreed through biological social prohibition. With a mechanism then essentially moral and social at the basis of the characterological reaction present in the neuroses, the logical adaptation for the neurotic patient would seem to lie in the direction of interests which permit the exercise of those faculties which subserve the highest moral and social ends.

It seems to me, therefore, that psychoanalysis ought to be accompanied by, or supplemented with, such re-educative influences as will stimulate our patients to an effective interest in the social and educational problems upon which depend the happiness and efficiency of the social community. Imbued by nature, as we have seen, with a love of truth, a respect for law, a sympathy for their kind, and a reverent sense of the value, the beauty, and the dignity of life, these neurotic men and women, who have faced unflinchingly the rigours of their own analysis, are, above all others, adapted to the high task of teaching and serving mankind.

Having learnt the organic truths of life through his own mental stock-taking, having recognised that his own neurosis consisted in the repression of these elemental truths, and having seen that his own mental conflict grew out of his unconscious and irrational adaptation toward moral and social inhibitions, certainly no one is better qualified than the patient who has undergone psychoanalysis to take an intelligent part in the moral and social problems of the community, problems which he must clearly see are approached from a standpoint of equally unconscious and irrational undercurrents of resistance on the part of the social polity, for, through his analysis, he has come to accept the truth that is in him, and, through the courage born of a great moral conflict, he is prepared to utter it.

CHAPTER THREE

The genesis and meaning of "homosexuality" and its relation to the problem of introverted mental states*

Negative or latent homosexuality enters so universally into the repression that underlies neurotic disorders as to be practically synonymous with a neurosis. Positive or manifest homosexuality, on the other hand, may exist quite apart from a neurosis. Here, the homosexuality, being applied, attains completion in its object. For, in manifest homosexuality, the libido is released, free and untrammelled. In the present study, however, we shall regard quite indifferently the homosexuality which is *entirely* latent and the homosexuality which is *in part* manifest, but devote ourselves for the most part to the phenomenon of repressed, unconscious homosexuality and its subsequent implications as regards the neuroses.

In considering the subject of negative or latent homosexuality, let us from the outset not forget that we have to do with a psychological situation. It might seem superfluous to remind an audience of psychoanalysts of the need of adhering to a strictly psychological interpretation of the problem at issue, and yet, from the very nature of life, such

* Read at the fourth annual meeting of the American Psychoanalytic Association, Albany, NY, 5 May 1914. Mss. received 2 March 1917.

is our enforced adaptation to external and objective criteria that even we, whose sphere is so essentially psychological, incline too often toward an external, mechanical method, and so are prone to bring objective bias to the solution of even the most subtly subjective of problems.

We are all familiar with the basic mechanism of homosexuality, as described by Freud in his "Drei Abhandlungen", and with the similar descriptions of Sadger. We are also indebted to Dr Brill's excellent paper on "The conception of homosexuality"[1] for a very complete *résumé* of the general interpretation of the homosexual complex as described by these authors, in terms of Freudian mechanisms.

According to this interpretation, the determining factors in the production of homosexuality are essentially two—the love for the mother and the love for one's own body. It is pointed out that these two components—the mother complex and the narcissism—are invariably present and stand to each other in a relation of contrast, the narcissism being a consequence of the repression of the mother ideal, that is, the individual rids himself of the mother image as object by identifying himself with the mother and replacing her with his own person as the sexual object.[2] Having thus established as his sexual object his own person, he later, through an association of similarity, extends his object to include other persons of a sex like his own, and thus is begotten *homosexuality*.

Thus, we have the mother complex giving way to narcissism as the first step, and narcissism yielding homo-erotism or homosexuality as the second. But this is not all. A more direct route from the mother to homosexuality is also described. This is offered through the immediate contrast mechanism whereby the homosexual (taking the male as paradigm) is assumed to have had recourse to the male object as a refuge from womankind. That is to say, he rebounds, so to speak, upon the man, because representing the opposite of the woman. Such are the factors and related mechanisms which have been offered to explain the development of the disposition to homosexuality.

Now, with regard to the actual components involved in the determination of the homosexual constellation—the mother complex, the narcissism, and auto-erotic elements—and with regard to the propriety of the theory of the relation of these factors to one another and of the mechanism of their interaction under special conditions, it seems to me that there can be no question, but I believe that we are compelled to assume yet further factors to account for the basic biological situation underlying this phenomenon. For while undoubtedly this interpretation is dynamically correct, it seems to me not sufficiently genetic to satisfy the demand for the broad, unitary principle such as must embrace the great mass of correlated mechanisms involved in the complex of homosexuality as envisaged by psychoanalysis.[3]

Instead, therefore, of three independent components causally interrelated one to another, as represented in the mechanisms just described, we ought, I think, to regard these three components as different developmental aspects of an original and basic biological principle. This principle we might, for convenience of designation, call *the principle of primary identification.*

We are not here speaking of the *process* of identification with the mother, to which we have just alluded, the dynamic process in virtue of which the individual represses the mother image as the love object by adopting the role of the mother and so constituting himself as the love object,[4] of this purposive adaptation, this process of means pursuant to an end we are not here speaking, but of a primary, biological, organic principle of identification inherent in the evolution of mental life. I would, therefore, urge that the distinction between the essentially mechanistic process of identification and the genetic *principle of identification*, which I shall here attempt to formulate and submit to the consideration of this audience, be very carefully borne in mind.

In an earlier paper on "Psychoanalysis and life",[5] I spoke of the original unity or identity of the offspring with the mother as the primitive, elemental state of the infant psyche. I said that, at its biological source within the maternal envelope, the infant's organic consciousness, as I called it, "is so harmoniously adapted to its environment as to constitute a perfect continuum with it". It is this psychic continuity and coherence, this organic homogeneousness of the infantile psyche with the maternal and its significance in later mental development upon the determination of homosexuality to which I wish especially to invite consideration.

Conscious life is determined by the organism's adaptation to the influences of its environment. As we go on in life, gathering to us new and untried experiences which more and more are vitalised through personal reaction, there is imbued in us an increasing predisposition toward a psychological constant. This gradually established bias in the individual's habitual tendency we call character, and the sum of qualities which go toward the determination of character we call the personality. Manifestly, the interest and significance of a personality depend upon the variety, the richness, and the depth of the experiences the individual has known. In other words, personality is proportionate to the obstacles incident to adjustment.

Now the newborn infant, and even the infant of the first several months of its existence, is, under this definition, not a personality; indeed, from the psychological point of view, it is not yet even an individual. Though physically a distinct and independent being, yet viewed from the aspect of consciousness, the young infant is as yet totally without identity, being, so to speak, but an outgrowth of the mother.[6] For there is, as yet, no condition making for adaptation, no adjustment to obstacle making for that sum of qualities which is personality. So, with regard to consciousness, the child is still neutral, quiescent, and undifferentiated. Having his exclusive experience as an organic part of the mother, the infant is, psychically, still of one piece, as it were, with the parental organism. And when we consider the tactual correspondence of surface quality and of bodily warmth that the child feels in its contact with the mother, we realise still more how its experience savours of the actual continuity and organic unity with the maternal organism which obtained during its prenatal life. Added to these general relationships of correspondence and identity there is the far more intimate and specialised relationship arising from the process of suckling. Here, again, is seen a relationship of correspondence and of unity, which still further correlates the post-natal with the original embryological relationship, the union subsequent to birth through the act of suckling contributing to replace the union that existed prior to birth through the umbilical connection.

Now, during these early months of the infant's exclusive relationship with the mother, organic associations begin to be formed which mark the beginning of the awakening of consciousness. Let it be remembered, though, that since the child is still in the subjective, undifferentiated phase of consciousness,[7] the associations of the first months of infantile life are entirely primary, subjective, and unconscious, and that, therefore, its early associations, being subjective, nonconscious, and undifferentiated, tend always toward the closer consolidation of the mother with itself, that is to say, they tend to the indissoluble welding together of the infantile ego and the mother image. Thus is strengthened from day to day the mental union, the psychic amalgamation between the mother and infant which establishes for him an organic bond in respect to feeling or consciousness subsequent to birth that is correlative with the organic correspondence prior to their separation at birth. It is this subjective continuity—this organic mental bond—which I call the *principle of primary identification.*

Now, among the experiences which come to the infant before its differentiation, by far the chief, it will be agreed, is the act of suckling. In the union of the offspring with the mother through contact of the lingual and labial mucosa with the erectile nipple, we have a reaction which, both from the implications of analogy and from the trend of psychoanalytic experience, may be most fittingly correlated with what we know later as the sexual impulse.[8]

Now, as has been said, during the period of suckling the infant consciousness is in the primary, undifferentiated phase, and its experiences are, therefore, primary and subjective, that is to say, they are experiences belonging to the early phase of primary identification with the mother. If, then, the act of suckling is analogous to the sexual impulse, the child's first experience of a sexual nature must be a subjective one, that is to say, it must be a sexual experience that takes place while the infant is still in the primary phase of homogeneousness and unity with the mother.[9]

We maintain, therefore, that though the act of suckling bears a sexual analogy, and though it is an act involving the mother, yet, because of the infant's subjectivity (its identification with the mother in this act pertaining to the sexual instinct), the mother cannot properly be called, at least in the beginning, the sexual *object.* For, as has been said, the infant consciousness, having in the beginning not yet attained the stage of outer adaptation, has no object in the accepted sense. He has, as yet, formed no associations such as may be said to constitute in any true sense the recognition of outer, objective reality, and, hence, he cannot yet be said to have any mental *object* in the sense in which he comes later to experience objects of consciousness. It is only later, through the gradually increasing demand for adaptation, that the infant begins to objectivise. When he does so, naturally being identified with the mother, he objectivates *as* the mother. His subjective consciousness being united to the mother, the child's first object of concern is the self-same as that of the mother. Now, the very special love object of the mother is the child himself—the child's own body.

That is to say, the child's primary ego or consciousness being united to and one with the mother, regards, along with the mother, its own body as the love object. With the process of weaning, the infant is thrown more and more upon himself. Being left more and more to the contemplation of his own body, it becomes the constant and insistent object of interest—his hands and feet, his navel, his alimentary and genito-urinary organs, and the functions pertaining thereto.

This is, in my opinion, the explanation of auto-erotism, my position being that auto-erotism is the psychological correlate of mater-erotism, or of primary identification with the mother. Now, auto-erotism, or the love of one's own body, is the love of that sex to which one's own body belongs and this, in the psychological interpretation, is precisely homosexuality.

We see then, in the principle of primary identification, the essential biological unity of the three above-mentioned components—the mother complex, narcissism, and homosexuality—and how these apparently distinct elements are really but different phases or aspects of this single, basic principle. As I shall try to show, this primary, genetic principle offers us, it seems to me, a distinct advantage over the dynamic process just outlined, in rendering a basic conception of homosexuality that enables us to refer the phenomena of homosexuality in general to a single, psychological law. The mechanistic explanation, as we shall see, does not fully measure up to this requirement.

For, when we come to examine the prevailing dynamic interpretation which accounts for homosexuality in the male on the assumption that homosexuality is due to a repugnance to the mother, the argument being, according to Sadger, that "with the repression of the love for the mother, there occurs a repression of love for all womankind", we at once come into difficulty. For, as soon as we apply this mechanism to the explanation of homosexuality in the female, straightaway the theory involves us in contradiction. In the female, a repugnance to the mother should, according to this mechanism, impel her toward the male as love object, which manifestly would not be homosexuality but heterosexuality—indeed, the more emphasised heterosexuality.

Again, when we examine the more indirect mechanism that explains homosexuality on the basis of an intermediate narcissism, we are in no better case. For here, too, it is explained, you remember, that the narcissism is a result of the individual's repulsion from the mother, that, for the purpose of defence against woman as love object, the individual identifies himself with the mother in order to love himself as she does.[10]

This explanation works well enough as long as we confine its application to the male homosexual, but, as before, as soon as we put it to the test in respect to the female homosexual, we are embroiled in dilemma. For, if the female attempts to rid herself of the mother through this mechanism, her plan is again immediately foiled, because, being herself a woman, she is afforded no escape from womankind through recourse to this dodge. And so it is seen that the mechanisms of homosexuality thus far described, while possessing a special application in special cases, fail to meet the test of universal applicability. These mechanisms are only partial expedients. They lack the basic solidity of a primary and inherent principle.

Indeed, it seems to me that the inadequacy of these mechanisms to serve as a general explanation of the psychology of homosexuality has been tacitly admitted by us. For psychoanalysis has hitherto failed to apply these mechanisms to the female, confining its observations entirely to the male homosexual; in illustrating these mechanisms, reference is made almost exclusively to the male, the detailed discussion of cases being limited to the male homosexual. So, to judge from the discussion of illustrative material, the non-psychoanalytic reader might well suppose that homosexuality was a maladjustment that is limited entirely to the male sex, whereas we know that homosexual trends are as prominent in the female as in the male neurotic. Besides, observation teaches us that in schools and other institutions in which sex seclusion is the aim, a sentimental interest for one another develops no less frequently among the inmates of establishments for girls than in similar institutions for boys. Rather the contrary, for the psychosexual inversion that is presented in the so-called "cases" or "crushes" occurring among girls, though a subtler manifestation of homosexuality, probably far exceeds, in point of frequency, the grosser homosexual practices sometimes occurring among boys living under like conditions of restriction.

Of course, we have explained the homosexuality of the female on the assumption of a recoil from the father analogous to that which takes place in the male with respect to the mother. So, the corresponding mechanism, having in view the repression of the father ideal, would, thus, consist of an identification of the female child with the father in order to replace him with her own person as the sexual object. This interpretation seems to me, from a biological point of view, untenable. Certainly, my own analyses have thus far revealed no such mechanism as the universal account of the homosexual complex in the female neurotic. Besides, there is ample *a priori* ground for rejecting such a mechanism as a sufficient causative factor. For we must admit that the intimate organic relationship between the mother and the female infant is no less strong or less significant than the relationship between the mother and the male infant. Why, then, should we disregard this organic attachment in the case of the female infant? On the other hand, the social relationship of the father is too remote and too little biological, or, from the standpoint of consciousness, too little *organic*, to constitute a factor correspondingly as potent as the mother factor.

That the father plays an important, and often a leading, role in the unconscious mechanisms elaborated by the neurotic patient, whether male or female, appears obvious enough, of course, upon analysis, but my position is that the role of the father as well as of the mother in this dynamic stage of pathological defence adjustments, the basis of which is *repression*, is a secondary role and that, while explaining the action and construction of the actual neurosis, it leaves out of account the native biological factor of a primary consciousness from which, as a sort of matrix, is developed the entire mental life of the normal as well as of the neurotic individual. It might be said that, in having given the place of primary importance to the reaction mechanisms, we began, as it were, with the anatomy rather than with the embryology of the mental life.

We claim, then, that the theory of the mechanism of repression through *replacement* is adequate to account for homosexuality in the male only, and is, therefore, lacking as a basic explanation of homosexuality in general.

It must now be asked: does the principle of primary identification meet this demand? Does the genetic theory here advanced afford an explanation of homosexuality such as proves equally satisfactory when applied to the homosexuality of the female as well as of the male?

With the principle of primary identification, we set out, as just said, with the postulate of an organic unity and identity of the infant consciousness with the mother. Now it is clear that if the original, subjective relationship of the infant in respect to the mother leads to its first objectivating, so to speak, from the standpoint of the mother, that is, *as* the mother with whom it is identified, and consequently leads to the infant's early regarding its own body as the mother regards it, that is, as the chief love object, then the result psychologically is in no respect different whether the child be male or female, for, in either case, since it loves itself, it loves the sex to which it belongs, and loving thus its own sex, it is homosexual.

Now we contend that if the principle of primary identification affords us an explanation of the phenomenon of homosexuality that is basic, uniform, and universally applicable, it offers us a basic and universal explanation of the neuroses themselves.

For, if our thesis is true, it follows that unconscious homosexuality is but an extension into adult life of the individual's original *identification*, and that the neurosis is, therefore, nothing else than a *heightened subjectivity*. It is an accentuation and a fixation of the original, subjective mode, in virtue of which the individual remains in an attitude of identification with respect to the mother, which leads to his objectivisation of himself. Hence, the statement which we set down in the beginning of this paper as a matter of observation we may now return to as the principle upon which the entire interpretation of the neuroses rests, which is that "negative or latent homosexuality is synonymous with a neurosis".[11]

According, then, to our interpretation, neurotic homosexuality presents an exclusively mental situation, and, it seems to us, if our view is correct, that it is incumbent upon the psychoanalyst to define his position more clearly than he has done as yet in respect to the psychological interpretation of the homosexual complex.

According to the original, tentative theory of Freud, the infant possesses a disposition to homosexuality as well as to heterosexuality, and this psychic ambisexuality represents the mental concomitant of the anatomical hermaphroditism presented in the rudimentary sex organs and their analogues.

Whatever validity this theory of concomitance may possess in the sphere of positive or actual homosexuality, investigation has more and more tended to weaken this theory of concomitance between psychic and structural sex ambivalence in the sphere of unconscious homosexuality, until it now appears that we have laid an altogether unwarranted stress upon anatomical sexual conformation in the study of this important psycho-sexual variant. Indeed, from the study of neurotic patients and the analysis of the homosexual complex as presented by them in a repressed and symbolic guise, I have come to feel that we shall only attain to a true conception of homosexuality when we have wholly repudiated a physical substratum in the literal, anatomical sense, and boldly adopt a radically mental point of view in the interpretation of this anomaly. Following this conception, I have come to disregard entirely the question of the sex of the individual from an anatomical point of view and to study the patient *per se* in respect to his greater subjectivity as opposed to his facility of external adaptation; in other words, to study the individual upon the basis of this principle of primary identification, quite apart from his physical differentiation into male or female.

With this conceptual background as a basis, we maintain, first, that the individual, whether male or female, in whom there exists a heightened subjectivity, that is, in whom the primary identification with the mother is strongly accentuated, the individual in whom the unconscious or the primary psychic system tends to persist beyond the average in strength and duration, is, on this account, strongly infantile, affective, introverted,[12] that is, he is the neurotic, actual or potential; second, that such a strongly subjective or autosexual individual, if a male, since he is in love with his own body, that is, with the body of the male, tends to develop in a mentally feminine way; and, if a female, being in love with her own person, that is, with the person of a female, tends to develop in a mentally masculine way. It seems to us, therefore, that, following these lines, we are forced to recognise a psychology of sex that is quite distinct from its biology. There exists, of course, in man as in other sexually differentiated animals, a biological sex attraction between the male and the female of the same species. This attraction we recognise as organic or instinctive. But in man there also enters a psychological factor in the choice of object. Now this factor we call *love.*

If we examine the sentiment that we know as love between individuals, we shall find that, in its essence, it consists of an *identification with the love object.* It is the seeing oneself in another—the recognition in another of that which one would himself be. We say that man and wife are "made one". Their "union" means oneness. This factor of identification is well shown in the acceptability of lovers toward each other even in respect to those manifestations which are ordinarily only acceptable in themselves—for example, the bodily odours, physical imperfections. Consider the tolerance of lovers to drink after one another, while to drink after any one else would be distasteful. Indeed, in this very connection is not the principle of identification celebrated by the folk unconscious in the established symbol of the "loving-cup"?[13] Besides, the very usage of our language sustains this interpretation. When we wish to express the especial attraction we recognise in the psychosexual affinity, we say "*in* love with".[14] To love, then, is not merely to appreciate, to esteem, but it is to find personified in an individual an unconsciously cherished image pre-existing in one's self, to identify one's self with, or, as we say, to realise one's ideal. It is because of the unconscious character of this ideal to which the love object must conform that the selection of object is entirely independent of conscious volition, love being an unconscious process.[15]

Now, normally the individual might identify himself with that love-object toward which he is sexually adapted, organically, instinctively adapted, that is, the opposite sex—the sex unlike his own. That is to say, normally the organic sex attraction meets with a capacity of identification, finds in the personality a degree of subjectivity such as permits of a complete and natural psychosexual union with an individual of the sex opposite to his own, but in the neurotic the primary identification is so intense, his subjectivity so persistent and overmastering, that he tends unconsciously to identify himself with an individual who is more like himself, who better personifies himself, who is of a sex like his own, that is to say, he is unconsciously homosexual.

It seems to me that upon this hypothesis we are enabled to explain much that is fundamental to neurotic processes, much that has long been obscure and perplexing in the psychology of this disorder. In the first place, as we said, the correspondence, the unfailing correlation between repressed homosexuality and a neurosis. Further, we may understand the universal concurrence of the mother complex and repressed homosexuality and the proportionate strength of these two factors in relation to one another and to autoerotism, as they are represented in a neurosis.[16] Here is explained also the infantilism which we know to be inseparable from homosexuality. Indeed, the genetic interpretation of homosexuality here advanced so far correlates and explains the various phenomena occurring in connection with it as would make necessary a separate discussion were we to attempt adequately to treat it.

But here it has been my purpose merely to urge the abrogation of the more mechanical, static, physico-biological theory of homosexuality, to modify somewhat the subsequent dynamic mechanisms by which, thus far, it has been explained and to invite in its stead a consideration of the more genetic and psycho-biological interpretation of this manifestation. Both from biological analogy and from the inductions derived from psychoanalytic experience, we are led to believe that in the formulation of the principle of primary identification—that is, the principle of monopsychism obtaining between maternal and infant organism—we are at the biological source of the phenomena of repressed homosexuality as well as of the neurosis itself.

We return to the text with which we set out: "Negative or latent homosexuality enters so universally into the repression that underlies neurotic disorders as to be practically synonymous with a neurosis". It is hoped that, in view of the foregoing discussion, we might have brought to this statement a somewhat clearer and fuller understanding of its import, and that because of the altered aspect in which we have ventured to present the genesis of homosexuality and its relation to the problem of introverted mental states, others may be stimulated to undertake the further investigation of this very difficult and important problem with perhaps a renewed impetus.

Notes

1. *Journal of the American Medical Association*, August 2, 1913.
2. Freud, *Leonardo da Vinci*, p. 65. Translated by Brill.
3. It will be remembered that in the early formulation of the above-mentioned mechanisms of homosexuality, Freud distinctly insisted upon the tentativeness of his theory and, with his characteristic open-mindedness, heartily welcomed the modifications which future study might suggest.
4. "The conception of homosexuality", A. A. Brill. *Journal of the American Medical Association*.
5. Read before the New York Academy of Medicine, 14 October 1913.
6. It is needful to consider the infant's many months of intrauterine life, during which it leads an entirely parasitic existence enjoying tranquil residence amid ideally equable surroundings. It is needful to consider the

many months subsequent to its passage through the birth canal, spent in an environment as ideal and as equable as adult ingenuity can devise. See Ferenczi's Entwicklungsstufen des Wirklichkeitssinnes, Internat. Zeitschrift für Aerzliche Psychoanalyse, 1 Jahrgang, 1913, Heft 2, März.

7. S. Freud, Formulierungen ueber die zwei Prinzipien des psychischen Geschehens, Jahrbuch für psychoanalyt. u. psychopathol. Forschungen, III. Trigant Burrow, "Conscious and unconscious mentation from the psychoanalytic viewpoint", *Psychological Bulletin*, *IX*(4).
8. To the great credit of Freud's scientific acumen, he early realised that the process of suckling pertains to the impulse of union, of correspondence, of conjugation, and, with a clear insight into biological analogy, he fearlessly allied the suckling instinct with the instinct of sexuality. Freud's followers, led by their own psychoanalytic experiences concur very fully in this position. The disparity of opinion that has lately arisen in respect to this fundamental theoretical position of Freud is due, in part, it seems to me, to a confusion of premises. For, in debating between the nutritional or the sexual interpretation of the suckling instinct, it is necessary, before deciding the issue, that we discriminate between the remoter end of evolution on the one hand and the immediate dynamic aim on the other, that is, between the purpose of nature and the purpose of the individual. While nature's directive aim in the act of suckling is undoubtedly nutritive, just as nature's directive aim in the act of copulation is reproductive, yet the primary incitement in the impulse of suckling, even though it mediates the nourishment of the individual, is directly no more for the purpose of nutrition than the impulse of copulation, even though it mediates the fertilisation of the ovum, is directly for the purpose of reproduction. In both instances the dynamic purpose or incitement of the individual is the immediate sensuous satisfaction. This being true, we are forced to recognise the teleological independence of these two factors—to distinguish between the immediate, individual impulse and the broader purpose of evolution which the individual impulse subserves. Thus, speaking figuratively, nature invests the act of suckling with a quality akin to the sexual to ensure the nutrition and growth of the individual, precisely as it endows the act of copulation with a sexual character to ensure the propagation and continuance of the species.
9. The bearing of this conception upon the theoretical interpretation of certain type-differences occurring in the neuroses will form the topic of a later paper.
10. Brill, "The conception of homosexuality", *Journal of the American Medical Association*, August 2, 1913.

11. Hence the infantilism that we know to be associated with homosexuality. This explains why it is that homosexuals, both actual and repressed, are so generally youthful in appearance. This youthfulness must often have excited the surprise of psychoanalysts. It is a circumstance, too, that is often remarked by the patient himself that, notwithstanding the intensity and duration of his sufferings, so often a question of years, he is still, strange to say, far younger looking for his years than his contemporaries. In his paper, Die Psychoanalyse eines Autoerotikers, Sadger says,

> Noch jetzt, mit 27 Jahren besitzt er bloss aüsserst wenig Schnurrbart und nur ein klein bisschen mehr, doch nur immer sehr wenig Backenbart und sieht ueberhaupt bedeutend jünger aus, als er wirklich ist. (*Jahrbuch für psychoanalytische und psychopathologische Forschungen, V*(II): p. 487)

12. Hence, the temperamental, intuitive, imaginative quality of neurotics.
13. Browning's lines are happily illustrative of this psychological identification characteristic of the sentiment of love:

> I would I could adopt your will,
> See with your eyes, and set my heart
> Beating by yours, and drink my fill
> At your soul's springs,—your part my part
> In life, for good and ill."

14. We say also *en*amoured of. The German expression is *verliebt in*; the Spanish, *estar enamorado de*; the Italian, *essere inamorato di*; the French *en etre amoureux.*
15. Consider the habitual expression "madly in love", and the proverbial obstinacy of " love" to the dictates of reason and prudence.
16. Perhaps nowhere is this relationship more strikingly observed than in analyses of patients representing the anxiety and cyclothymic types of reaction. The evidence from actual psychoanalytic data that is specifically most convincing is the frequent convergence in the patient's dreams of the mother-image and the homosexual object.

CHAPTER FOUR

Notes with reference to Freud, Jung, and Adler*

Among the psychoanalysts who have dissented from the teachings of Freud, the most prominent and significant figure is Jung, and next in importance, Adler. More than any others, these two writers have contributed to check the necessarily difficult progress of the Freudian tide. But, for all the criticism and defection that these deprecating voices have aroused in the professional and lay mind, I hold that their positions are not essentially irreconcilable with Freud.

That which is subsumed under the term "Freud" is a scientific observation relative to the genus man. It denotes the tabulation of a phenomenon. It marks a discovery. I am speaking now of Freud entirely from the point of view of the dogma of science. The question as to whether Freud is humanly acceptable with respect to his observations is not in order. This is not the concern of the scientific observer. It is the man who is advocating a cause, expounding a theory, or exploiting a doctrine, who has to be "right" in this sense.

* Read at the 8th Annual Meting of the American Psychopathological Association, Boston, 26 May 1917. First published in *The Journal of Abnormal Psychology*, Boston, August, 1917.

But Freud is merely observing a fact, and the man who observes a fact is preserved in his integrity by virtue of his fact.

In a discussion of the relative views of Freud and Jung, we are apt to overlook an important point which will largely assist in clarifying matters with respect to the difference between Freud and those who diverge from him. It is one thing to disagree with Freud, the observer, and in so doing to deny the criteria of science, and quite another to offer palliations intended to mitigate the poignancy of unwelcome consequences inseparable from the observations of Freud. It is my feeling that this has been the essential aim of Jung's teaching, and if, in his impatience, he has been led into fundamental disagreement with Freud, his inadvertence has been due to his eagerness to propitiate unacceptable alternatives.[1]

I maintain, then, that Jung's digression from Freud is of the nature of a difference, rather than a disagreement, and, if this is true, it puts Jung's position in a changed light. I think this distinction cannot be overemphasised. I know that for myself I agree with Freud unequivocally, but I also know that in certain respects I unhesitatingly differ from him. I differ from Freud, for example, when he says that sexual repression is due to the interdictions of society, but I differ from him not because of disagreement. On the contrary, it is rather through the fuller agreement; it is, rather, that in this position Freud does not seem to me Freudian enough, so to speak. One must discriminate, then, between a divergence from Freud that is due to a difference in point of view and one that is due to a disagreement.

From this standpoint, it seems to me that Jung and Adler are, in the main, quite right in their general principles, and that their error consists in the dissent from Freud which they have assumed to be inevitable in the modifications of his principles as embodied in their respective teachings. Had Adler, for example, stated simply that an inherent egotism underlies the manifestations of neurotic states, had he pointed out that in certain types of reaction, as in stammerers, there is present an exaggerated self-assertion, a disproportionate overvaluation of the self, and had he recognised that this reaction in these patients is just another expression of the manifold forms of vicarious sexual manifestation, I think no psychoanalyst who is familiar with these cases would have taken issue with him.

Substitutive reactions of an analogous character—those in which the ego is overemphasised as a result of repression of the libido—had been long ago recognised by Freud. Such has been precisely the mechanism to which he long ago drew attention in his interpretation of paranoia, with its self-references, its ideas of persecution, its delusions of grandeur and its hypertrophy of the ego generally. The mechanism underlying the psychology of stammering is really identical with that of paranoia. In both, there is the desperate recourse to egoistic overvaluation in the effort to evade a powerfully determined subjectivity of the sexual libido, or so-called unconscious homosexuality. The stammerer represents in reality a *somatic paranoia*. Instead of the construction of the mental system seen in the elaborations of paranoia, the ego complex of the stammerer shows itself in an overcharge of the affective life, which manifests itself in connection with the social adjustments as specifically mediated through speech.

The situation is similar with Jung in his hypothesis of a presexual mode. As I understand it, his sense of the term presexual implies the existence of a mode that is not only presexual in that it precedes the pleasure mode, but that is presexual in the sense of a generic contrast—a contrast which assumes a non-continuity with the sexual mode. Here, it seems to me, is an instance in which Jung is entirely defensible in his view, but unwarranted in the manner of it and in the subsequent implications it entails.

In positing a presexual mode of consciousness, I am heartily in accord with Jung. The whole significance of the sexual phase of consciousness and of the unconscious is inconceivable to me in the absence of the conception of this presexual phase. To state it figuratively, the whole notion of the sin of sex as symbolised in the expulsion of the first man from the Garden of Eden is, to me, unthinkable in the absence of a Garden of Eden. I call this phase the preconscious, but in this term as I use it there is implied, as the name indicates, no such distinction as Jung's "vital energy", but a distinction that is based solely on a developmental difference, my conception of a presexual mode being not only compatible with Freud, but, as it seems to me, a requisite correlate of his teaching.

The unconscious of Freud is the sphere of repression, or of sex inhibition. If one prefers, he may denote the Freudian conception of sex as the sphere of the pleasure aims, as Freud himself does when he speaks of the "pleasure principle"; or he might sum up the unconscious as the *desire life,* in its broadest, most basic sense. For that which is inherent in sex is the covetous aim. It carries essentially the notion of attaining satisfaction, of possessing for one's self. Thus, desire is the essential element in the aims of sex. Of course, desire presupposes an element of assessment. Desire is to look upon an object and pronounce it good to have. Such is the meaning of "desirable". And so, in this reaction of desire there is involved a judgement. It is a process of cognition, and, however complete or incomplete, however frank or repressed, an act of cognition is an act of consciousness.

Now, there is a period covering many months before cognition may be predicated of the infant, in which the organism is the subject of a condition of comfort or repletion. That is, before it may be said to experience satisfaction in any conscious sense, the organism does at least embody satisfaction as a condition of being. It is this state of tranquil quiescence, representative of the infant's existence prior to the inception of cognition, that I call the *preconscious*. It is, thus, a prejudicial, a pre-conative, a pre-covetous phase of consciousness—a phase of consciousness which precedes the desire or the sexual phase.

For, if the primary, conative phase of consciousness (what is known in adult life as the repressed unconscious) is sexual, then the preconscious—the phase which precedes this sexual or desire phase and out of which the sexual evolves with the onset of cognition—is surely also presexual. If I have made my position clear, this conception of a genetic presexual mode to which the trend of my investigations leads me, entails no dissent whatsoever from Freud and the unconscious as envisaged by him.

Now, the point is that the presexual mode as conceived by Jung does, on the contrary, assume features which demand an entirely altered conception of the unconscious and of the fundamental teachings of Freud. I might go on citing other instances of Jung's divergence from Freud and in general point out in them, as in the instance just mentioned, the unessential disparity of his hypotheses. More than that, it could be shown, I think, that Jung's conceptions could well have assumed a quite complemental position with respect to Freud, and with entire consistency with regard to their fundamental import.

I think, for example, that Jung is correct in saying that there is contained in dreams, as in life, a non-sexual clause. I think there is in life a factor that is preclusive of sex. I do not mean the repressive factor, exhibited in the censorship of social inhibition. This is a quite secondary, artificial proscription, reacting in response to an external agency. But I mean a primary and inherent non-sexual tendency, the biology of which is traceable to the embryonic matrix of consciousness represented by the preconscious mode.

In my view, it is only after clearing away the interpolations of sex as represented in the antisocial demands belonging to the furtive unconscious mode that the native presexual mode becomes assimilable with adult social aims. But, when Jung advances the hypothesis of unconscious trends aiming directly toward constructive social goals, it seems to me we are carried along by an over-hasty optimism that leaves us quite breathless and dismayed. Here, too, Jung's assumptions are made at the cost of Freud's objective observations. Again, it is Jung's manner of approach that seems to me mistaken.

My position is that it is sheer blindness not to recognise that Freud has held faithfully to deliberate observation in reporting the exclusive assertion of sex as disclosed in the symbolic disguises of the unconscious. Yet, I feel that a patient study of life, such as is given the psychoanalyst to pursue, brings to light yet deeper-lying factors, beside which the intense craving for self-satisfaction expressed in sex, notwithstanding its insatiate affirmation, is revealed as an anomalous exaggeration, a sporadic miscarriage of affectivity representing the distortion of an originally harmonious principle of life. We think that repression is the result of sex. But we are mistaken. *Sex is the result of repression*. I believe that when child-life shall be permitted to develop naturally and joyously, its growth unfolding simply from the harmonious setting in which life has its inception, we shall have gone far toward mitigating the driving, obsessive mania that now, whether covertly or frankly, is universally accredited under the name of sex. The principle upon which this position is based is embodied in my conception of the preconscious.[2]

Without this rudimentary principle of consciousness, I am utterly at a loss to formulate satisfactorily the psychoanalytic conception of sublimation. Without this genetically unitary principle as a background of consciousness, what are commonly called sublimations seem to me mere substitutive forms of repression, subsisting under the patronage of social sanction. These socially acceptable "sublimations" seem but cunningly disguised forms of moral adaptation. They are a sort of buying-off of sex—hush rewards, as it were. And, thus, it is sex again with the cover thrown over it. The informing principle is absent.

But after all, man is new to life. That sex or its vicarious palliations should have become for him the affirmation of existence is due to the novelty and immaturity of consciousness itself. It is but natural that, having come suddenly into the franchise of consciousness, man should employ his liberty of action in the wanton aims of personal satisfaction, or in the tedious propitiations of vicarious conformities. But there is something deeper still, more native to man, than all this. It is expressed in the social merging of personalities into each other in the pursuit of the common good. It is that quality in man that ever goads him to search and strive to the utmost benefit of the race. It is this quality of harmoniousness and unity inherent in the social aims of man that is, it seems to me, the strongest principle of man's consciousness. This it is that men have called love. This, it seems to me, is the true affirmation of life, and its prototype is the harmonious principle of the preconscious.

I fancy that it was some such perception as this that animated Jung in his divergence from the rigid scientific formulations of Freud with respect to the sexual libido. But it is unfortunate that in the pursuit of some such modification as this, the temperamental quality in Jung, coupled with his natural impatience of dogmatic prescription, should have driven him to exceed the bounds of moderation and have led him to challenge the actuality of Freud's untempered observations. I shall not believe that the breach is an irreparable one. It would indeed be a calamity if Jung's genial perspectives have misled his splendid genius into an irrevocable disagreement with the clear, steadfast, disinterested observations of Freud.

Notes

1. After all, observation is not the only duty of science. Presentation is no less important. To communicate one's findings aptly and appropriately and, thus, gain the sympathy and acceptance of one's audience is a task that seems to me to rank equally with that of faithful observation itself. Apt presentation invites a sympathetic understanding through assimilating the new with the customary aims and methods out of which the new has taken its growth.
2. "The preconscious or the nest instinct", read at the 7th Annual Meeting of the American Psychoanalytic Association, Boston, 25 May 1917.

CHAPTER FIVE

The origin of the incest-awe*

EROS

"They put their finger on their lip,
The Powers above:
The seas their islands clip,
The moons in ocean dip,
They love, but name not love"

(Emerson)

If it were asked which of the manifold items that psychoanalysis has unearthed had been shown to be the most vitally important factor, the answer would be, without hesitation, the mental revolt against the sexual implication involved in the primary relation of the infant in respect to the maternal organism—the reaction recognised under the name of the Incest-Awe (*Inzest-Scheu*).[1]

Because of the basic significance of this factor in relation to disordered mental states, perhaps no subject can engage the study of the psychopathologist with larger offers of reward than this of the genesis

* Mss. received 4 March 1918 [Ed.] Read at the fifth annual meeting of the American Psychoanalytic Association, New York City, 4 May 1915. First published in *The Psychoanalytic Review*, *V*(3), July, 1918.

of the incest horror, the reaction technically known as the Oedipus complex.

Referring to this moral repugnance inherent in the idea of incest, W. G. Frazer says that "the origin of incest is a mystery". I do not believe it. I do not believe that this biological phenomenon is beyond the range of comprehension. I believe that if we will follow to their ultimate conclusion the genetic data of consciousness which have been made accessible through the dynamic psychology of Freud, we shall not only reach a solution of the innate repugnance represented by the incest-awe, but we shall find that the solution of this phenomenon possesses an almost self-evident simplicity.

With regard to this problem of the incest revolt, certain students have been content merely to affix the generic label of "instinct" and there to let the matter rest, but if the incest revolt is a problem that is pertinent to psychoanalysis, we cannot be satisfied with any such inclusive generality as is connoted by so broad a concept as that of biological instinct. For the problems before the psychoanalyst are, of their very nature, concrete mental problems. They are problems of phylogenetically recent adaptations of consciousness. The aim of psychoanalysis is to determine the *reason why* of every reaction. However basic and original might be the source of a mental reaction, as psychoanalysts our task is to discover the dynamic *wherefore* of it.

Hence, to invoke the oceanic concept of biological instinct is inadequate to the criteria of psychoanalysis. Besides, if I understand the meaning of the term "instinctive", it refers to an inherent, integrative trend determining the specific reactions of organisms with reference to their particular species. Now certainly the primary attachment of the child to the mother is instinctive. In its characteristic manifestation we are all agreed in speaking of the "instinct of suckling". If, then, the revolt due to the recognition of this primary fixation, or the incest horror, is instinctive, we are driven to the conception of two elemental and inalienable instincts which are essentially opposed to one another—of two genetic, cosmic impulses set at cross purposes. Thus, it is to erect towards an inherent urge of nature herself a no less inherent counter-urge.

At the furthest extreme from this biological position there is the more widely accepted psychological statement. According to this account, the incest-awe is due to the interdictions of society, to the universal ban of convention and of civilisation. That is to say, the incest revolt is regarded as the individual's response to a general social prohibition. This seems to me merely begging the question. To appeal to custom is to proceed from mouth to source. Such an account is certainly not genetic. Social custom is a derivative, not an elemental factor. The dynamic and inherent process of organic law precedes the mere consideration of social bias. Indeed, to cite social proscription as the account of a reaction as biological and inherent as the incest-awe is comparable to a process of reasoning which would ascribe to ecclesiastical ordinance the origin of the religious impulse. That an argument so superficial should have found adherents among us is, of itself, proof, it seems to me, of our remoteness from the true interpretation of this reaction—that is, from the genetic account of this phenomenon.

I cannot help feeling that the vicarious rationalisations which have been thus far accepted indicate that the psychoanalyst is, here, face to face with an almost insurmountable resistance within himself, that here is presented a crisis in the handling of which psychoanalysis has very nearly met its Waterloo. I cannot otherwise account for the general acceptance within the ranks of psychoanalysis of an explanation which is not only utterly inadequate from the point of view of logic, but which so entirely abrogates the sworn aims and methods of the psychoanalytic ideal.

I believe we shall gain a distinct advantage if, in studying this mental problem, we will, at the outset, separate our notions of what is primary, subjective, and biological, from what is secondary, objective and psychological, if we will separate our conception of unconscious, biological *unity* from our conception of conscious sexual *affinity*, isolating from our conception of the conscious sexual life (the so-called "unconscious", when subjected to repression) a conception such as envisages a *preconscious* mode of consciousness, representing the original state of the infant psyche. With this distinction in view, let us for the moment leave the consideration of psychological mechanisms—the dynamic reactions we have studied in the analysis of our cases (reactions which I feel more and more are effects rather than primary causes) and proceed to the study of an antecedent stage of consciousness, the original phase of mental life or the preconscious mode, as I have called it, from which, as I believe, such mechanisms are a later outgrowth.

The relation between the mother and the suckling infant is primary and biological. It is unitary, harmonious, homogeneous. For the infant, the relationship is an essentially subjective one. It exists simply, without conscious arrangement or adaptation. It is the one single instance of inherent biological union—the one perfect, complete phase of conjugation. It exists simply and of itself, being exclusive of choice, of calculation. It is spontaneous, disinterested. Existing without object, it is, so to speak, one with life, like the course of the planets or the growth of trees. Being preconscious, it is in the truest sense unconscious. As I elsewhere expressed it, "the infant's organic consciousness is, at its biological source within the maternal envelope, so harmoniously adapted to its environment as to constitute a perfect continuum with it".[2] Such is the character of this original biological union with the parent soil, this mental oneness of the infant with the maternal organism.

This unity with the mother, however, exists only in respect to the affective sphere—to the primary feelings and instincts. That is, it belongs to the subjective life of the organism, for there is as yet no cognition, no objectivation, no contrasting of the ego with the outer world, of the self with other selves—no *consciousness* in the habitual sense. In other words, this original mode, representing the primary glia of experience, consists of an essentially unitary, homogeneous, subjective, non-differentiated state of consciousness.

Now, the demands of the world of outer objectivity or of consciousness proper entail increasing outrage to this state of primary quiescence. They more and more disturb the organism's vegetative repose. Thus, our primary nature shrinks from the intrusion of those outer impressions which disturb its elemental sleep. And so it may be said that *Nature abhors consciousness.* But with the increasing importunities of reality there begins the gradual increase of outer, objective consciousness. Slowly, there is the establishment of that *rapport* between the organism and the external world, which constitutes individual adaptation. Observe that the process of adaptation is essentially outward tending, away from the ego, that it is inherently a process of *objectivation.*

With increasing objectivation, this outer *rapport* is later established in respect to the organism itself. Objectivation returns upon the very self from which it set out. The self becomes its own object and consciousness is, as it were, infolded. Being thus turned in upon itself, the mental organism has attained a state of mental development which distinguishes the human species from the rest of the animal world—the stage of self-consciousness.

As long as the consciousness of self, even though a process of infolding, remains within the mode of cognition, it is but the more inclusive process of objectivation, and self-consciousness proceeds smoothly, uniformly. Even though there is the recognition of the self in respect to conduct, the relating of the ego to the outer act, as long as the process remains objective, consciousness maintains a constant course and the result is a uniform process of adaptation. But when this cognitive function applies itself to the primary affective sphere, when this objective principle is turned in upon an essentially subjective mode an inherent discrepancy arises, for the subjective and the objective spheres being essentially opposite and unassimilable, there is here an attempt to unite opposed and mutually exclusive principles. It is to turn about upon the essential self. It is to attempt to reconcile two phases of consciousness which are inherently incompatible—the phase of consciousness that arises from the primary pleasure-principle and the phase of consciousness that belongs to the secondary and adaptative reality principle.

This disparity between trends that pertain respectively to the subjective and objective spheres of experience is illustrated upon every hand. The difference lies in the fact that that which we *feel* (the subjective) flows from within out, while that which we *apprehend* (the objective) flows from without in.[3] In the first is represented the immediacy of affectivity, in the second, the circumvention of cognition, rationalisation, reflection. The one expresses the world of feeling, the other the world of thought.

My position is that these two components of consciousness are mutually incongruous. Pure cognition or reason impairs the processes of pure affective perception and vice versa. The essence of the affect of enjoyment is its spontaneity. In the presence of beauty, one is caught up by the feeling it invites and forgets to think. When asked to think about it, one is, as we say, "brought down to earth again", that is, he has left the realm of feeling and encountered again the world of "hard" fact.[4]

Everywhere there is seen this discrepancy between consciousness as feeling and consciousness as thought—that is, between the subjective and the objective spheres of consciousness.

The intuitive, artistic, inspirational type of personality—the subjective individual—senses his world through a process of subjective identification with it. The critical, scientific, objective type of personality compasses his environment through a process of calculation, of comparison, of contrast. It is the nature of enjoyment that one yields oneself completely to it, that he does so, that is, nonconsciously. Conversely, experience is robbed of enjoyment, of its affective quality, when it is too consciously objectively experienced. It is so with music, with painting, with poetry, with all forms of art appreciation, such appreciation being a process of feeling, sympathy, and *identification.* If this is true of affective appreciation in respect of art, of nature, of the harmonious elements about us, how much more is it true of the harmonious principle within ourselves, of those organically subjective states of experience we know as the reactions of love?

For love is unity, participation, understanding. It is simple, harmonious, unquestioning. Love is one with life itself. It is life in its subjective relation. Cognition, on the contrary, pertains to contrast, demarcation, distinction. Knowledge is ulterior, consciousness strategic. Cognition is close kin to pride. It is one with *self* as an end. In other words, it is synonymous with acquisition, aim, calculation. Hence, it is kin to self-interest, to desire, that is to say, to *sex.*

It is my thesis that the irreconcilable mental conflict represented in the incest revolt is the expression of the inherent discrepancy that is due to this reversal of life when the objective mental principle is turned in upon the essentially primary, subjective phase of consciousness. It is the conflict embodied in the opposition between love as aspiration and life on the one hand, and sex as covetousness and self on the other. Thus, in my interpretation, the incest-awe is the subjective reaction resulting from an affront to an inherent psychobiological principle of unity. It is the revulsion due to the impact of an organic contradiction.

Such, I maintain, is the meaning of the horror of the incest revolt. I contend that the incest-awe is unthinkable except as the objective consciousness of an inherently subjective mental mode, that incest is the mind's recoil at the rending in twain of what was before biologically simple and indissoluble—the primary homogeneous, subjective ego. Thus, there is no incest but thinking makes it so. I have said that nature abhors consciousness. I might add that nature will not tolerate the encroachment of consciousness within the sphere of that primary, affective preconscious, which pertains to the original subjective unity and identity of the organism with the maternal life source.

In this view, then, the incest revolt is the shock due to the impact of consciousness with its inherent self. This is the meaning of sex. This is the meaning of repression. This is the meaning of sin. Sin consists not in nakedness, but in the knowledge of nakedness, not in the genital organ, but in the fig-leaf with which it is concealed. It is to *behold* our nakedness. It is to objectivate and render conscious an inherently preconscious, subjective state of being. This is why sex is "impure". Convention does not make it so. It is, of itself, impure. That is, it is not simple, not unmixed, not unalloyed.[5]

I repeat, incest is not forbidden, it forbids itself. It is the protest of our organic morality. Its prohibition is inherent. It is primary and biological.

Let us look at the testimony of the folk unconscious, as recorded in history, in literature, in religion, and in language. The Biblical usage "to know a woman" means to have sexual intercourse with her, and there is the legal term "to have carnal knowledge of a woman". Moreover, it is the highest commendation of virtue to say that a person is "innocent", but though this word means "not guilty", if we enquire into the real implication of the term, we find that what is actually conveyed by it is "lack of worldly knowledge". That is, we are identifying virtue with ignorance, we are convicting knowledge of sin. If we search for the genesis of sin, if we trace sin to its psychobiological source, we find that this usage is borne out by the facts connected with the origin of the moral sentiment, as, of course, it must be, for the language of man cannot be else than the expression of the mental biology of man.

No better proof is to be found for the psychobiological identity of knowledge and sin than in the sources of philology. Through a comparative study of language, we find that the word "sin" traces its origin to Latin, Gothic, and Anglo-Saxon roots which signify "truth". The Gothic word *sunja*, from which the word "sin" is etymologically derivable, means "truth". "Sin" is also related to the Anglo-Saxon *soth*, which means "sooth" or "truth". Similarly, a comparison with the Latin and Icelandic forms reveals an etymological kinship between words which mean "being" or "being so" and our English word "sin". Thus, we see that the psychobiological theory which relates sin with consciousness or knowledge is actually substantiated by the records of man's earliest forms of expression.

Consider, too, how all *knowledge* has had to struggle for advance against the universal prejudice of "sin"; how from Pliny and Galileo to Darwin and Freud the progress of knowledge has had to contend against a superstitious implication of evil. Consider how far more violent has been the outcry against the "knowledge" introduced by Freud, by reason of the direct outrage to the subjective ego which his investigations have occasioned, investigations which force the primary mind from its pleasant immanence of quiescent unconsciousness into the boldly disruptive actuality of consciousness. But why this ban upon knowledge? Because knowledge is sin. Because through knowledge is begotten the *realisation* of those organic reactions which constitute sex.[6]

The fall of man consisted in his having eaten of the tree of the *knowledge* of good and evil. Here again, knowledge is sin. This is what is meant by man's "original sin". Thus, again, the folk mind records in unmistakable symbols its intuitive realisation of the inherent sin of knowledge. If we will read between the lines of the Book of Genesis, the latent thoughts that underlie the manifest content of this symbolic legend, we cannot fail to see the identity between the idea of sexuality and the objectivation of the primary consciousness. In Chapter II, verse 16, it is written, "And the Lord God commanded the man saying, Of every tree of the garden thou mayest freely eat; but of the tree of the knowledge of good and evil thou shalt not eat of it. . . ." And again, in reference to Adam and Eve, we read, "And they were both naked, the man and his wife, and were not ashamed". Later, in Chapter III, verse 7, relating the consequence of the disobedience of Adam and Eve, it is said that "The eyes of them both were opened, and they knew that they were naked, and they sewed fig-leaves together and made themselves aprons". Again, Chapter III, verse 9, "And the Lord God called unto Adam and said unto him, Where art thou? And he said, I heard thy voice in the Garden and I was afraid because I was naked; and I hid myself. And God said, Who told thee that thou wast naked? Hast thou eaten of the tree whereof I commanded thee that thou shouldst not eat?"

Essentially similar to the Hebrew tradition of the fall of man, as told in the story of Adam and Eve, is the Greek account of the fall, as related in the story of Prometheus and Pandora. In both, the Gods impose a prohibition upon just one thing. In both there is an act of transgression precisely in regard to this one command. "That is to say, the conscience of the Greeks and Jews, intent on solving the mystery of pain and death, convicted them alike of sin."[7]

This prohibition imposed upon hero or heroine against the doing of some one thing that, if done, will bring evil is the central theme of the folk unconscious as shown throughout the legends of mythology. In the legend of Psyche and Eros,[8] Psyche must never see Eros. If she does, he will not return. She contrives to see him and so he is lost to her. So of Zeus and Semele. Semele is beloved of Zeus, but must never ask to see him in all his godlike glory. She does ask, and is withered by his glory. In the story of Orpheus and Eurydice, you remember that Orpheus can bring Eurydice back to life if, leading her from Hades, he will refrain from turning to look at her. He turns and looks at her and loses her forever. Again, Elsa must not ask the name of Lohengrin. She does so, and he must depart. There is a like motive in the story of Pandora's box, in that of Lot's wife, in the story of Proserpine, and others. In countless varieties of setting this same theme, with its ever-recurring prohibition motive, is presented over and over again the allegorical symbols of the race unconscious.

That the folk mind should be imbued with so deep a conviction of sin, as indicated by this general prohibition motive inherent in its earliest and most durable legends, must indicate some deeply biological principle within human consciousness. It seems to me that this principle is nothing else than the innate abhorrence of the primary affective sphere of consciousness toward the ruthless incursions of an alien objectivity.

It is, I believe, from this source that has arisen the widespread perversion of the human spirit which has caused the hideous distortion of human values embodied in the repressive subterfuge and untruth of our so-called moral codes and conventions. I cannot see the expressions embodied in these reactions of the social organism as other than vicarious representations of an organic law of life, as the feeble efforts of man's immature consciousness to compensate his essential nature for the frustration and denial of his inherent life. These distortions of life represent the organic outrage to this innate principle of unity within him occasioned by the enforced encroachment of conscious objectivation upon his original spontaneous subjectivity and oneness.

Thus, man's "morality"—the code of behaviour that represents psychologically the zealously courted standard of conduct he designates as "normality"—is, in my view, nothing else than an expression of the neurosis of the race. It is a complex of symptoms representing the hysterical compensations of society that are precisely analogous to the compensative reactions manifested in the hysteria of the individual. As morality is essentially the pain of the neurotic due to an intuitive sense of his inadequacy to the demands of his own individual code of behavior, so morality expresses equally the pain of the social organism because of its inaptitude to the requirements of the generic social code. The "hysteria" of the one is the "normality" of the other, but in both the inherent psychological mechanism is identical: the mechanism in the one as in the other representing vicarious compensations due to the frustration of principles of organic truth. So much for the morality representative of "normality".

Among the lower animals there is no recognition of sexuality; there is no sin. There is no "morality". For they have not consciousness, they have not eaten of the tree of the knowledge of good and evil. That is, consciousness has not yet ousted them from their Eden of unhallowed innocence, for the vital separation within the psyche through the birth of objective consciousness has not been imposed upon them. It is this extraneous interpolation in the consciousness of man, this innovation causing a violation of the primary mind principle, or the essential preconscious, which I believe to be the psychological interpretation of the horror entailed in the incest-awe.

"Cursed is the earth in thy work," said God to Adam. This is the universal world tragedy; this is the conflict indigenous to the mental life; this is the doom under which man labours because of his attainment of the knowledge of good and evil. Such, in a word, is the curse of life embodied in the repressed, distorted reactions constitutive of *sex* and its disguised equivalents. Hence, the parable which represents the first man as an outcast, a wanderer sent forth under a life sentence of hard labour, to toil by the sweat of his brow and reap in the end a harvest of thorns and thistles. It is the allegory of the world's neurosis, the prodromal of that universal anguish popularly interpreted as life!

The ban under which sexuality is represented as sin and the consequent repression of this sphere in order to remove it from the light of acknowledgement and deny it objective recognition in consciousness is to none so evident as to the psychoanalyst, for it is within the soul of the neurotic patient that this tragic conflict has entered most deeply and with most vital consequences.

We who study the riddle of the neuroses from day to day and from hour to hour have learnt at least that these disorders are essentially exaggerated states of self-consciousness, that they are due to a confusion of the subjective and the objective spheres of mind, and when we have penetrated to the innermost fastness of the disquieted minds of our patients, to the repressed unconscious, we find unfailingly that this conflict is synonymous with the consciousness of sex and with the horror embodied in the incest-awe.

Notes

1. At the reading of this paper, the question was asked upon what ground the term "incest" could be made coterminous, as I here apply it, with the conception of biological repression in general, it being objected that incest is restricted to sexual relationship between members of the family of a necessarily opposite sex determination, for example, between mother and son, father and daughter, brother and sister.

   In the anti-Freudian days, such an objection to the implication of my usage would have been quite in order. But, with the general broadening of the connotation of sex through Freud's demonstration of biological sex ambivalence, the conception of incest is correspondingly expanded to include the reaction of revolt against the implications of sex with respect to all the members of one's own family, whether they be of the same or of the opposite sex character. Here, then, the term incest-awe is used to express the revolt against the intimations of sex in relation to the members of the individual's family irrespective of a differentiation as to sex.
2. "The genesis and meaning of homosexuality", *Psychoanalytic Review, IV*(3), July, 1917.
3. The reason why the conventional, scientific student of medicine so generally misconceives the nature of the psychological problems of individual life lies in the fact that the objectively trained expert lacks access to the subjective sphere of perception through which alone any possible glimmer of understanding of these intricate processes is made manifest.
4. For example, see Rupert Brooke's poem, "The Voice".
5. It frequently happens that young men, possessed of the popular prejudice in favor of "sex-functioning" per se as a requisite test and verification of "manhood", find themselves inadequate to the act when favoured with such opportunities as are conceded by the promiscuous type of women who render themselves available for such enterprise. A conflict is the outcome. There is apprehension in regard to their "potency" and they consult a doctor.

I know that the popular view is in favour of sex functioning as such; that in these cases it is customary to assume the existence of a pathological condition calling for immediate treatment—"treatment", whatever its method, having in aim the patient's encouragement to successful cohabitation.

In the light of the conceptions this paper attempts to set forth, I am at variance with this whole tendency of interpretation. If such individuals are impotent to satisfy the sex demand presented in such commercial arrangements, they are, in my observation, by so much the more adequate to fulfil the requirements of the larger and deeper affiliations based upon the permanent unions of love.

Even a so technically skilled psychoanalyst as Ferenczi (Ferenczi, *Contributions to Psychoanalysis*, p. 19) and a so faithful adherent of Freud as he to the contrary notwithstanding, I cannot but feel that a psychoanalysis is of a very shallow and short-sighted order that fails to recognise, in this situation, upon which side lies the alternative of health and upon which that of pathology, and that does not assist the more constructive, conservative, integrative process that is shown in the individual's instinctive repudiation of these dissociated and perfunctory trade arrangements. It seems to me that, in this instance, the perplexed youth is *biologically* truer to form than his professional consultant.

6. This inherent discrepancy in human, values which identifies truth with "sin" is nowhere more blatantly shown than in the naïve inconsistencies of our public censorship of "morals".

In the theatre, we are presented with up-to-date "Reviews", contemporary "Passing Shows" which, as everyone knows, owe their success to the carefully conceived sexual appeal they furnish. With their hints, innuendoes, and *double entendres* these popular spectacles are made in the fullest sense "suggestive", as we say, though of what no one, of course, by any chance suspects.

But let some intelligent, earnest, clean-minded student of life attempt to present upon the stage a thoughtful drama of human conduct in which the reactions of life embodied in the perversities of sex are dragged from their habitual retreats and thrust openly before the public consciousness, shorn of their hypocritical cloak of respectability and pretence, and straightaway a cry of protest is raised that is not silenced until the doors of the theatre are closed and darkness again reigns in the playhouse and in the spiritual consciousness of its proletariat audience.

Thus, while "art" productions of the genus "leg-show" are quite permissible, such presentations as Henry Arthur Jones's *Hypocrites* or Witter Bynner's *Tiger* are not to be tolerated because of their "immorality". What could afford a prettier illustration of the true, psychological significance of "immorality", of "sin"? It is precisely the forthright drama that dares to show the truth of things that is pronounced immoral. Verily, sin and truth are synonymous!

7. *The Greek Poets*, by John A. Symonds.
8. See the charming narrative by Walter Pater in *Marius, the Epicurean*.

PART II

PSYCHOANALYTIC ESSAYS IN THE NEW PERSPECTIVE OF GROUP ANALYSIS

Editors' note

From 1918 to 1924, there is a six-year hiatus during which, having questioned the theoretical basis of the Freudian psychoanalysis, Burrow suspended his psychoanalytic practice in order to dedicate himself *in toto*, through the innovative group analytic method, to the research and clinical testing of the social principles included in his first psychoanalytic formulations.

In 1924, on the basis of his six years of group experimentation, he broke his silence and resumed writing, starting this new cycle with two noteworthy theoretical works ("Social images versus reality" and "A relative concept of consciousness: an analysis of consciousness in its ethnic origin"), wherein he exposed the new foundations that should constitute the theoretical structure of group analysis as a social conception of the human being. Both are astonishing: in the former, the concepts of "social unconscious" and "social images" are introduced for the first time and connected to the assumption of roles; the latter subverts the process of observation.

In the other papers of this second set, he dealt with the most relevant theoretical–technical topics of classic psychoanalysis by rethinking and reworking them, through sharp but constructive criticism, in the light of the new perspective of group analysis: that is, by "an interpretation based upon a social conception of the consciousness" (Burrow, 1927a) and of the social unconscious.

CHAPTER SIX

Social images versus reality*

Thinking is a biological process, its manifestation is a function of the social organism. Thought and action are coterminous and the measure of consciousness is its productivity. The builded piles we construct into cities with all their intricate mechanism and design are the outward expression of a concomitant thought process. With the widening relationships of men and our closer national contacts, man's thought has come to encircle the earth and simultaneously it receives outward demonstration in the physical activity of the radiogram. Today, through the genius of the relativists, the consciousness of man has predicted the course of the remotest light waves, and in the motion of the stars his calculations have been vindicated to an infinitesimal measure. Man's thought tends, thus, to dispose the universe but is by it in turn disposed. This agreement in terms between mental processes and the physical universe is explicable only on the basis of the organic accord between those processes and the physical world about us.

* Paper read at the fourteenth annual meeting of the American Psychopathological Association, Philadelphia, 7 June 1924. First published in *The Journal of Abnormal Psychology and Social Psychology*, *XIX*(3), October–December 1924.

Through the discoveries of Einstein, we have been led to outlooks that must inevitably bring into closer alignment the objective phenomena occurring within the physical universe and the subjective reactions that occur within the sphere of consciousness. In the past years, I have come to feel more and more that a relative basis is as indispensable in computing values pertaining to the realm of man's conscious processes as in reckoning evaluations that occur within the objective universe of the physicists. In one respect, at least, the formulations of the relativists have a fundamental bearing upon the interpretations of the psychologists. In respect to the physical universe, Einstein repudiates Newton's basis of absolute evaluation and posits a frame of reference that is variable or relative. In respect to the mental sphere, it becomes correspondingly necessary that a frame of reference that is fixed shall be replaced in favour of frames that are variable. Consciousness offers an infinite variety of frames, but we, in our unconscious limit of outlook, are confined to the position of observation that is our own petty viewpoint.

Under the impetus of our race intelligence, the course of man's thought, like the course of the planets, is onward, and its reach, like theirs, is limitless. Unlike the cosmic revolutions occurring within the planetary system, however, our thought is embarrassed in its progress by the traditional accumulations of much needless impediment. In the process of man's reflection of the observable universe, within his own consciousness he has inadvertently caught sight of the wonder of his own statue and it has come about that, to the serious exclusion of the actuality of the world around him, he is now unconsciously occupied almost entirely with his own image and its reflections. This preoccupation with our own image would seem to entail a mechanism in accordance with which we unconsciously substitute the private satisfaction of arbitrary social[1] images for the largest interests of the race as measured by its activities as a concerted functional unit.

For some time, I have been deeply interested in this form of unconsciousness, which one may see in the tendency among us to substitute social pictures in our quest for personal satisfaction. I have been the more interested in this social recourse of the unconscious because of the vital circumstance that these mental pictures within the social mind appear to present the same mechanism that actuates the dream images within the individual mind. Upon analysis, it may be shown that the social image is prompted in every instance by the same tendency to substitution, symbolism, and indirection which, through Freud, we have found to underlie the dream. Indeed, a relative or inclusive analysis of our mental life reveals a parallelism that shows step by step an unbroken correspondence between the psychic manifestations characterising the individual's unconscious and the psychic manifestations that comprise the unconscious of the race.

The first characteristic common to both of these reactions is an eminently practical one. If we are to proceed upon our enquiry with analytic disinterestedness, we shall do well to give it the place of first consideration. I refer to the hidden, furtive, self-protective nature of all unconscious processes, individual and social. We know, of course, that the unconscious of the individual is exceedingly chary of disclosure. We know that it is quick to obstruct every avenue to self-recognition. So, too, our social unconscious. Indeed, the results of experimentation in group analysis show that it is equally characteristic of the social unconscious that its processes are cunning, self-protective, and secretly suspicious of every approach to self-discovery.

Certain of the social images belonging to our generic unconscious are matters of daily, hourly preoccupation among us. Such images constituting our own social self-reflections present myriad of [*sic*] facets. We rise from the sleep images of our individual unconscious only to enter the no less unconscious reflections of our social mind in its waking activities. Each of us, for example, occupies a position professionally, politically, economically, personally. Each has his special relationships to this one and to that. There is his relationship to his wife, to his child, to his mother, his friends, his servants, and to every class and condition of the people that come within his casual daily contacts. In all these relationships, the individual is constantly measuring his behaviour according to the estimate of those in front of him. Unconsciously, he is at every moment taking stock of his reactions as they appear in the eyes of others. In this way, the persons about us have come to represent unconsciously a sort of social foil against which we watch the outline of our own image. Thus, in his social relationships, the individual *sees* himself in the light in which these relationships reflect him. All of them give back his personal image in the social mirror they present to him. To the servant, we play the master; to royalty, we play the slave. To the persons who admire us, we play the heroic role; to those who regard us trivially, we play a correspondingly insignificant part. Accordingly, our so-called social consciousness becomes but an unconscious exchange of personal images based upon habitual covenants of social reciprocity. The more we consider this self-reflective tendency, the more we may realise how readily we fall into the adoption of this, that, or the other charactero-logical role in response to the image or role that is unconsciously being played opposite us.

With every individual, as we know, the image opposite him that is most important is the image of his earliest and most intimate association. The image, in short, which every individual carries in the locket of his unconscious is the image of his mother. It is this image that he treasures throughout life as beyond price. From Freud, we have learnt the far-reaching influence of the mother-image upon the affective life. But there is the need to recognise that the mother-image becomes the underlying criterion of every judgement that the individual forms. Its impress is the emotional substrate of all the thoughts and activities of his life. And so the individual's guiding principle in life becomes centred upon the single issue involved in the praise or blame he receives from this, the mother-image. With this image held constantly before him he must ever sue for favour. Winning it, his cup of happiness is overflowing; failing it, he is cast down into inconsolable dejection.

But what is the nature of this mother-image? Or what relation has the mother-image, as existing within the mind of each of us, to the personality of the mother as actually existing in the world of objective experience? If we will observe our data from a basis of relativity or from a point of view that includes our own processes within its own envisagement, we cannot fail to recognise, as we observe the outlines of this early implanted image, that *what is called the mother-image is but the sum of the impressions reflected by the mother from the social environment about her, and that these impressions are again transmitted by us to others through their reflection within ourselves.* If this is true, then the mother-image bears no relation whatever to the mother organism and our impression of this early association of our childhood is totally unconnected with the personality from whom we receive it. Indeed, it would seem that this unconscious idolatry of the maternal image is throughout but a replacement for the organic personality of the mother.

We shall be helped if we will keep in mind the organic significance of this replacement. Much of the confusion of psychoanalysis is due to our failure to realise that there is this distinction between the mother-image and the mother organism. The image we unconsciously cherish is not the image of the mother's personality. It is the image of the social suggestion that has surrounded the mother. For I think we must ultimately come to see that the child automatically replaces the biological reality of the parent organism with the *social image* that is artificially reflected to him by the parent. Following the investigations of the past years, it has come to my definite conviction that it is this element of the socially pictorial as reflected in the parent image that is the chief impediment to consciousness. But, still not recognising this fanciful image, we arbitrarily call it "love for the mother", and under this popular misnomer it continues to be apotheosised by us as from time immemorial.

With the social mind, the important image is the immediate community about it. The community occupies the central position within the social unconscious that the mother image occupies within the individual unconscious. Like the latter, the absorbing desire to which the social image prompts us is the approbation of the community. Our every effort is bent toward winning its favours. In its propitiation, we count ourselves fortunate. In its disaffection, we are discouraged and unhappy. Thus, it would seem that the community is but the projection or extension within the social unconscious of the mother image within the individual unconscious.

As with the individual image of the mother our sole preoccupation is love or the mother's approval, with the image of the social mind about us, our daily and absorbing preoccupation is success or the community's approval. As in our individual fixation upon the image of the mother, our constant affect oscillates between the issues of fear or favour, praise or blame, so in the social fixation upon our cherished image of the community, as it exists under our various institutions, economic, political, social, and personal, our constant preoccupation vacillates perpetually between the dual issues represented by our success or our failure, our private profit or our private loss. But if the social image represented by the community possesses the same underlying psychology as the mother image, then this social image can have no more relation to the reality of the social organism than the image of the mother has to the reality of the mother organism. If true, such a conclusion deals a stunning blow to our social as well as to our personal pre-possessions. It means that we shall have to reckon altogether anew with the unconscious factor that is of central importance in psychoanalysis—the factor of the mother-complex—and that, if we are truly to comprehend its significance in its inclusive meaning, we shall have to alter the very foundations of its present interpretation, individual and social.

What we call "love for the mother" is, then, upon analysis, but love for ourselves as reflected to us in the image of the mother, as this same self-love was reflected by her in turn from the social environment about her. For, in all our human relationships, we have been diverted from the organic reality of these relationships and have substituted for them the mental pictures formed by our own artificial projections.

This fetish of our social image worship is no more recognisable by us in the absence of conditions that make possible an analysis of the social mind as it exists within each of us than it is possible for us to recognise the fetish of our personal images as they exist within the unconscious of our individual minds. If we are to be free and uninhibited in the expressions of our social consciousness, it is as necessary that we bring the images underlying our folkways and our folk symptoms under the scrutiny of analysis as that we bring to analysis the unconscious images that underlie the symptoms and reactions of the private individual.

Thus far, in dealing with the arbitrary images to which the individual neurotic is subject, our function as psychopathologists has unwittingly led us also to the substitution of social images that are no less false. We have not recognised that everywhere dissociation is essentially the substitution of the image for reality and, in our presumably analytic work, we, too, have been content if only the image shall have the basis of social approval. But an analysis that is based upon discovering and realising the complexes of the individual in his personal adaptation is in no way competent to discover and realise the complexes of the individual in his social adaptation.

The time is not far distant when the psychopathologist must awaken to his wider function of clinical sociologist and recognise his obligation to challenge the neurosis in its social as well as in its individual intrenchments [*sic*]. Once we discard the absolutistic basis of evaluation upon which our mental processes at present depend, it will no more be possible for us to blink the social than the individual implications of the neurosis. Vicarious images, however much they may enjoy the protection of social convention, are still vicarious images. However general their acceptance by the current and institutionalised mind, they are, none the less, impediments to consciousness and growth.

To form a conception of our unconscious mass mind and its social condensations, it is required that we forego our present absolute basis of evaluations residing in the private judgement of the individual and that instead we assume a basis which, being relative to, and inclusive of, our mental and social processes, will envisage both on the basis of a more universal and encompassing evaluation.

Note

1. In my use of the word "social", I have not in mind the customary acceptation of the term, either scientific or popular. It should be understood that the usage in the present paper is in no way involved in the general usage surrounding the objective concept "social". Rather, I have in mind a group or syndicate form of mental imagery as contrasted with the isolated mental imagery of the individual. Examples of social images in this connotation are "the church", fashion, property, the absolute, democracy, insanity, "The North and The South", civilisation, caste, money, equal rights, and so forth. My meaning will be best understood through the fuller statement contained in a thesis of mine soon to be published.

CHAPTER SEVEN

A relative concept of consciousness. An analysis of consciousness in its ethnic origin*

In presenting a psychological discussion that presupposes the altered basis of the relativists, I am under no illusion as to the wide disparity between the mathematical conception of the relativists in regard to the universe and the clinical preoccupations of a psychoanalyst. It is now conceded, however, that the theory of relativity is not without its revolutionary influence upon our scientific thought processes generally. And so, though I am not competent to an appreciation of the theory of relativity in the objective sense of the physicists, I hope I shall not seem presumptuous in attempting a discussion of consciousness that demands as its basis a viewpoint that is analogous to theirs.[1]

As I understand it, the inadequacy of the Newtonian system of astronomy is its autogenous exclusion of data requisite to a principle which presupposes a basis of universal applicability. Assuming an unqualified absolute to reside within the limits of its own circumscribed area, it posits a principle which fails to take account of factors

*The following essay forms a chapter of a larger thesis, to be subsequently published, representing the outcome of a practical experiment in group or social analysis. First published in *The Psychoanalytic Review*, *XII*(1), January 1925.

operating within the larger constellation wherein its own system is but a contributory element. So that in estimating the components requisite to a more inclusive scale of computation, the Newtonian postulate omits to reckon with the principle of the time–space element constitutive of the extension intrinsic to itself and, hence, mathematically indispensable in an encompassment of the universal and all-inclusive astronomical purview with respect to which its own system becomes but relative and extrinsic.

Little by little, the necessities of a widening outlook have demanded a gradual broadening of conceptual principles generally. Of late, I have been led to views that appear to warrant the conclusion that, in the sphere of psychic phenomena no less than in the realm of physics, a system of absolutism preclusive of data existing outside its own autogenously circumscribed principle wholly dominates our presumably conscious world. Accordingly, if we are to reckon with consciousness upon a true and inclusive basis, it is required that the system of absolutism thus embodied shall give way to a conception of relativity in the conscious sphere comparable to the principle of relativity in the physical universe.[2]

I do not see why, in the sphere of his mental and emotional reactions, man may not so far free himself from the traditional superstitions of imbued inference as to recognise at last that there is a difference between the values that *seem* and the values that *are*, even with respect to conceptions that are the basis of his own mental operations. I do not see why he may not recognise that processes which he has hitherto regarded as habitually inevitable are not by any means organically necessary, but that the two might, in fact, be essentially contradictory one of the other. If, in the objective world, man may ungird himself of the accustomed limitations of a hitherto accepted Euclidean geometry, may he not, within the sphere of his subjective consciousness, also rid himself of prepossessions which, though they appear to us now as no less basic, may ultimately prove equally non-essential?

We have recently waged a world war that, according to the *state of mind* of its participants prior to its occurrence, was the admittedly inevitable recourse, but which, in the opinion of thinking men subsequent to its enactment, is now equally admitted to have been a wholly unnecessary eventuality. How, then, upon our present basis of mentation, may we conclude what is an adequate criterion by which we may determine a dependable process of thinking? If we may know our states of mind only after we have vented the emotions that first incited them, of what use is it to know them? If states of mind can produce calamities that gather their toll of human life by the millions, and we can by subsequently taking thought come to regard them as unnecessary, what must be felt toward states of mind that have produced such calamities? Surely it is not the part of intelligence to feel regret of a disaster only after the disaster has befallen. If disaster need not befall, would it not be wiser to deplore it beforehand and so avert the disaster? This would seem the logical course, but the truth is that the logical course is not accessible to man in his present state of unconsciousness. Man may think logically, but he cannot be warranted to act logically. For, in his present stage of development, his actions are predominantly under the guidance of his emotions and his thought can, therefore, only follow after.

Consciousness is the individual's acquiescence in sequences that are determined by the necessities of organic law. Unconsciousness is the individual's resistance to these organic processes. As consciousness is anterior to its own realisation, so unconsciousness ever follows in the wake of its own event. We think today only in terms of what ought to have been yesterday, and the event of tomorrow embodies again the reaction to the issues of today. Thus, our actions are always but the unconscious reflections of the day preceding, and in our unconsciousness it is only in the aftermath of the morrow that we interpret the omens of to-day.

If man's judgement is competent to apprehend the data of events subsequent to their occurrence, why may it not be equally possible, through our prior apperception of the mental states leading up to them, to envisage the same events with the same clarity anteriorly and, thus, forestall the useless mistakenness and destruction that now follow inevitably with their enactment? Surely it is clear that in continuing to preserve unaltered this same state of mind whose world-wide consequences we have just witnessed, we may be at the present moment preparing a similar, if not a yet greater, catastrophe, the while we are at the present moment as completely oblivious of it. Indeed, from a position that is anterior to the emotional inducements to which our mental states are inevitably subject in our present absolute view, it will be seen that an unconscious and destructive disposition toward life is as inseparable from an absence of self-cognisance on the part of the social mind as the factors of disintegration and unconsciousness are inseparable within the life sequences of the individual unit.

In its intrinsic limitation with respect to the relativity of consciousness in its universal compass, the constellated system of processes which at present comprises the sphere of the mental life will, in my view, ultimately appear analogous to the traditional system of Newton with respect to the universe of relativity in the encompassment of objective mathematics. As in the intrinsic principle of absolutism comprising the Newtonian system of gravitation, so in the self-determined principle of absolutism comprising our present system of psychology a dimensional factor has been left out of account, the inclusion of which completely shifts the basis of former calculations and so distorts our habitual reckonings as to demand the fundamental reconstruction of accepted values.

But while the principle of relativity envisaged by the objective formulae of the physicists is mathematically beyond my reach, the conception of relativity within the subjective life appears to me not only compellingly clear, but organically necessary. Indeed, in the absence of this conception of the relativity of consciousness, it is no longer possible for me to reckon adequately with the processes of the mental life. For, in default of a working basis broad enough to encompass the dimensional element of the system, individual and social, whereof we ourselves are a component part, there is lacking the scientific inclusiveness requisite to a universal principle of evaluation.

It is worthy of note that between the objective or mathematical theory of relativity of Einstein and the subjective or organismic[3] theory of relativity here envisaged, there is to be traced, however inconclusively, a philosophical parallelism that is significant.[4] It is my feeling, though as yet it is little more than an intimation with me, that this cosmological parallel between the subjective and objective spheres of relativity marks a concomitance that is consistent throughout. I do not see how it could be otherwise, since the subjective and the objective spheres of life, embodying the bipolar aspects of the phenomenal world, represent but obverse phases of one and the same universe. The analogy that interests me here, however, has to do with the feature that is equally the basis of the two modes of relativity, which is the feature that entails the abrogation of absolute standards of evaluation and the recognition of the kinetic factor that is organic to both. In the objective envisagement of astronomy this factor comprises the mathematical space–time coefficient of the physicists' fourth dimension, and, in a subjective envisagement of consciousness, it comprises correspondingly the kinetic element that determines the functional coefficient of the organic life as a whole.

What is envisaged by the organic life as a whole is, like the inclusive scheme of the physicists, to be understood only by exclusion, that is, by exclusion of a point of view that is *not* organic, or by exclusion of the absolute system, individual and social, comprising our present static basis of consciousness. As this organismic conception of consciousness is relativity itself within the subjective sphere, its encompassment can no more be apprehended in the scheme of evaluation represented by Freud and his predecessors than the relativity of the physicists can be apprehended on a static Newtonian basis.

Just as Einstein's theory of relativity is not intelligible on the absolute basis of the older system of astronomy, of which conception the newer mathematical theory is, by reason of its wider inclusiveness, the logical replacement, so the theory of subjective relativity or the organismic conception of consciousness cannot be understood on the basis of the absolute principle resident in the Freudian conception of consciousness, of which principle the organismic conception is, by inclusion, the more encompassing formulation.

Hence, this organismic conception of consciousness subsumed under the postulate of relativity will be understood only as we discard entirely the absolute conception envisaged in our present system of psychology. Because of our own absolutistic basis we do not realise that the absolutism intrinsic to the dynamic system of our present individualistic conception of consciousness maintains a position that is relatively not less static than the older descriptive systems of consciousness in relation to the dynamic psychology of Freud. The Freudian system is dynamic in respect to the system it has superseded, but static in respect to the principle by which it must now in turn, I believe, be superseded, precisely as our own Newtonian system is dynamic with respect to the older Ptolemaic system of astronomy it has transcended, but static with respect to the mathematical principle of relativity which now in turn has transcended it.

Of course, the fact that the intrinsic limitation of our astronomical systematization has led us arbitrarily to regard time and space as absolute entities rather than as the functional coordinates of matter has no immediate bearing whatever beyond the need of adjusting a quite infinitesimal error in the astronomical reading of certain minimal deflections. It does not in the least alter the practical conduct of human affairs. For the grocer and the apothecary, our standards remain undisturbed. So also, in the more intimate adaptations of our human relations, the absolute basis of mensuration that has actuated our reckonings with respect to the objective world about us has not for a moment touched our subjective mode or the affective sphere of our living. But when this artificial basis of self-determined absolutism operates within the organic sphere of man's affective life, wherein is the very centre of his being, there are recorded errors whose consequences reach to the core of life itself. It is here in the absolute system of evaluations pertaining to the affective reactions of human conduct that consists the needed correcture in reading the deflection, both individual and social, that comprises man's unconsciousness.

We have yet to learn that it is in the common affects of men that there resides the basis of their collective biology. Only in the affective reactions comprising the native, organic continuum of life may we trace the menstruum of our human consciousness. And so, in approaching the affective or organic implications entailed through the arbitrary systematisation that is our own absolutism, we are entering upon the study of the distorted sensations and reactions in which is embodied, I believe, the essential pathology of consciousness represented in neurotic disharmonies.

In considering the conception of the relativity of consciousness, we shall acquire a clearer insight into the more comprehensive scheme subsumed under it, if we will begin with an analysis of the rudimentary processes comprising our personal judgements and consider the elements into which our primary impressions may be resolved.

Our judgements are formed from the material of our impressions, or, as we say, we reason from observation. This being so, what must be the substance of our observations and what the nature of the processes of reason thus derived? To observe is to stand apart from and record the impressions reflected to us from the object observed so that, upon consideration, our observations are seen to consist of the reflected *images* or mental *pictures* of the world of objects by which we are surrounded. That is to say, impressions of objects consist of the aspect or surface which is reflected to us from them and which is, thus, mirrored in the reflecting surface of our own perceptions.

But in this very process of observation, an unwarranted assumption has already been posited in advance—the assumption that the position intrinsic to the observer is an all-inclusive and authentic one. Already, it presumes a universe of which the onlooker's own self-limited position is the basis. It does not account for the integral component that is the observer's own organic dimension. In brief, the very point of view of the observer lays claim to the prerogative of an absolute cosmogony whereof he is himself the unconsciously static, self-determined centre. Whatever the point of view, it is invariably "the point of view" of the observer. So that, in constituting ourselves perceptual foci from which, according to our self-appointed terms, we look out as from a background upon the phenomena of life, we have unconsciously become artificially detached spectators of a merely static *aspect* of life. This is what I mean by the autogenous exclusion of data extrinsic to the self-determined system of which we ourselves are only a part, but which, in the encompassment of the relativity of consciousness as a whole, is revealed on the contrary as an arbitrary system determined by our own static absolutism. Regarded from the point of view of relativity, to adopt such a detached, observational outlook toward life is to view it in the merely flat, bi-dimensional plane of the image. It is not to experience life through participation in the inclusive extension of its full dimensional actuality.

Upon analysis, then, our world of subjectively tabulated impressions becomes but an artificial world reflecting the artificial systematisation that is our own detached observation of it. Our unconsciousness is our failure to realise that bi-dimensional reproductions of actuality are not actuality. Our own organisms, as well as the surrounding objects of actuality, are elements that are equally to be included in the organic continuum of our human experience. The mental pictures comprising our bi-dimensional *impressions* of them, however adequate as pictures, are not adequate as expressions of actuality in the sense of the dynamic extension comprising our own organic inclusion.

Contrary, therefore, to the casual assumption current among us, we do not apprehend the objects about us as they exist in their cubic actuality, but only in the bi-dimensional "foreshortening" that is our own mental or pictorial impression of them. Our so-called objective apperception of the world of actuality is, in fact, superficial and unreal. Our presumable world of impressions is pictorial rather than actual. It is static rather than kinetic. In consequence of the bi-dimensional visual plane in which our objective fields are reflected, it is inevitable that our environmental actuality should appear in the form of pictures before us. Looking out upon the actual world from a bi-dimensional basis, we can perceive it only in terms of the reflected image formed upon our own bi-dimensional mental background. It is due also, then, to this contributing factor of a flat or reflected visual image within ourselves that there is registered within ourselves a flat or reflected mental image of the world about us. For, in virtue of the bi-dimensional picture in which our impressions are necessarily reflected, our mental perception of objects is likewise necessarily pictorial and bi-dimensional.[5]

Such is the probable ethnological account of this misconstruction of actuality that underlies our mental world. The significance of such a pictorial and artificially foreshortened representation of the objective world and its mental influence in foreshortening the tri-dimensions of actuality in general cannot be overstressed. We need to realise the circumstance of our remote or bi-dimensional position of merely mental or impressionistic observers. From this position, the mentally reflected and artificially pictorial outlook with which the world of solidarity is individually envisaged by us represents but the portrait of life, whereof the reality is the inclusiveness of life as experienced through our subjective continuity as functional elements in the organic whole. So that, while it is most true that we reason from observation, yet, if our observation is imbued with a bi-dimensional or superficial bias, then our reason is also influenced by this same bi-dimensionally imbued bias. If our observation is not subjectively inclusive of the objective world about us, in the same measure, our judgements are not inclusive of it.

It is this non-inclusiveness of consciousness that constitutes our mental systematisation. In this perceptual relationship to life, due to our detached basis of interpretation of it upon grounds of the apparent aspect rather than of its solid actuality, consists the arbitrary absolutism of our present system of consciousness. Due to this organic misconception of consciousness, we habitually prefer the picturesque semblance of the aspect to the pragmatic inclusiveness of the actual. This is why we tend to explain life rather than to live it. This is why the adduced hypothesis of life counts with us more than life itself. But an account of life that does not include the consciousness that is our own kinetic function and repudiates the static pictures of life arbitrarily projected by us does not compass life in the full orb of its rounded actuality. A principle of life that does not embrace the principle arising out of the bias of our own self-made systems of personal absolutism and unconsciousness is not adequate to encompass life in the rounded sum of its functional inclusiveness. It is needful to recognise that, in the unconscious absolute underlying the personal relatedness of each of us to every other, there is involved an organic *resistance* or a mutual repulsion among the elements of the societal personality that forms an impasse to its concerted function. On the contrary, in the mutual inclusiveness of our individual organisms as elements within the confluent sum we thus compose, there is embodied the organic continuum that underlies the societal organism of man as a whole. It is this homogeneous substrate of man's consciousness in its totality that is envisaged in the principle of the relativity of consciousness.

If, however, an ethnological account is adequate to explain the remote, pictorial relation in which we stand with respect to the world of objective actuality, such an account is not adequate to an understanding of the pictorial view we have unconsciously come to assume toward the world of subjective actuality or in relation to the organisms with which we constitute a common species and with which, being subjectively akin, we are organically identical. If phylogenetic theory accounts for the deflections from reality of the reactions of consciousness in the large, it does not account for the deflections of consciousness in the particular reactions of the personality that determine our relations to our individual fellows. Thus far we have considered this absolute system comprising our personal basis only in relation to the objective world or to the world of things; we have not yet considered it subjectively or in relation to the individuals with whom a common affectivity renders us organically identical. It is only within the subjective sphere of our affects representing man's organic racial continuum that this distortion of our outlook is manifested in its deepest poignancy.

It is, therefore, only in its ontogenetic mode that we may fully realise the organic deviations within the consciousness of man due to his bi-dimensional and unreal apperception of his fellows and to his consequently false inferences resultant upon an artificially remote and pictorial attitude toward them. It is here alone, I believe, that is to be traced the philosophy of the deflections observable in the above mentioned reactions of personal resistance as it appears not only in the difform reaction characterising the isolated personality of the neurotic individual, but also in the uniform reactions presented in the *relatively no less deflected group expressions comprising the collective personality of the social consensus.* It has become more and more clear to me that it is this error of our mental refraction, due to the subjective deflection comprising the bi-dimensional judgement of each in assuming a pictorial, rather than a real, relationship to others, that is the essence of our resistances. In this surface reflection that is the personal attitude of each toward every other and that embodies the psychology of our resistances is represented man's traditional systematisation, both individual and social. For, in judging or viewing life on the *absolute* basis of how it appears to *me,* I automatically render it beholden to my personal interpretation of it. In my autocratic attitude of onlooker, I necessarily repudiate the inherency of the individual or object looked on. Thus, as the self-assumed centre of the universe, the individual is completely detached psychically from the organic actuality of everything within his observation and, in his present mental attitude, whatever he thinks he knows and feels is unconsciously constrained by the illusory supremacy of his personal wish. It is this that is the insidious fallacy of the reflected aspect. It is this that constitutes the personal absolute or systematisation which, in dominating our present mode of consciousness, completely distorts the universe of reality. It is such a reflective attitude of personalism and unconsciousness that is our exclusion of data that lie outside the system intrinsic to ourselves, and that may be included only in the fuller envisagement of an organic relativity.

This reflective attitude entails an autocratic interpretation of life on the basis of one's own personal evaluation, and its effect is to sever the natural bond between the elements of the societal body. Mental dissociation is the inevitable concomitant of this habitually reflective attitude toward life, rather than an assimilative participation in it such as may only be realised in the inclusiveness of consciousness as an organic whole. Only an organic coalescence in our common affectivity, as contrasted with our present attitude of detached, bi-dimensional perception of one another, will open the course to spontaneous development in yielding the natural way to the instinct of mating and reproduction wherein alone is the basis of a constructive societal life. For resistance is of the affective life. It is a phenomenon that is essentially organic, in that it marks an obstruction within the societal personality of man in the relation *inter se* of the elements, individual and social, of which our societal personality is composed. In our blind inversion of the inherent processes of life, we fail to recognise that there can be no healthful growth of the organism apart from the soil to which it is indigenous. If isolation and an artificial medium are death to the growth of vegetation, they are death no less to the societal instinct of our common consciousness, in which is found the natural medium for the growth and activity of man. In the measure in which we allow ourselves to participate in and become intrinsic and contributory elements in the world of organic actuality about us, will our pictorial mode of envisagement yield place to the subjective experience of a dimensional inclusiveness that is complete in its actuality. To view the world of actuality in its merely static, cross-sectional appearance is to know only the photography of life. Its kinetic reality may be known only through the subjective inclusion of our organic participation in it.

We cannot return too often to original sources in repudiating conceptions whereof they are the basis. We experience reality only in the measure in which we disavow the symbols of unreality. In proportion as we apprehend subjective fallacy may we encompass the reality underlying it. It is where our conceptual constructions of life leave off that our constructive conceptions of life begin. We have seen that the mathematicians have come to regard as theoretically worthless those objective calculations whose standards of evaluation are not measured in accordance with the principle of an inclusive relativity. Likewise, a formulation of values in the subjective sphere of consciousness lacks an adequate principle of evaluation if it does not rest upon the relative principle comprising the organic and inclusive conception of consciousness in its societal totality.

If, in the dissociation of the consciousness of man from his organic individuality, he is unconsciously assuming a personal absolute that is merely a reflection of the mass absolute assumed by the collective social unconscious about him, then what we call the consciousness of man, with its presumable function of dependable evaluation, is at all times but a system of images, and his mooted prerogative of a personal absolute is only a dissociative reaction due to his own secondarily adaptive systematisation. Upon this basis, what we call our opinions are, after all, not our opinions, and our so-called beliefs are not beliefs at all. For all our formulations and systematisations with respect to human consciousness are but rationalisations serving as convenient foils for the blind assertion of the personal absolutism that is but the autocratic prerogative of our own dissociation, both individual and social.

While theoretically the objective findings of Freud are throughout of unquestionable validity, as has been fully corroborated through the repeated investigations of those of us who have studied the manifestations of the unconscious in ourselves and in others, my researches within the past years have convinced me that our objective finding is not the point, that what we have called the objective evidence has been all along but our personal or adaptive evidence, and that, being unconsciously based upon habitual bi-dimensional inference, this basis has no relation whatever to life in its organic inclusiveness. The system of Freud is, thus, adequate only on the adaptive basis of normality. *By normality, I mean the consensus comprising the personal absolute vested in the unconscious of the collective mind determining the social average.*

It is disconcerting, I know, now that the psychoanalyst has but recently settled himself to enjoy in comfort the established principles of Freud's psychology, to think that he may be compelled through the requirements of wider accommodation to seek other ground. Nevertheless, if the position in which we have settled to study the complexes of men is itself just another complex of the social mind whereof the individual mind we would study is but a reproduction, it is clear that we have no choice but to recognise the autonomy of our absolutistic values of reckoning and to readjust our measures of consciousness in accordance.

Surely, if the whole meaning of our mental orientation is a disorientation, if our rationality is everywhere but irrationality, if, with all of us alike, the vicarious image comprising the reflection of our systematised selves takes precedence over the native reality of our primary organic individuality, there is no other course than that we wipe the board clean and approach the problem of consciousness completely anew. For, clearly, since our present process of mentation is not spontaneous or from within out, it is necessarily adaptive or from without in. Hence, as the reflection of the absolute principle that is the personal basis of each, it can never lead to a realisation of the relativity of our conscious life or to the acceptance of the organic individuality that is the encompassing life of man in the inclusive principle wherein alone his consciousness truly resides.

It is the position of this thesis that when we neglect to take account of the *organic mass consciousness of man*, to which the personal systems of men, single and collective, are but relative, we fail to reckon with a significant dimension entering into the determination of the subjective life of man. On the basis of the time–space extension of the astronomers' fourth dimension, it is possible to compute errors of deflection only through a conception of the universe which regards our own planetary system as a function of, and, hence, relative to, a more encompassing programme of planetary motion. Concomitantly, it is possible to evaluate accurately man's place in the subjective scheme of consciousness only through a conception that regards his present personal and social absolute as itself relative to a more encompassing background comprising the relativity of man's consciousness as a whole. There is the need to recognise that in the sphere of consciousness, as in the realm of physics, it is in the kinetic dimension comprising the organic participation and inclusiveness of life itself that consists the functional component which actuates the other three dimensions and which, in uniting all, embodies the relativity of consciousness as an organic reality.

In this transition from bi-dimensional picture to tri-dimensional actuality, from contemplation of aspect to participation of function, a gulf is spanned that bridges a most significant hiatus in the course of man's evolution. It is no less an interval than that which separates the mode of man's unconsciousness from the mode of his consciousness. For the transition is one in which we are no longer dealing with the mere static dimension of the pictorially reflected *image* of actuality, but there enters the kinetic extension of an organic inclusiveness corresponding to the functional or space–time extension of the physicists' universe of relativity, a universe which, in the psychological no less than in the physical sphere, entails the abrogation of our prevailing system of absolutism and its replacement through the conception of the relativity of the conscious life as a whole.

Notes

1. "To free our thought from the fetters of space and time is an aspiration of the poet and the mystic, viewed somewhat coldly by the scientist who

has too good reason to fear the confusion of loose ideas likely to ensue. If others have had a suspicion of the end to be desired, it has been left to Einstein to show the way to rid ourselves of these 'terrestrial adhesions to thought.' And in removing our fetters he leaves us, not (as might have been feared) vague generalities for the ecstatic contemplation of the mystic, but a precise scheme of world-structure to engage the mathematical physicist" (Arthur Stanley Eddington, FRS).

2. It is, of course, not possible to trace through mathematical intricacies detailed analogy between the cosmic theory of relativity as it bears upon the objective data of an abstruse calculus and the organic theory of relativity as it bears upon the subjective data of the all-inclusive principle of psychology here regarded as the basis of a universally comprehensive scheme of consciousness. The comparison has significance for me merely in the aptness of its theoretical alignment with a conception of consciousness in whose envisagement are encompassed data extrinsic to the habitual psychological system that is intrinsic to ourselves and that is commonly accepted by us a the totality of consciousness.
3. By organismic, I mean the feelings and reactions common to the social body regarded as a coherent, integral organism. The term organismic, as I use it in its social application, is identical with the term organic in its individual application, so that the connotations organic and organismic are here used interchangeably.
4. Newton observed the universe from the point of view of his fixed position upon the earth. Einstein observes the universe from the point of view of all possible positions within the universe. Likewise, the prevailing psychology regards the conditions of life from the position of observation that is one's individual point of view toward them. In the conception here advanced, these conditions are regarded from points of view that are socially relative to, and inclusive of, all possible positions of observation.

The reader will recall that the conceptions of the physicists first led them to a theory of special relativity through their calculations of uniform motion, while their deductions came only later to embrace data pertaining to difform motion, or to motion that is not uniform, as envisaged under the conception of general relativity. With regard to the theory of relativity in the subjective sphere, it was upon noting the habitual deflections from a predictable organic constant observable in the erratic reactions of the neurotic personality that the conception of relativity in the sphere of consciousness first occurred to me. It was only subsequently that the relativity of consciousness as applied to the uniform reactions characteristic of the collective social mind came to shape itself into the organismic conception of relativity here outlined as the underlying principle of consciousness.

While representing in no sense a detailed correlation between them, there is, nevertheless, a certain analogy not only in the manner of inception of the objective and subjective theories with respect to the observation first of difform or abnormal deviation and later of discrepancies of normal or uniform reactions, but there is also this further concomitance between the two aspects of the principle. The Newtonian hypothesis takes account of motion or reaction in the planetary system only in the large, while the theory of Einstein is adequate in contemplating the motion of planets both in the large and in the small. Conversely, our present Freudian theory of the unconscious takes care of the reactions of the personality in the small or in an individual or particular sense, while the theory of relativity of consciousness envisages personality not only individually or particularly (whether regarded singly or in its collective social expression), but also societally, or in the sense of consciousness in its universal or organismic encompassment.

5. Our psychobiological misconception is doubtless also aided in large measure by the physiological conditions of our visual organs of perception and to the bi-dimensional surface upon which our impressions of objects are received. Because of the disposition of the nerve terminals of the retina upon a flat or bi-dimensional area, our visual perception of objects is limited to impressions of a flat or bi-dimensional plane. If, by means of binocular accommodation, objects present to us the appearance of "depth", it is, of course, not to direct visual perception that we owe our sense of perspective, but to stereoscopic inference, seconded by our stereognostic experience of tri-dimensional solidity. Hence, what is actually "perceived" upon looking at an object of three dimensions is a visual facet, as it were, due to our own mentally flattened "cross-section" of the solid object before us as determined by the particular aspect of it that is momentarily presented to view. I think it cannot be doubted that this mechanism of our visual perception is a contributing factor in influencing our tendency to "see" mentally. One says "I see" when he means "I understand". There is the same implication in saying that one "sees" the logic of such and such a statement So, too, we speak of a "mental point of view" or of "intellectual vision". This illusory character of our mental percepts probably owes its explanation also in part to the fact that our visual sense is the sense that best permits a distant and detached observation *of*, rather than a contact *with*, the surrounding world.

CHAPTER EIGHT

Psychoanalytic improvisations and the personal equation*

"'Tis with our judgments as with our watches,—none
Go just alike, yet each believes his own"

(Alexander Pope)

There are two grand divisions of psychoanalysts. There are the psychoanalysts proper, that is, those who have attempted to enter understandingly into the intimate processes of individual life, and there are the psychoanalysts who have been too proper for any such intimate undertaking. In the latter class may be counted the great majority of psychiatrists. They probably got an inkling of things in early life and decided that curiosity was a propensity not to be lightly encouraged. But the psychoanalysts proper were of a more adventurous spirit. Of course, they did not suspect what they were adventuring upon—but that is the element that makes adventure. And, accordingly, the mess so commonly substituted for human life

* Paper read at the Fifteenth Annual Meeting of the American Psychoanalytic Association, Richmond, Va., 12 May 1925. First published in *The Psychoanalytic Review, XIII*(2), April, 1926.

presented no terrors to them. The rosy apple of our human curiosity tempted them and they did eat, whereupon the trouble began to brew. The problem now, it seems to me, is for the psychoanalyst proper to realise the mess in which unconsciously his overweening curiosity has embroiled him and to get out of it, and for the psychiatrist to realise the mess from which his habitual apathies have unconsciously preserved him and to get into it.

I remember many years ago having spent the long hours of a summer afternoon arguing with Sherwood Anderson as to the merits of the psychoanalytic aim. Anderson argued that human life was not a thing to be delved into with surgical probes—that it was not to be got at that way. Needless to say, I argued as stoutly that the surgical probe was the most wonderful of all human inventions and that it was the only way to lay open to health and growth the sick personalities of our human kind.

Said Anderson, "You blind fool. Men like you are fools. You cannot go along that road. It is given to no man to venture far along the road of lives . . . You are no more and no better than myself. You are a dog that has rolled in offal, and because you are not quite a dog you do not like the smell of your own hide. . . . The illness you pretend to cure is the universal illness. The thing you want to do cannot be done."

Said I, "You cannot be so definite without missing something vague and fine. You miss the whole point. The lives of people are like young trees in a forest. They are being choked by climbing vines. The vines are old thoughts and beliefs planted by dead men. I am myself covered by crawling creeping vines that choke me. . . . You come from the West. You have kept away from people. You have preserved yourself—damn you! I haven't—I have entered into lives. I have gone beneath the surface of the lives of men and women. . . . You think you understand but you don't understand. What you say can't be done can be done."

I was so sure that I was right that I felt nothing would show how right I was but Anderson's analysis. Anderson was so sure that he was right that he wrote the essay, from which 1 have quoted, to prove it.[1] As I look back from the experience of the intervening years, it is not difficult for me to realise that, as is always the case with two people who are sure they are right, both of us were wrong. But that was fully ten years ago, and ten years ago we were both very young for these times. In the personal equation, represented in the private predilections of us both, each of us was out for himself. I in my egotism was in for understanding life and helping humanity (God help it!). Anderson was out for "many marriages" and for helping himself. Our positions were those of the circumspect psychiatrist and the inquisitive psychoanalyst proper. Nothing but the phrenological bump of curiosity lay between us and our opposed interpretations of life. As with the psychiatrist who has kept himself out of the mess and the psychoanalyst who has got himself into it, the result of our differing enquiries seems to me merely to have left us both on conflicting sides of the same dilemma. We were both the unconscious instruments of private improvisations. In both, the theme we used owed itself, though unacknowledged, to the personal equation that secretly actuated our separate positions.

This element of the personal equation has become for me the most significant element in all my psychoanalytic studies. It actuates not only the interpretations of the artist and the layman, but it actuates also the interpretations of the psychoanalyst and the psychiatrist. It is quite generally acknowledged that this element of the personal equation is exceedingly subtle. But, after all, this is mere concession to our demand for a quiet corner by the fireside where we may hug our own infirmities without being intruded upon. The fact is that the personal equation, however subtle, is, in its self-flattery, a thing desirable and wished for. It is not a hard necessity; it is a coveted disease. In the layman, it is so commonplace that it passes unnoticed. In the artist, it is cultivated to a point of refinement and is conceded to be a prime requisite for all artistic interpretation. But, in a social interpretation, the personal equation is but another term for the personal vanity that actuates all conflict. It is another term for the personal greed that constitutes our mental blind spot and that actuates all private prepossession. It is the instigation to private improvisation, artistic and scientific. It precludes all thought of a social consideration of a social disease.

I have no wish to enter here into a systematic analysis of this social element of the personal equation and attempt to amass the meticulous details of findings in evidence of this unconscious social factor. I have recently undertaken this task in another paper of somewhat similar trend.[2] I want here merely to state the problem as I see it, and, having presented it in its broad lines, to leave with this society the responsibility, which I feel rests upon us, to deal with this problem or to dismiss it, according as it sees fit. Perhaps it will seem to this audience that Mr Anderson is quite right, that the illness to be encompassed is a universal one and that nothing can be done about it. I concede that the illness is universal in the sense that it has laid hold of man's consciousness on every side. But I am obstinate enough to believe that meeting it is a thing that can be done when there is a scientific consciousness to cope with it. Of course, if we who are psychologists and educators are ourselves as personally constellated in our own private equation as the sick society whose disorder it is our function to remedy, then certainly the outlook is not a bright one. But it seems to me a not too extravagant expectation that the social neurosis or the private basis upon which the social mind everywhere rests its judgement might be met on the basis of a consensus that permits its conscious recognition as a scientifically controllable process.

Man's private preconceptions were dispelled in regard to the physical universe through the introduction of laboratory methods in the observation of physical phenomena. From this moment, our esoteric philosophies were snuffed out. Elective interpretations were no more. In the laboratory of science, mental and spiritual improvisations became obsolete and were consigned to the discard of ancient myth and religion. 1 think it can be plainly disclosed that the element we call unconscious is only the personal equation actuating each of us and that naturally it cannot attain acknowledged recognition except as science bars this element of the personal equation through recourse to the consensual technique of an objective laboratory observation of it.

In the domain of chemistry, the fundamental principles of chemistry are not altered in their basic elements, be the laboratory here or in Timbuctoo. Biology is biology whatever the subjective prejudices of the observer. For, in these spheres, there exist certain scientific principles of stabilised recognition resultant upon the controlled and consensual observation of definite observable sequences.

One may say, without flattering it, that the laboratory invariably minds its own business. The materials at hand are its uncompromising monitors and it has no concern outside of this. In its procedure, it is bound to the processes of direct objective observation. No latitude is granted to the element of the personal equation. There is, in the laboratory, no room for private improvisations based upon the esoteric interpretations of the particular observer. For the laboratory has no other purpose than the observation of the materials provided under the scientific routine of the laboratory in question. Of course, in the clinic, our acknowledged purpose is to help the individual. But any notion of helping the individual is wholly foreign to the purpose of the laboratory. The laboratory proceeds with the unbiased observation of its materials and the individual may take it or leave it according to his will. Its observations are its own authority and it does not seek for individual favour in support of this authority. If the individual is not interested in the processes of the chemist, it is the individual's loss. This characterisation of the laboratory is common to laboratories everywhere throughout the world of objective phenomena. The individual might strenuously object to the findings of the physical laboratory. In point of fact, very many individuals and institutions do object to them. For these findings often interfere seriously with the private prepossessions of early training, family predilection and religious sentiments. It is no matter. In the laboratory, the consciousness of man is brought into organic alignment with the events of the physical universe and the price of consciousness is man's inevitable submission to inexorable physical sequences through his enforced acknowledgment of their authority over him.

Within the mental sphere, however, in which there should prevail no less the scientific processes of the laboratory, the personal equation constitutes a distinct barrier to observation. This element has been slowly building from year to year through gradual accretions of the materials that embody the privileges of private sentiment and interpretation, so that the personal equation can only preclude within the individual the scientific recognition of these subjective materials. Sentimental indulgence, private interest, inhibiting memories, and endless hidden compensatory images definitely enter in to bias the clear observation of what are presumably the psychoanalyst's objective materials of observation. Where he would observe, he interprets. He embellishes where he would record. Where the situation calls for scientific tabulation, he interposes the fanciful, artistic touch of unconscious improvisation. He does not intend to do this. He does not know he is doing it. That is the point. He cannot know it. The student of the unconscious has himself unconsciously yielded submission to the personal equation. He has withheld his conscious concession to controllable observation, so that the discipline of observation characterising the uncompromising method of the biological or physical laboratory is utterly lacking as soon as science enters upon the so-called mental field of enquiry.[3]

In the observation of physical phenomena, the scientist's personal equation is entirely subordinated to the authority of exact data. But such a process of mental alignment with observable data presupposes a consensus of agreement among the observers. Such a consensus is the necessary sequence of a strict adherence to the materials observed. Accordingly, no arbitrary interpretation may interfere for a moment with the stabilised routine of scientific laboratory enquiry. Through the organic consistency of the materials observed, there can only be an organic consensus of observation among the several observers. But, in the mental sphere, there has been no such consensual observation of consistent laboratory materials because there has been no consistent laboratory material. Our laboratory material has not been recognised as being precisely man's own inconsistency. It has not been recognised that our material has been our own personal equation, that this has all along constituted the mental processes requiring observation. The result has been that the personal equation, the private interpretation, the unconscious improvisation have fairly honeycombed our psychoanalytic formulations. And yet, we go on innocently unsuspecting our own embroilment in the very inadvertencies we are presumed to study in our patients.

In the isolated neurotic patient, the condition presented by such an organism is a lack of a consensual basis or of an organic concurrence among the elements of the patient's personality. His discrepancy represents, to use the classical phrase, a conflict within his personality. Of course, the individual cannot remedy his own condition. For, in his own division and conflict, there is lacking the consensus of understanding requisite to a scientific observation of himself. His recourse, therefore, is to the physician or psychotherapist. But the physician, in his own lack of an organic consensus of observation, can only meet the patient's compensations and improvisations, based as they are upon a system of personal equations, with compensations and improvisations that are equally dependent upon a system of personal equation. In brief, there is an unconscious covenant that exists within the individual's personality in accordance with the terms of which certain elements within his personality are peremptorily barred from communication with other elements within this same personality. It is my position that, within the organism represented by groups of individuals, there exists a social covenant of repression that is as definite as that existing within the single individual, and that, in accordance with its terms, certain elements within this social personality can under no circumstances communicate on terms of a common consensus with other elements within that same social organism. To bring the matter home, we might realise how discrepant our own psychoanalytic organisation is when we observe the wide disparities which have always separated its various members severally among themselves. Let any two psychoanalysts come together long enough for a heart to heart talk and before parting they will have damned the methods of every other psychoanalyst extant. Were there a truly consensual basis of organic terms upon which we might repose our conclusions, there would not be such mock agreements between any momentarily paired individuals among us or the prevalent wrangling and division that exist throughout our presumably scientific ranks as a whole. Were there a scientific unity of observation, such a shocking absence of definite data of accord as exists among us would not be possible. But there needs no dissertation to prove that as yet psychiatry and psychoanalysis do not rest upon sound scientific principles. . . . In the esoteric tenets of Jung and his disciples, in the unconsciously recessive birth fantasias of recent innovation, and in the many popular interpretations of the psychoanalysts proper, one may discover, through a technique of laboratory observation, mere improvisations based upon the personal equation private to each. Among other theoretic improvisations looking to the therapy of neurotic patients, the marriage state has been seriously advocated as a panacea for these ills. But this happy ending is too naïve to deserve sober mention. We know very well that for all the young doves who go in quest of mating affidavits, there are as many old birds who want them revoked. Neither are the improvisations offered by Rank and others competent to do the trick. This novelty has neither the merit of getting the psychoanalysts improper out of their mess nor of putting the psychoanalysts too proper into it. Such psychoanalytic discrepancies are an index of our social neurosis and are inseparable from our consensual disagreement in organic social terms.

For clinical material illustrative of this tendency to private improvisation we need seek no further than our own psychoanalytic group. There are, plainly observable within ourselves, all the substitutions and improvisations that characterise the social mind elsewhere. But we do not challenge these compensatory improvisations as they are represented among members of our own profession. These unquestionable marks of an ill-concealed social neurosis existing within individuals of our own immediate social group are naïvely passed over by us, and the private and obviously compensatory improvisations that characterise the coloratura interpretations we presume to offer as scientifically controlled data meet with complete acquiescence on the part of this social group as a whole. Of course, there are individual comments following the meetings, private exchange of criticism and whispered asides out of hearing of the meeting as a whole. But there is no concerted group observation of the private and substitutive improvisations characterising the separate individuals composing this group. The reason that there is not a group observation is that there is not a unity or consensus within the societal organism underlying all groups as well as individuals. Only such a unity makes possible a scientific consistency with respect to the observable materials. In the absence of this unity or consensus, there is excluded the consensual scientific observation that characterises the laboratory method. *In sum, the fact that we all disguise is that the neurosis is social and that a social neurosis can be met only through a social analysis.*

These concerns are of wide social import and belong to the social community in general. No medical or psychological specialty can, from the vantage coign of the mere remote onlooker, appropriate to itself the treatment of the mental frailties of our human kind. Our human kind is answerable for its own frailties and these maladjustments cannot soon enough be brought to book by the rank and file of men as the real sponsors for these disordered states. The situation is serious. Its ramifications are national and even international. The matter is not one of professional, but of public, responsibility. There has been too long the tendency to restrict such problems to the limited sphere of an arbitrarily assumed medical or psychiatric syndicate in the alluring belief that there is here a responsibility that stands quite apart from that of our social life as a whole. In this way, the layman finds an easy way to thrust upon others the responsibility for problems that are of his own making. The individual might go to the psychoanalyst or the psychiatrist on behalf of his individually sick mental system, but when it is a matter of a socially ill mental system, the psychoanalyst and psychiatrist are as much a part of that sick system as the patient who turns to them for aid. If the neurotic illness is universal, a remedy must be found that will be universal also. We cannot leave to the individual and the clinic the solution of problems that are social and that properly belong to the laboratory of the sociologist.

Psychoanalysis needs to be up and facing its social involvement in complexes that are as definitely neurotic as the personal complexes it now presumably attempts to analyse in the neurotic individual. Our emotions are as like as our blood cells. Repression is a diathesis common to us all. Tap any number of individuals in the right place and the same secret will come out! Under our present social system, there is no individual who is not neurotic. If his neurosis does not appear, he has merely climbed behind barriers which you and I, as members of that social system, are assisting him to keep before him. Not only has every individual a neurosis, but every individual has within him the rudiments of every neurosis with its concomitant deviations in the emotional and sexual spheres. But, though these discrepancies are clearly observable on the features of all social groups, they are only admittedly present within the textbooks we write to hide them. At political conventions, amid our annual Chautauquas, at the racetrack, on the boards of charity organizations, and in our own psychoanalytic gatherings, one may readily detect beneath the protection of the social repression the veiled features of mankind at large. . . . For individualism preserves its individualistic secret and necessarily bars all consensual approach to these anomalies. No one, in short, dares stand socially for the mental obliquity he secretly cherishes individually. Of all our organic distortions, however, the most vitally significant and the most carefully disguised are the frequent conjugal combines under which society affords protection for every form of sexual deviation known to psychopathology. But whether single or in combination, as unseemly as they are, under our present social system society must have these anomalies. They are the symptoms of our societal repression. And, in the midst of a secret social order, under whose covenant it is death to reveal the secret that is common to the members of that social order throughout, naturally the individual is going to hold his peace. Nevertheless, as everybody knows (but prefers to keep "unconscious") every deviation we isolate in the clinic is represented in obvious outline within the various members of every social assemblage that comes together. But no one of us observes any other, because each of us has from earliest childhood agreed not to observe anyone else upon the solemnly accepted condition that everyone else shall agree not to observe him. This is the earliest lesson we have learned from our parents and, barring the little episode in the Garden of Eden, our parents have been all of them without exception innocent people.

After all, the mother of us all is the same proper old lady—to wit, the social system—and under her maternal discipline we are all one and the same family of repressed and subservient children.

The naughty pranks to which the more refractory of this family of repressed youngsters are often driven is taking on serious proportions in these days of futurism and jazz. In the midst of this futuristic hubbub, what our artist-psychoanalysts, for example, are perpetrating in the direction of unconscious psychic improvisation is a sorry commentary upon our scientific schools of analysis. . . .

Where there exist compulsive acts socially hidden under the guise of artistry, the only freeing approach to such ineptitudes is a laboratory analysis. These unconscious mechanisms of art have been called sublimation, if you please. But a laboratory analysis of sublimation reveals it to be but another name for repression. I recall one such sublime impropriety recently perpetrated and exposed to view in one of our American studios. It is supposed to be the subtle and searching story in bronze of a particular individual. In truth, it represents nothing else than the blithe and chubby unconscious of the vicarious artist who conceived and gave it birth. If you will draw closer and examine this obstetrical improvisation, you will discover that the cherubic voluptuousness is purely autogenic, that its offspring has been unconsciously sired by the personal equation of the artist. . . . Such interpretations, resting, as they do, upon an unconscious projection to another of what is repressed within oneself, need to be brought to book through the intermediation of a more encompassing survey of man's psychosocial life than our present individualistic improvisations will ever make possible.

But, aside from the psychopathologist and those presumably initiated, what the world is getting away with in the way of unconscious substitution based upon the personal equation is really too preposterous for words. These expressions exist not only individually, but *en masse*. For example, the whole reason why prohibition is not a success and never will be is precisely the personal equation of the prohibitionists. It is this element of the personal equation that makes for the fanaticism of the prohibitionist. The underlying principle of prohibition is temperance. But fanaticism is as intemperate as alcoholism. In fact, alcohol may be used without intemperance, but fanaticism is always intemperate. . . .

My position is that there exists a dissociation that is as systematised *socially* as its isolated expression in our patients is systematised *individually*. Until a social analysis permits each of us to recognise the presence within himself of all the substitutive anomalies and mental digressions which he now represses (a condition for which there is required the earnest collaboration of serious students in the method of stabilised laboratory technique), psychiatrists and psychoanalysts must continue to substitute the tedious ratiocinations and private improvisations that are based upon the personal equation inseparable from our common societal repression.

We need to face the truth that is concealed beneath such connotations as "social" and "normal". We need to recognise that normality means working off socially the neurosis that everyone cherishes individually. As we psychopathologists are members of this large and imposing class called normal, naturally we are not going to give it away. We shall be the more loath to do so if it is true that unconsciously we are actually capitalising the vicarious inefficacies of the less fortunate neurotic individual whose social ineptitudes have ostracised him from the enviable social position occupied by ourselves. On this basis of assumed differentiation, we can only continue to speak as now with tremulous reverence of a patient's "restoration to normality" . . . And so, like good psychopathologists, we prudently lie low.

The neurotic is the spoiled child. And what the spoiled child preeminently wants is attention. The one thing, however, he ought not to have is precisely the attention he wants. For this attention the neurotic patient wants represents but his own personal equation. Giving attention to neurotic patients on the basis of their personal equation, that is, on the assumption that their condition calls for special consideration on the part of science, is a fallacious procedure. What the neurotic needs is a laboratory consensus that will afford him the opportunity to observe his condition as part of a social expression that is universal and to bring his processes in line with such mature methods of observation as shall quite obliterate the basis of personal equation on which he rests his claim for attention.

It is this element of the personal equation that has not received the attention it deserves. It probably deserves all the attention we can give it. I am not sure whether, throughout all our varied psychoanalytic preoccupations, any other element merits attention except this. It might even be that this secret element of the personal equation that has so far eluded our attention is the secret occasion for all repression and unconsciousness.

As in pathology, so in psychopathology; the difference between the clinic approach and the laboratory approach is significant. The psychiatric clinic is interested in the individual from a supposedly established basis of normality. The psychiatric laboratory can be interested in the individual *and* normality only from the basis of the biologic continuum composing the social organism common to both. The clinic is interested in curing people. The laboratory is interested in its investigations and results. What is, in the clinic, an occasion for attention to the individual, becomes, in the laboratory, an occasion for social observation precisely *because* of the claim for attention which the individual attempts to secure. The clinic is interested in the study of mental conditions represented to it on the basis of the unconscious personal equation. The laboratory, on the other hand, aims to discover the universality of the subjective occasion for these mental conditions and finds it to consist in precisely the personal equation which occupies the attention of the clinic in response to the patient's personal demand.

As it is not the purpose of the physical or chemical laboratory to render help to the individual, neither can it be the purpose of the psychiatric laboratory to help him. There is need of a psychiatric laboratory that will present as sane a basis for the observation of our mental processes as has been offered in the physical laboratory for the observation of objective phenomena. When this scientifically controlled method shall come into its own, our patients who are suffering from an organic discrepancy of outlook will have no choice but to learn through proper laboratory experience the consensual method of observation that characterises its uncompromising procedure. In the absence of a social consensus of laboratory technique based upon such a consensual agreement in terms, I am convinced that psychoanalysis and psychiatry can only be a purely arbitrary improvisation based upon the personal equation of the particular observer and not a truly scientific observation based upon the accepted symbols of stabilised recognition.

I have spoken of the seeming division between the methods of interpreting our human values as these values were seen from the differing angles of Mr Anderson and myself. At that time, I did not see that, on the basis of the personal equation, the interpretations of the psychopathologist were as inevitably the improvisations of unconscious artistry as the improvisations of the admittedly creative artist. In this view, the positions of Mr Anderson and myself were really the same. Anderson was as bent on understanding life and on the service of man and his personal relationships as I, and I was as bent on the sheer experience of life and on helping myself to such personal relationships as custom doth not stale in their infinite variety as was Mr Anderson. I have written so psychologically mistaken a thesis as "Conceptions and misconceptions in psychoanalysis".[4] Anderson has drawn so artistically mistaken a portrait as "The man who became a woman".[5] Mine had been the better psychology had it treated of conceptions and misconceptions in and out of psychoanalysis; Anderson's the better art had he discovered the fundamentally lacking touch in his drawing and recognised in his portrait the woman who became a man. I do not hesitate to say that there are artists who are quite as able analysts of human character as any psychoanalyst I have ever known. I do not hesitate to say that there are psychoanalysts who are quite as subtle artists as any artist I have ever known. But, with analysts as with artists, as long as our expressions arise from a basis of personal equation, in the end they can only result in the compensations and improvisations of mere artistic projection.

The psychopathologist in his isolated clinical view, weaving romance as he does into the materials of his analysis, is, from the standpoint of a group analysis, in precisely the same unconscious position as the artist who weaves romance into the pages of his novel. This situation merely brings us back to the psychoanalyst proper, that is to say improper, and to the psychoanalyst too proper, that is to say the psychiatrist, the one improvising because of the mess he has got into, the other improvising because of the mess he has kept out of. As it is, the course of both is mere artistic touch and unconscious improvisation. We do not intend to do this. We do not know we are doing it. But, as I said, that is the point. The need is for the psychoanalyst and the psychiatrist to unite in the mutual observation of their own processes as they involve their own personal equations and to bring their several improvisations to a common analysis through the consensual method of observation offered through an organised laboratory technique.

Notes

1. "Seeds". In: *The Triumph of the Egg*, Sherwood Anderson, B. W. Huebsch, 1921.
2. "Psychiatry as an objective science," paper read at the Fifteenth Annual Meeting of the American Psychopathological Association, Washington, D. C., 7 May 1925. *British Journal of Medical Psychology, V*, Part 4.
3. "The laboratory method in psychoanalysis", paper read at the Ninth Congress of the International Psycho-Analytical Association, Bad Homburg, Germany, September, 1925. *The American Journal of Psychiatry, V*(3): January, 1926.
4. Paper read before the Huxley Society of the Johns Hopkins University. See "Contemporary Science," Modern Library Series, Boni and Liveright.
5. See "Horses and men", Sherwood Anderson. B. W. Huebsch, 1923.

CHAPTER NINE

Psychoanalysis in theory and in life*†

Now that the excitement following the inundation of psychoanalysis has died down and the clinical territories most affected have been once more built up and restocked, it is interesting to witness the changes wrought in different quarters as a result of the general havoc to habitual prepossessions. There is no question, as we stand amid the debris of past conceptions, but that the sudden descent upon us of Freud's postulates has destroyed many old landmarks that shall not be restored and that it has brought in a wealth of new material that has altered no little the configuration of the old.

As I happen to have been of those who were carried in upon the current of the general onsweep of new interpretations ushered in by Freud, my experience forms the record of a reaction to that movement that is internal because from the vantage ground of a participant in it.

* First published in *The Journal of Nervous and Mental Disease*, *64*(3): September 1926.

† The following essay is the introductory chapter of a larger work, to be subsequently published, representing the outcome of a practical experiment in group or social analysis.

As the position to which I have gradually come differs today so essentially from the followers of Freud, as well as from his dissenters, some account of the development through which my conceptions have passed might be of interest to others who, like myself, have earnestly tried to bring order and a permanent coherence out of the large mass of conceptions that cluster about Freud's dynamic idea, so many of which are of epoch-making significance in their envisagement of mental disharmonies, so many of which, in being immature and unsound, only obstruct the passage that Freud has contributed so splendidly to open.

The theory of psychoanalysis rests on the conception that nervous disorders are the substitutive manifestation of a repressed sexual life; its basic position is that this substitutive factor is responsible for neurotic processes and that it is the sexual impulse for which recourse is sought in the process of substitution. This position of psychoanalysis is, in its essential significance, now generally accepted—the position, namely, which affirms the factor of replacement as the essential account of nervous manifestations and posits the urge of the sexual instinct as the element replaced.

While, with other psychoanalysts, I am in full accord with this thesis, my finding in regard to the relation of these two propositions to one another is so entirely at variance with the prevailing psychoanalytic view and alters so fundamentally for me the ultimate interpretation of psychoanalysis in its bearing upon the problems of consciousness, that I shall make clearer the ideas expressed in this essay if at the outset I may state briefly in what manner my interpretation of this relation differs from the accepted conception.

The difference lies in the fact that I do not regard this replacement as *primarily* a replacement for sexuality as we now know it. On the contrary, sexuality, as manifested today amid the sophistications of civilisation, is itself a replacement for the organic unity of personality arising naturally from the harmony of function that pertains biologically to the primary infant psyche. This original preconscious mode[1] I regard as the matrix of personality. The spontaneous process of the organism's unhindered growth through the gradual development of experience or awareness from this unitary mode as a basis is, in my interpretation, the meaning of consciousness. The whole meaning of sexuality, on the other hand, is substitution, compensation, repression. In a word, sexuality, as it has come to exist today, is identical with the unconscious, while a unification of personality is alone to be found through eliminating the recourses of substitution and sexuality and, thus, reuniting the elements of the conscious and organic modes now kept asunder through the interposition of the unconscious mind.

Hence, the modern substitutions existing under the name of sexuality, whether repressed or indulged, are but a symptom of this organic denial of the inherent life of man. Sexuality is not only utterly unrelated to sex, but it is intrinsically exclusive of sex. Sex is life. It is life in its deepest inherency. Sex is the spontaneous expression of a natural hunger. In the instinct of sex, there is felt a yearning from the depths of man's soul for mateship and reproduction, while sexuality is the personal coveting of momentary satisfaction in mere superficial sensation. By sexuality, then, I mean something very different from sex. I mean the restless, obsessive, overstimulated quest for temporary self-gratification that everywhere masquerades as sex and is everywhere substituted for the strong, simple, quiet flow of personality that unites the organic and the conscious life in a single stream and is the expression of personality in its native inherency.

With this altered conception, other modifications have followed which necessarily entail a distinct departure from the accepted psychoanalytic position. As this organic denial and the restless compensations and substitutions comprising the unconscious are, in essence, the psychology of the mental reaction average known as normality, it is no longer possible for me to accord with the popular analytic view which places a premium upon this manifestation of the collective unconscious and assigns the criterion of normality as the desired goal of adaptation for the neurotically repressed personality.

I cannot accept this view. For an analysis of the social unconscious shows that the collective reaction embodied in the adaptations commonly accepted as "normal" betrays a tendency to repression and replacement that is no less an indication of disease-process than is the reaction presented in the individual neurosis. Indeed, from the point of view of constructive consciousness and health, our so-called normality is, of the two, in many respects, the less progressive type of reaction. For, in truth, many of our normal reactions, in evading the issues of the unconscious, envisage less the processes of growth and a larger consciousness than the neurotic type of reaction, which, however blind its motivation, at least comes to grips with the actualities of the unconscious mind.

It is the hallmark of normality that, suspecting nothing, it takes itself completely for granted. In the spirit of true conformity, it accepts its expressions of the vicarious at their face value and assumes the burden of its self-inflicted compensations with entire complacency. The neurotic, on the other hand, at least senses the inherent discrepancy in his life. He at least demurs in so far as to withhold assent from the mass compromise embodied in the substitutions and connivances of the social unconscious. In a word, it is the distinction of the neurotic personality that he is at least consciously and confessedly "nervous".

This, as far as I can see, is the chief distinction between the condition represented in normal adaptations and that represented in the neurosis. It is a distinction that lies merely in the greater weight of numbers. Normality, in its numerical strength, concedes acceptance to the average reaction and so yields it right of way. In normality, the unconscious carries the day, while in the neurosis it is pushed to the wall. The distinction psychologically lies in the successful compromise of the one as contrasted with the enforced doubt and self-questioning of the other. It is the compact security of the social polity on the one hand, compared with the more sensitive isolation and uncertainty of the individual unit on the other.

It is my position, therefore, that, from the point of view of life, many of our normal reactions are psychologically as truly a manifestation of the distorted and substitutive as are those more isolated manifestations we commonly stigmatise as neurotic disharmonies. I cannot see but that the element of the repressed and substitutive, on which is based Freud's theory of the neuroses, is an element that underlies the expression of consciousness in all phases of its manifestation and that, hence, underlies also the phase represented in normality. In brief, many so-called normal reactions too are nervous. Normality, too, since it is actuated no less from motives of the ulterior and vicarious, even though it supposedly represents the criterion of adult consciousness, is no less an expression of the distorted and symbolic. This distortion is to be seen upon every hand in the restless greed and self-seeking that underlie the national, industrial, political, social, and religious possessivism and competition which are the typical psychology of the normal mind, notwithstanding its plausible exterior of human progress and universal good will. Universality and good will are not there. These are but the manifest symptoms represented by the social personality after it has undergone the distortion represented in the substitutive reactions characteristic of the societal neurosis, that is, after it has been subjected to the mechanism of diplomatic repression and modification. What is there in reality is the will-to-self and the particular aim that best serves the egoistic advantages of the individuals comprising the social unit in question. The mechanism is identical with that which underlies the individual neurosis: the covert aim toward the satisfactions of self constitutive of unconsciousness.

Normality, too, then, might be neurotic. Normality, too, might have its repressions and its substitutions, its secret symbols and equivocations. The difference is that as normality possesses the warrant of the institutionalised and current, it enjoys the protection of the consensus. And just as the neurotic fails to comprehend the meaning of this vicarious manifestation in its individual expression within himself and is a prey to the inscrutable symptoms in which his organism finds its compensations, so we who are accounted normal as little suspect the meaning of this same symptomatology as it exists in its social expression within ourselves. The neurotic resolutely defends his unconscious duplicity behind an ingenious charade of unconscious symbolism, and we no less resolutely defend ours through recourse to an identical device. But, if we will look beyond the narrower confine of the clinic and face squarely the logical issue of Freud's thesis, we cannot avoid the conclusion that it is an indictment of man's consciousness in its entirety. Hence, normality, too, must make answer for its complicity in the unconscious ruse of substitution and evasion which we observe in its more intense reaction as the introversions of personality presented in the obviously arrested expression we call neurotic.

If anyone is disposed to question this view, let him consider but one symptomatic reaction recently manifested throughout the social organism. Could there be anywhere imagined an unconscious reaction more wasteful and destructive, or one of wider scope or severer intensity than the symptom reaction represented by the war that has recently convulsed the world? Or consider the equally unconscious expression presented in the tendency to religious emotionalism that has followed in its wake with its corresponding effort towards compensation and self-propitiation through recourse to the sentimental and spiritualistic. Yet, all the while, the existence and the significance of the unconscious motives that are latent in the two extremes of emotional reaction underlying these manifest expressions have not yet begun to be suspected and reckoned with on any clear, conscious, analytic basis.

What, then, is the meaning of this tendency to substitution as shown in the reaction of the social as well as of the individual organism? If sexuality is the element substituted for, what is the psychology of this factor called sexuality? What is its meaning? In analysing the unconscious of the neurotic personality, it has become gradually clearer to me that the factor underlying and actuating the conflict Freud describes as repressed sexuality is nothing else than the personal desire of ascendancy or the lust of acquisition *concomitant with the organism's unconscious reversion upon its own image.*[2]

Sexuality, then, is but a larger word for self. It is the effort to limit life to the ends of personal aggrandisement. It is the greed of the self-limited personality to compass the whole, as contrasted with the societal personality that is encompassed by the whole. But, since the unconscious is the same under all forms, self or sexuality, with its pride of possession, its lust of gain, is no less the unconscious element underlying the psychology of the normal reaction average. And precisely as in the individual reaction these unconscious wishes are manifested only in the disguised symbols and substitutive equivalents portrayed in neurotic symptoms, so too in the social organism these egoistic interests antagonistic to consciousness and growth venture to express themselves only in the corresponding substitutions of the mass unconscious.

Thus, the unconscious represented in the social reaction we call normality is no whit different from the unconscious represented in the individual reaction observable as the neurosis. We are habitually deceived by the give-and-take policy of normal adaptation with its secret covenant of good manners and outward forms. But the apparent difference between the social and the individual neurosis consists merely in the fact that the poignancy of the conflict underlying the symptomatology of the social personality is largely mitigated and condoned by reason of the wider numerical distribution of the social organism and the consequent freer dissemination of the elements involved.

But, though of wider distribution, there underlies the expressions of normality no less of conflict and repression than exists in the acuter expression seen in the individual neurosis. In the personality of the more sensitive or affective type we think of as neurotic, this tendency to self-acquisitiveness or sexuality and its organic incompatibility with the quiet inherency of life become, as it were, stalled and impacted within him, while in the societal organism the discrepancy of personality occasioned by its sexuality or pride of ascendancy apparently entails no such organic blocking as that occurring in the individual. But the pain and impacting are present nevertheless, and are betrayed no less in the recourse to the substitutive and symbolic, characteristic of our prevalent social hysteria, not to mention the more violent disorders that crash upon the world in the reactions of political and industrial dissension and in the fiercer paroxysms of war.

Such is the meaning of our so-called normality. To a degree that is quite unsuspected by us, its psychology is unconsciousness, and the psychology of unconsciousness is the psychology of the self-image secretly worshipped under the habitual guises of symbolism and replacement. It is time we should recognise that this recourse to the vicarious image is the psychology of many of the reactions of the normal as well as of the neurotic that in ourselves no less than in the neurotic there is the putting forward of that which *stands for*—the exploitation under countless different aspects of that which may be adroitly put *instead of* rather than the simple acceptance of that which *is*.

It is part of the purpose of the present study, however, to try to bring into clearer light a substitutive reaction that is much nearer home. As psychoanalysts, whether educational, sociological or medical, we need to take into account a distortive process that has a much closer bearing upon ourselves and our responsibility toward the problems of our common social consciousness. For of all the forms of substitution to which normality has recourse, the form that seems to me of deepest significance for us, and that presents the most vital need of analysis and understanding within ourselves, is the vicarious expression growing out of the tendency to an objective approach toward the problems of consciousness that has come to be embodied in the formulated *system* of psychoanalysis.[3]

In the whole symptomatology of normality, with its societal expression of the vicarious, there is no symptom complex that is of greater significance than that embodied in the attempt to apply to the actuality of human life the *system* of human life offered in psychoanalysis as it is today interpreted and applied. For a system of psychoanalysis is itself but a substitution for life, a theory of life in place of life itself. The theory of psychoanalysis sets out with a premise; life does not. Psychoanalysis offers a solution; life is its own solution.

It is not theory as theory at which I demur; it is theory as application to the needs of human growth. From the point of view of the theory of psychoanalysis, this therapeutic recourse in the treatment of nervous disorders seems to me completely adequate and true; but from the point of view of life, I have come to regard the application of the system or theory of psychoanalysis to the problems of individual needs as an utterly futile procedure. I have come to feel that what is here of value in the textbook is utterly worthless in our daily relation to human personality.

I would not, of course, be understood as repudiating theory as such. Seen clearly as the extrinsic expression it is, theory undoubtedly has its place, but its place is not in the earnest relationship of one human being to another, such as obtains in the confidence and communication offered in the actuality of psychoanalysis. It has not yet been recognised, however, that we who are psychoanalysts are ourselves theorists, that we also are very largely misled by an unconscious that is social, that we too are neurotic, in so far as every expression but that of life in its native simplicity is neurotic. Our disharmony, however, is a phase of that widely diffused neurosis that exists under the prevailing social consensus represented in the normal adaptation. And so, as I now see it, there is no more subtle form of substitution or one that is more successful in its capacity to evade the censor of consciousness and obtain the stamp of genuineness than the symptom represented in the *theory* of the reactions of human beings as a replacement for the actuality of these reactions in life itself. Personal experience compels me to concede that it is such a symptom that is comprised in the theory of psychoanalysis as it is widely operative in the consultation rooms of psychoanalysts today.

It has been assumed that, in envisaging the unconscious, psychoanalysis presupposes a more inclusive position than is presumably characteristic of the theoretical or systematised clinician. But it is a far-reaching commentary upon the analyst's capacity of discrimination that he still presumes to analyse another on the basis of a system or theory, as though a neurosis, which is an essentially subjective condition, were of the nature of an objective bodily lesion. A dissociation within the personality might find its analogy in a bodily lesion, but never a basis for its understanding. An objective analogy is necessarily a thing apart from a subjective dissociation. In the sphere of objectivity, the formulated system or theory occupies a very different place. The theory of an objective phenomenon is entirely commensurate with its application. After all, the theory of a mechanism is but the description of the principle of its operation. In the objective world, such an objective description presents no discrepancy. It is the application of the objective method to an objective principle. The theory of the hydraulic press is perfectly consistent with its application. Between theory and application there is here complete conjunction. No disparate element intervenes to mar the transition from the descriptive to the practical. So too with the theory of psychoanalysis as long as it pertains to the objective viewpoint of the textbook. But in the subjective sphere a totally different situation is presented. In dealing with life in its actuality, we are not dealing with the descriptive and objective. Human life is subjective. It is something experienced, something felt. It is not theoretical; it is actual. It is not descriptive; it is dynamic. Human life *is*; it is not a *theory* of what is. Life, as it is felt, is our ultimate subjective actuality. Subjectivity or feeling is the very basis of life. As such, feeling is life's reality and no theory of feeling is an adequate substitute for this reality. And so the objective theory of psychoanalysis, or the objective theory of the motives of human life, is wholly inapplicable to the subjective experience or the actuality of human life as it is felt in individual personality.

We do not begin to reckon in the least understandingly with the nature of the subjective as contrasted with the objective sphere of life. We are, in fact, quite naïve in our attitude toward the whole subjective field, preferring to adopt toward it either a mood of beatific reverence and mysticism, in which we conjure unwarranted images of "psychic phenomena" that are allied with man's pseudo-religious vagaries, or we adopt a "scientific" attitude which repudiates as nonexistent or regards as unworthy of serious thought any phenomena that do not lend themselves to objective observation. Neither position seems to me tenable. We might dismiss at once the attitude of the occultists, for mysticism entertains no argument. But there is the need to consider very seriously the subjective field of scientific reasoning and to keep clearly before us the distinctive and impassable interval between the subjective and the objective domains of scientific enquiry.[4]

The basis of this essay is precisely the recognition of this impossible breach between the condition of consciousness produced through a knowledge *about* feeling and the condition of consciousness that is the *feeling itself*, between the state of mind that is *commentative* and the state of mind that is *functioning*. The former is objective; the latter is subjective. The failure of our psychological methods to recognise this intrinsic distinction is, to my mind, the failure of our entire approach to the problems of mental and social disharmony. It is this unwitting substitution of the *theory* of human feelings for the unannotated experience of the feelings themselves, as recorded in our interactive functioning as human beings, that is the impossibility of our present "method" of psychoanalysis.

This position is, for me, an all-important one. Upon the acceptance or rejection of it, I believe, depends the growth or the decline of psychoanalysis as an agency of release for the intrinsic needs of the neurotic personality. Today, under the impetus of an objective psychoanalysis, or of psychoanalysis in its theoretical or vicarious form, we are carrying theory to the point of absurdity. There is now, for example, the psychoanalytic theory of the nursery.

Anxious young mothers are running about looking for texts that will serve them as guides in the love of their children. They are diligently searching upon every hand for the latest approved theory of maternal love. And, in response to the demand, the popular literature is supplying them with full details. But there are no librettos of the nursery. Baedekers to motherhood are not to be had. The motherhood that is true is a subjective relationship, and it is only subjectively that it can be felt and understood.

I shall not forget the experience told me by a patient whose mother, actuated by the theory of motherhood in its highest "scientific" interpretation, undertook to enlighten her upon the significance of sex. The incident left the most painful impression upon her. The mother, having gathered courage for the performance of her maternal duty, delivered her errand with a punctiliousness that, from the point of view of technique, was irreproachable. She spoke out of the strictest regard for the theory of motherhood. But, unfortunately, her theory left out of account an item that needs to be reckoned with, which is the native simplicity of the consciousness of childhood. The woman spoke out of the theory of a truth, but her child listened with the organic susceptibility of truth itself. The mother had not accepted within herself the actual significance of life, and so, in accordance with the formality of a theory, was vicariously imposing its acceptance upon her child. But childish perception pierces the veil of pedagogic finesse. The rigid demeanour of her instructor readily disclosed the discrepancy between the verbal recital and the utter lack of conscious acceptance within herself. For the child, now a middle-aged woman, the moment was an unforgettable one. She had witnessed in her mother an outrage to organic truth, and the shock of that experience caused a psychic disunity between mother and child from which there resulted an introversion of personality that covered half a lifetime. And so, while the theory of the nursery is from the point of view of theory wholly irreproachable, it is from the point of view of the nursery wholly absurd.

It is a lesson that parents have yet to learn, that the child is closer to the inherency of things than the grown-up, that the consciousness of childhood stands in a far more truthful relationship to the actuality of life as it is than the consciousness of the conventionalised and sophisticated adult. For years it has been my feeling that beneath the conflict of the neurotic personality there is iterated an urge toward the expression of this primal inherency of consciousness. Today, it is more than ever my view that in the neurotic reaction there is expressed an inherent plea for the native simplicity and truth of this organic consciousness. It becomes more and more clear to me that the pain of these personalities is due solely to the organic discrepancy of an unconsciousness and indirection within themselves, and that inherently their urge is to bring themselves again into harmony with the law of their being by reuniting the needs of their consciousness with the needs of their organic life.

As Nietzsche says, "May there not be—a question for alienists—neuroses of health?"[5] This question for alienists is indeed a vital one, but it is one which, as far as I am aware, has not as yet even dimly occurred to them. There is nowhere, it may be noted, a clearer argument for Nietzsche's hypothesis than Nietzsche's own neurosis. Unfortunately, however, alienists are still as little interested in the positive processes that bespeak the organism's conscious health as physicians in general are interested in the positive processes that ensure the organism's physical health. But as long as the collective social mind remains the collective unconscious mind, it is not to be expected that we shall envisage the unconscious of the individual, in either its psychic or in its somatic aspect, from the basis of an inclusive consciousness and health. The question so often asked is whether insanity will ever become curable. The answer can only be that the insanity of the individual cannot be curable as long as there exists the insanity of the social mind about him. It is not humanly possible for the psychiatrist to remedy conditions of dissociation as long as he himself is part of a dissociated group mind.[6]

If the psychoanalyst, in applying to the lives of his patients a theory of life, is himself unconsciously resorting to the self-protection of the substitutive and symbolic, if the blocked personality of our patients meets with a blocking in ourselves, with a compromise, a theory, a something which stands as a *sign for* rather than that which *is*—a situation which offers a compromise mechanism identical with that for which they have sought aid from us—then clearly the way is not yet open for the release of the conflict within these personalities. For a patient may be only in so far untrammelled as the analyst is himself untrammelled.

In taking this attitude, I do not make any personal claim for myself. This position is not one to which I have come through the success of my work, but, rather, through its failure. For in the measure in which I have adhered to the dictates of a preconceived normality, in just that measure has my work defeated itself. Though I have for some time theoretically disavowed the mental status represented in the normal reaction, I have tended unconsciously all the while to ally myself with this standardised brand of unconsciousness and thus, in my own work, have inclined to hold to a theory of life rather than to its actuality. Not, then, with the neurotic alone, but with us all, it would seem that consciousness is mainly employed in efforts of self-protection and evasion. Truly, consciousness makes cowards of us all. But this is not consciousness in the sense of life and growth; it is consciousness in the sense of retention and self. It is not a free consciousness; it is consciousness with a reservation. It is not true consciousness; it is unconsciousness.

In accordance with such a mode of consciousness, each of us is elbowing for a place for himself. Each is seeking more territory for his own expansion. Each of us is an unconscious overlord striving to secure the supremacy of his own personality. Universal and normal as this reaction is, its tendency is obsessive and ill. I do not believe that life is aggressive and that growth is concerned for itself. Personality is impersonality. What is needed is the quiet acceptance of life in its actuality. In it and it alone lies the opportunity for freedom and growth.

We hear much today of the technique of psychoanalysis. In truth, there is no such thing. It is just another defence mechanism, just another resistance to life in its actuality. As in all instances of therapeutic specialisation, the technique of psychoanalysis has become a fetish with us. It has become a veritable complex, a disorder from which I find patients actually suffering. The situation is quite ridiculous. The more I think of it, the more I am convinced that the so-called technique of psychoanalysis is but another hobgoblin wherewith the unconscious tendency of professionalism, with its egoistic striving for preferment, contrives to preserve its own separateness and distinction. I confess to having, in my own unconsciousness, more than once laid stress upon the importance of the analytic technique. But let us not be misled by what is called the technique of psychoanalysis. It is but another subterfuge for the reality of life. A technique of psychoanalysis is no more possible than a technique of love, or of friendship, or of motherhood. There is a technique, and a very difficult technique, of the *theory* of psychoanalysis. But that is quite a different thing. Psychoanalysis itself or, as its name implies, the loosening or freeing of consciousness, is nothing else than the conscious acceptance of life. As such, it is the exact contrary of the objective and technical. Life is not a technique. It does not express itself in terms of technique. Technique is an objective instrument. Life is a subjective experience. It is a joy or a sorrow, a disappointment or an aspiration, and it can no more be handled from the point of view of technique than it can be handled with the scalpel of the anatomist.

From these and similar reflections, I have come to regard the formality of applying a system of psychoanalysis to the life of an individual as an actual hindrance rather than as an aid to the true expression of his personality. It is but an added repression. It blocks the very way it attempts to open. It is to meet the unconscious of a patient with unconsciousness within oneself. It is to answer symbolic substitution and indirection with the same substitution and indirection in an altered, more subtle, socially plausible form.

The whole meaning, therefore, of an analysis that is actual and not theoretical is the realisation and acceptance on the part of the analyst of the utmost unconscious symbolisation and distortion within himself. The analysis of a patient is the analysis of oneself. It cannot be otherwise. And when I say analysis, I do not mean an analysis that is a mere unconscious concession to normality, a giving vent to the egoistic erotism of the individual by diffusing it among the widely distributed elements of the social personality in the manifold distortions of sexuality. I mean an analysis of personality in its widest expression, an analysis through which the individual comes into the conscious acceptance not only of the repression or distortion that is personal and that is comprised within the individual introversion we know as the neurosis, but of the distortion or substitution of personality that is social and that constitutes the confederacy of unconsciousness popularly endorsed as normality.

It is my unhesitating position that the prime requisite for clear, free, untrammelled work in the analysis of human personality is the unqualified rejection of the unconscious compromise embodied in the social reaction of normality. Repudiating the attitude of the healer whose criterion is the restoration of his patient to a condition of normality, the medical analyst who is not himself capitulating to the concession of the social unconscious will take his stand against any recourse that is based upon a programme of compromise and habituation. He will see that what is often considered as normality is merely unconsciousness on a co-operative basis and he will not be deceived by its insidious offers. It is only through such an attitude of complete freedom within oneself that it is possible to offer the opportunity of freedom to the personality of the neurotic patient, the very heart of whose disharmony lies in an inherent repugnance, however bewildered and confused, to the untruth of the social unconscious comprising his milieu. Viewed analytically, normality can become but the self-flattery through which we pretend we are not unconscious. By so pretending, however, we are only furthering our tendency to deeper unconsciousness.

As long as there is self-protection, there is self-limitation; as long as there is self-limitation, we are necessarily setting a limitation to the possibility of growth and consciousness in our patients. It is only through rejecting such protection that we may come to accept the testimony of the unconscious within ourselves. Otherwise, we ourselves become the inhibitors rather than the liberators of consciousness; we who are psychoanalysts become mere guardians of disease processes instead of the willing repositories of these unconscious factors as they exist in others, through our understanding and acceptance of these processes as they exist within ourselves. For consciousness grows upon the medium of consciousness. It cannot be nourished upon an extraneous soil. Theories of consciousness are extraneous. In the presence of the actuality of life, theories of life become mere intellectual snobbery. Being wise, sophisticated, and remote, they are inadequate to meet life in its native simplicity. Bearing the testimonials of authority, the credentials of office, they do not come low enough. These insignia of rank only tend to intimidate personality in its inherent simplicity. What is needed for the release of the neurotic individual is the personality who imposes nothing of his own and, thus, allows the completest opportunity for the unfolding of the repressed and introverted personality of another.

But there enters here a consideration of vital importance and one that has not yet been adequately reckoned with and understood. If the psychoanalyst is to be the recipient, there must be those who stand to him as recipient also. If he is to understand, he must be understood. If the life of the analyst is to be a reality and not a system, he himself must in reality participate in the life in which he invites others to participate. If it is his thesis that human life cannot subsist alone, that communication is life, that it is the very meaning of consciousness, neither can he subsist without communication. And so there need to be in the life of the analyst the personalities with whom he may share, with whom he may communicate, who accept him and are accepted by him in turn. For to analyse is to be analysed, to understand is to be understood.

These are conclusions to which I have not come alone. I could not have. They are the outcome of my own opportunity of participation and expression, as the need of communication has come to unfold itself in my own experience.

It is needful, then, that we who stand as the promoters of a new and untrammelled consciousness look carefully into our own lives to discover whether we ourselves, as part of the social consciousness, are not theorists rather than unified personalities actuated solely by the law of understanding and of growth within ourselves. It is needful that we realise the completely vicarious and repressed element underlying the expression of unconsciousness embodied in the social unrest within and about us, and that, fearlessly repudiating this collective reaction of substitution and evasion, we break completely with the popular policies of compromise and untruth underlying it. In this course, we shall take our stand for the freedom and clarity of a mode of consciousness that aims solely toward the growth of self-understanding and communication. For life is not a system, it is not a technique. Life is simple, and its course is one of quiet flow. In so far as psychoanalysis is technical, it is not life. In so far as its aim is the systematised, it is not free.

The choice is an unequivocal one. It is a choice between expediency and truth, between fixity and growth. For the habitual mind whose criterion is expedience, the choice is already determined, but for the personality that is sensitive to the inherency of life, the choice of growth is no less inevitable. It is organically so. Hence, it is for each of us to make his choice on which side he will take his stand: whether, adhering to a theory of life, he will blindly protect himself against the recognition and acknowledgement of the vicarious element of habituation and compromise within his own unconscious, or whether he will stand for a mode of consciousness that flings away every habitual protection and accepts only the conditions of life as they unfold themselves in the development of his own personality as well as in that of others. The outlook is really not ambiguous. The question is whether life will be a theory or system corroborated by the technical outfit of the clinic, or whether it will be the deeply fulfilled experience that comprises consciousness in its organic reality.

To sum up, the definite biological concept on which this thesis rests posits a societally organismic continuum as the essential basis of consciousness. To understand this concept, it will be necessary to replace the more or less arbitrary divergences of personal outlook with a conception that attempts to stand far enough removed from our personal mode to envision within its more ample formulation this personal outlook as well. It will be necessary to recognise our tendency to personalistic delimitation due to the unconscious systematisation of the restricted individual unit and, in this way, to envisage consciousness anew from the more inclusive basis of its societal meaning. The activities of the small group with whom I have worked in association during the past years give promise of the inception of a more comprehensive psychoanalytic technique applicable to social units as well as to the single individual. Through the study and analysis of our human moods and complexes, as actually observable within the reactions of groups, there has at least been made a beginning of an actual laboratory approach to the study of our social consciousness.

Notes

1. "The preconscious or the nest instinct", paper by the author read at the seventh annual meeting of the American Psychoanalytic Association, Boston, MA, 25 May 1917.
2. "Social images versus reality", *The Journal of Abnormal Psychology and Social Psychology*, *XIX*(3): October–December 1924.
3. "The laboratory method in psychoanalysis", *American Journal of Psychiatry*, *V*(3), January 1926.
4. "Psychiatry as an objective science". *British Journal of Medical Psychology*, *V*(4).
5. "Giebt es veilleicht—eine Frage für Irrenärzte—Neurosen der Gesundheit?" *Nietzsche's Werke. Erste Abt, Band I. Die Geburt der Tragödie*. Leipzig, 1903.
6. "Our social evasion": Presidential Address before the mid-year meeting of the American Psychoanalytic Association, New York City, 27 December 1925. To be published in a forthcoming issue of the *Medical Journal and Record*.

CHAPTER TEN

Speaking of resistances*

The chief inconsistency in our psychoanalytic basis is the lack of a broad biological definition of what that basis is. In the absence of such a definition, there is lacking on our own part a clear concept of our own basis. In this situation, a helter-skelter vernacular has come to take the place of sober formulations such as should stand for a scientifically accepted concept, and with this loose tendency in our basic conceptual usage, our psychoanalytic superstructure must necessarily be loose also.

The basis of psychoanalysis is the individual's resistance, and an entire system of psychology has been built around this phenomenon of resistance. But just what a resistance is biologically, we have not yet enquired. In response to this question, we psychoanalysts have, in effect, merely replied, "A resistance is an objection to *my* interpretation of your reaction." This is certainly not a position calculated to give edification to our scientific *confrères* in other fields of biological investigation, for, in this position, we advocate a system of psychology

* In its original form, this paper was read as an address before the Sixteenth Annual Meeting of The American Psycho-analytic Association, New York City, 10 June 1926.

based upon presumably definite elements, although upon enquiry, it turns out that we have never yet thought it necessary to define in clear, biological terms what these elements are.[1] This quite esoteric, non-biological definition of a resistance is, I think, inseparable from our present individualistic and uncontrolled basis of interpretation. The private, individualistic basis is, it seems to me, necessarily unbiological, and yet this position represents, in the present stage of our psychoanalytic evolution, the position of us all. We might not like this. It might cause us to feel very uncomfortable, but the fact remains that this circumstance is significant, and that as psychoanalysts, it becomes our special function to analyse the significance of just such lapses in our own mental processes. For it is only too apparent that in not defining a resistance, we have been ourselves the dupes of the very resistances which it was our business to define.

Consistent with this scientific *faux pas*, there is among us the prevailing notion that there exists some inherent relation between an attitude of resistance and an attitude of antagonism. This view has its correlate in the contrary assumption that an attitude of acquiescence and mutual endorsement is somehow *not* a resistance. In fact, as we all know, despite our naïve protests to the contrary, we unconsciously make it our business to induce in our patients precisely this attitude of acquiescence and conformity, and this we label "the overcoming of resistances". When, in his mental imagery toward the analyst, the attitude of the patient is one of trusting devotion, the analysis is going nicely. The mental attitude of such a patient is: "I will tell you of my sexual inadvertences, fanciful or actual, because you alone are so understanding, so sympathetic, so wise and good and what-not, that I can confide in you." It is this attitude that we commonly presume is not a resistance. But thereby hangs a tale.

In a less personal, less individualistic interpretation of resistances, I think we must come to see that, biologically, a resistance is based upon the artificial situation prevailing under a system of social images in which the family album, so to speak, is the unit—a social system which arbitrarily subjects the individual to the parent as a mere sadistic *image* of authority.[2] Like the parent who prefers the docile child, we analysts have failed to see that childish docility is but the necessary and opposite reaction to this parental sadism, and that the patient who is acquiescent to this parental image is no less resistant, in his intrinsic organism, than the patient whose reaction takes the counter-sadistic form of antagonism. It is my position, therefore, that, organically, the individual's subservience to this individualistic image authority—it matters not whether it takes the form of acquiescence or opposition—is equally a resistance from the viewpoint of his biological integrity, that is to say, of his relation to the species as a whole.

In the analytic situation, of course, there is rehashed the family situation once more. Like the patient of the hypnotist of old, if he "comes under readily" he is a good and docile subject—that is to say, he is a good subject from the point of view of the image- or transference-authority now vested in the person of the analyst. But my point is that subordination to an image authority, be it parent or analyst, as definitely involves a resistance as the attitude that opposes this image subjugation.

Were there not present an inherent resistance in this benign and seemingly harmonious filial situation with its note of loving submission, how does it happen that, after many years of such gentle *rapprochement* between a father and son, let us say, some stimulus such as a money conflict or an inept marriage can cause two such people to fly apart in violent and lifelong antagonism one to the other? Is it not apparent that the resistances were already there when so arbitrary an occasion can provide tinder for so violent an outbreak? If the family is really united in so great a love, as we say, why could it not brook this momentary interruption to the habitual tenor of its ways? Or if the proverbially absorbing devotion of the newly married pair is so deep and real, how does it happen that its ardour is so soon dampened? How does it happen that it so soon cools into indifference or even aversion? It is, I maintain, because love (I mean by that the unconscious manifestation we are wont to call love in our present purblind narcissistic interpretation of it) is itself man's major resistance. If this is so, we are merely hoodwinking ourselves when we apotheosise this most naïve of our human frailties and fail to see that in it lies the very essence of our human resistances.

It must be clear that there is some serious unconscious factor operative within us that we could all this while have been so taken in by our popular personal and social interpretations of love. It must be clear that it is our own social involvement in our own socially involved family images that has permitted us all this time to regard a resistance as something opposed to our own interpretation, and not to have seen that our own interpretation is likewise a resistance. It is only on the ground of our own naïve family images that we can account at all for our having failed to demand of ourselves long ago a sound biological definition of a resistance. This individualistic or family *naïveté* is truly a significant commentary upon our own family or individualistic basis of analysis.

Now, whether we like this or do not like it, as I have said, it is certainly very interesting. I, for one, frankly confess that I do not like it. It is an imputation that I find extremely uncomfortable. Nevertheless, it does interest me. In fact, it quite fascinates me to find myself one of a group of scientists advocating a system of psychology that is based implicitly upon a resistance, when it has never occurred to us to enquire what is the biological nature of this phenomenon called a "resistance". Humiliating as this circumstance may be for us individually, yet, from a more inclusive basis, I think it is not impossible for us to derive quite a deep satisfaction in the attempt to account honestly for this extraordinary phenomenon occurring within our own mental processes. I venture to say that we not only do not know what a resistance is, but that we have not the ghost of an idea to whom or what the resistance is. The situation is really too naïve. The Freudian says, "The resistance is to me and to my system." And so do you and I. . . .

I venture to submit the proposition that, in the private capacity of interpretation claimed by Freud and by you and by me, the authority for our interpretations rests upon as unwarranted and as wholly gratuitous an *image* of private privilege.[3] . . . Again I do not like this. I feel sure that you do not. Unquestionably, it reflects upon our mental processes, if it can really be shown that all this while we have been chasing a will-o'-the-wisp in what we have called the authority of our interpretations, in contradistinction to what we have been claiming are the incorrigible resistances of other people. Nevertheless, I find myself completely captivated by the absurd spectacle of my own presumptions and quite unaccountably incited to investigate the matter. What gives yet keener zest to this situation is the recognition that the position of you and me is not peculiar at all to the systems advocated by the devotees of these systems, namely, by ourselves. Not at all. For all these incorrigible folk who, we say, have resistances to us on the basis of our interpretations—that is to say, who object to our interpretations of their reactions—claim no less stoutly and, as far as I can see, with no less authority, that we have resistances to them because we object to *their* interpretations of *our* reactions. So, this phenomenon of resistance would seem to be the reaction of every individual to every other individual, and in each it would seem to consist in the claim to an indisputable prerogative in judging the reactions of others. This phenomenon of resistance would, then, appear to be a socially universal reaction, and, accordingly, its biological meaning becomes, I think, an investigation that is the more imperative for us.[4]

Setting out from the basis of a laboratory consensus, I should like to attempt tentatively to define resistance as a social phenomenon due to the universal presence among us of spurious (transference) social images, and to the compulsion on the part of each individual or collection of individuals to enforce upon all other individuals an authority that is arbitrarily *vested* in him by virtue of his original image of the parent. That is to say, an authority that is not based upon observable facts, but that rests its sole claim upon the personal or social image.[5]

A social group represented by our own psychoanalytic unit or family affords a conspicuous instance of this factor of social resistances. As we all recall, Jung was, in the beginning, the very apple of Freud's eye. In Freud's album of cherished images, Jung was unquestionably the scion of the family. But Jung found himself unable to accept the interpretations of Freud. He had interpretations of his own which he liked better. Likewise Adler, Stekel, Wittels, and others. True to form, Jung and the rest say that it is the Freudian who has resistances to *them*. And, for the life of me, I cannot see that their claim rests upon any less demonstrable authority than that of the Freudian who in turn says, "Not at all, it is they who have resistances to *me*." Could anything be more typical of a family squabble? Could anything more clearly illustrate the absence of a scientific definition or basis determining just what a resistance is?

Now, it is obvious that in this situation our only solution would be to take sides with one or the other faction, that is, with the father or with our errant brothers. But what has science to do with taking sides with the private prejudice or private interpretations of any individual or collection of individuals? We do not have sides or resistances elsewhere in the sphere of biology. We do not hear one bacteriologist talking about the resistances that another bacteriologist has to his interpretations. And why? Because the bacteriologist does not reserve to himself the privilege of having private interpretations. Faithful to scientific traditions, the bacteriologist submits material to a consensus of observers, and that consensus and the biological sense perceptions shared by them commonly constitute the inherent authority determining the facts before them.[6] There is no place for autocratic presumption, no possible chance that observation shall be arbitrary because of any influence upon our evaluations of a private or esoteric prerogative.

This muddle, occasioned through our not having defined the very first principles upon which our whole system of psychoanalysis reposes, necessarily occasions a very difficult situation for our confiding patients, as indeed for a naïve and confiding community at large.[7] In our present position, the practical question is simply, has or has not a patient insuperable resistances to my interpretation of him? And the only earthly way to discover is to subject the patient to my interpretations. Very nice for me, but what about the patient? Such an ultimatum might be clever and it might even be useful, but by no stretch of the imagination could we call this type of legislation scientific or sound. Yet, this is the test to which the patient is arbitrarily subjected: has he resistances to me or has he not?

As we know, there exists an infallible test for determining whether certain fungi, presumed to be mushrooms, are or are not poisonous—to eat them. But, however decisive this test, it can hardly be called scientific, because as many times as not the investigator succumbs in the process of his investigation. Such a test, it seems to me, is identical with that of the patient approaching the psychoanalyst who cherishes a private basis of interpretation. Does the personality of the patient agree with that of the analyst? Can he accept, can or can he not assimilate the analyst's interpretation of him? If he can, well and good. If not, the patient is in a sorry pass, and as often as not must either accept permanent invalidism, insanity, or suicide. Beyond question, this is a most decisive test as regards the fitness of the analytic diet for the particular patient, but, like the test of mushrooms, it is had at a high cost to human life.

These reflections lead me to feel the complete inadequacy of an analytic technique that artificially separates the individual patient from his natural soil or social setting. An analysis that does not take into account the resistances that are manifested socially toward the patient as well as the resistances he manifests toward others includes but half of the picture. Our resistances are social. An observation that takes account only of the individual's reactions and leaves out of reckoning the interreactions existing between him and his social environment is necessarily biased and one-sided. Our resistances are physiological. To interpret this phenomenon apart from its neural biology is to talk in the air, and again we have reverted to the arbitrary prerogative of the religionists. My position is that, in our own resistances, we have not yet sensed the social and physiological value of a procedure that retains intact the physiological and social conditions of the organism. In our failure to recognise the biology of resistances and their social physiology, we have been labouring under a misapprehension, and our private method of analysis has necessarily been hampered in its efficiency in the measure in which we have been restricted to its personal and exclusive use. A modification of the private analysis and its supplementing with a social or group basis of technique will, I think, be found to constitute the only logical—because it is the only physiological—condition of observation competent to cope with civilisation's pandemic of resistances.

It does seem to me that it is clearly time that this organisation cease to point out the resistance as though it were something outside and opposite itself, and that we realise that our problem is a social one in which we are all participants in a social *system* of resistances. To look at a patient before me and say that he has resistance because he does not agree with my interpretation of his reactions, is a method that really must go by the board. As one psychoanalyst of more than usually broad perspectives recently wrote to me, "this [the private basis of interpretation] refers to a situation from which I have suffered the deepest 'feelings of guilt' over botches in psycho-analysis. And what is the remedy?" And the writer adds, "A consensus of sincere acceptance of certain objectified results obtained from a group of interested workers."

With individual psychoanalysts awakening more and more to the unsoundness of a basis that is private because it excludes a consensus of co-workers with respect to the data under investigation, it seems to me that psychopathologists generally will be led inevitably to adopt a basis that is as obviously scientific and controlled with respect to data within the mental field as the basis obtaining in respect to data within other spheres of biology.

Notes

1. Some months ago, there appeared in one of our popular magazines an article purporting to be an authoritative repudiation of the method of

psychoanalysis by a former advocate of it. This statement, however, was anonymous, and an anonymous contribution in the sphere of the subjective sciences is, by its nature, scientifically untrustworthy. The objection so popularly felt that there is something essentially unsound in the system of psychoanalysis has doubtless its warrant in certain structural lapses within that system. The fact is, there is something in the psychoanalytic position that is decidedly unscientific, and there is definite need of its scientific reconstruction. But pointing the finger at this situation, being critical of it, and holding oneself superior toward it—and especially where it is done behind the screen of anonymity—is not to the point, and will avail us nothing.

As one of those questionable beings known as a psychoanalyst and possessing the vantage ground of a long experience in the use of that method, I feel in some measure qualified to speak of the very grave defects of the psychoanalytic basis as now applied, without in any sense discrediting its scientific possibilities, or for a moment disdaining the Freudian formulation as offering a position that cannot be, with proper scientific controls, adequately met and adjusted.

2. "Social images versus reality": paper read at the Fourteenth Annual Meeting of the American Psychopathological Association, Philadelphia, PA, 7 June 1924; *The Journal of Abnormal Psychology and Social Psychology, XIX*(3), October–December 1924.
3. "Psycho-analytic improvisations and the personal equation": paper read at the Fifteenth Annual Meeting of The American Psycho-analytic Association, Richmond, VA, 12 May 1925; *The Psycho-analytic Review, XIII*(2), April 1926.
4. "Our mass neurosis": paper read at the Fourteenth Annual Meeting of The American Psycho-analytic Association, Atlantic City, NJ, 3 June 1924; *The Psychological Bulletin, XXIII*(6), June 1926.
5. "The heroic role—an historical retrospect": paper read before the Section of Historical and Cultural Medicine of the New York Academy of Medicine, 26 March 1925; *Psyche, VII*(1), July 1926.
6. "Psychiatry as an objective science": paper read at the Fifteenth Annual Meeting of The American Psychopathological Association, Washington, DC, 7 May 1925; *The British Journal of Medical Psychology, V*(4), 1925. "The laboratory method in psycho-analysis": paper read at the Ninth Congress of the International Psycho-analytical Association, Bad Homburg, Germany, September, 1925; *The American Journal of Psychiatry, V*(3), January 1926. "The group method of analysis": paper read before the Washington Psycho-analytic Society, 14 November 1925; to be published

in a forthcoming issue of *The Psycho-analytic Review*. "Die Gruppen-methode in der Psychoanalyse", *Imago, XII*, 1926, Heft 2/3.

7. "Our social evasion": Presidential Address before the mid-year meeting of The American Psycho-analytic Association, New York City, December 27, 1925; *Medical Journal and Record, CXXIII*(12), 16 June 1926.

CHAPTER ELEVEN

The problem of the transference*[1]

For some time I have wanted to discuss the problem of the transference. My reason for wishing to do so is not only that I regard the phenomenon of transference as the major problem in psychopathology, but that I do not think that throughout the field of psychopathology there exists any other problem except the transference phenomenon. In short, it is my view that the neurosis and the transference are one.

This position calls for explanation. It calls for it the more because a right account of this wider acceptation of the transference affords also a right account of the essential basis of group analysis—a basis upon which my entire position in psychoanalysis rests.[2]

As technically described, the transference is the unconscious response with which the neurotic patient reacts toward persons of his environment and specifically toward the personality of the psychoanalyst. This response (attraction or repulsion) represents a replacement for early affectional memories, most particularly for the early

* First published in *The British Journal of Medical Psychology, VII*(II), 1927.

impressions that cluster about the parent. Once a relationship of close confidence is established toward his physician, these early impressions surge back to the patient and automatically fixate his emotional interest upon the analyst. But, under conditions of group analysis, one finds this description far too narrow for the scope of the phenomena embraced under it. One can only attribute so restricted a definition to the limited tendency of interpretation to which one is necessarily confined upon an individualistic basis of analysis. As the presumable therapeutic efficacy of the transference and its axiomatic conditioning of the analysis grow precisely out of this restricted conception of it, it is the more urgent that we expand our outlooks and define more broadly the phenomenon of the transference.

In the first place, I cannot any longer regard the transference as a specific phenomenon. I cannot feel that it is a process that has been given clear scientific definition or that it has, as yet, received a definitive analytic handling from us. As far as I can see, the transference is by no means a phenomenon that distinguishes the state of mind of a particular patient sitting in front of me, but is a condition of the social mind generally. Upon analysis, this state of mind proves to be, in essence, an unconscious condition of dependence on the part of each individual toward every other, and it invariably shows itself in an unconscious attitude that alternates constantly between favour or placation on the one hand and irritation or complaint on the other. In a mood of placation, for example, our contentment is but a reflection of the "niceness" of those about us. In a mood of irritation, we demand that others shall so acquit themselves as to appease our displeasure. Such a quite normal and everyday attitude is nothing else than the transference, or a dependence upon another individual for one's own state of mind. This mood dependence, existing socially and shifting constantly between love and hate, happiness and pain, is, I maintain, operative at all times and is as completely automatic and unconscious as the unconscious mood we habitually observe in the individual patient.

This process of the transference can best be studied if we will observe it as it first arises in early childhood. As we all know, the social attitude of mind surrounding the child is such that there is straightaway placed a premium upon an attitude of behaviour in him that is called "good". This moralistic attitude, however, invariably rests upon a referred affect. For this social attitude of mind that stands opposite the child summons the mind of the child over to itself, as it were, and bids him regard himself from a position opposite to him. From this dissociative position, the child is counselled to see to it that his conduct conforms to a socially standardised pattern designated as right or commendable. This mechanism, whereby the mind of the child is placed in a position of criticism opposite himself, induces in the organism of the individual a dualistic or disparate basis of action. Under the influence of this dissociative social mood, the individual is led to identify himself with a criterion that is opposite and outside of himself, and, henceforward, he is bidden to measure his every action in the social mirror in which his action is thus reflected. In this way, the individual's every mood is bound up in a social image that is based upon a referred affect.[3]

This social image and its original psychogenic incitement is interesting in relation to the mood alternation we find represented in the two poles of the transference—complacence or complaint, pleasure or pain, love or hate. For this referred or dependent mood is, according to the finding of the group analysis, directly traceable to the early inducement in the child of this social image of himself as inculcated by the parent. This dualistic condition by which the child measures his best interest according to how his image is reflected by others is called the knowledge of good and bad. It is called the early training of the child. It is, in fact, a completely unconscious inducement in the child of a transference or image relationship based upon dependence upon others and is the reflection of an equally unconscious attitude of transference or dependence on the part of others with respect to him. This image relationship, with its referred affect, establishes a purely adventitious connection between the parent and the child, between the world of image and the world of function. It sets before the child an artificial basis of comparison or contrast between himself and his social environment. In so doing, it places a bar to the natural unity or physiological mood through which the individual is organically continuous with others. For, through the transference existing in the social milieu surrounding the child, he early imbibes this social transference basis also. In this way, there is artificially induced in him a secondary and disparate mood which replaces the spontaneous relationship comprising the natural function between the parent and child organisms, or between the individual and the social world about him. Such is the essential cleavage or division concomitant with the social induction in the mind of the child of his own image or self-reflection. Such is the embryonic origin of the phenomenon of transference.

As this social image is phyletic in its source, its distribution is phyletic. As it is general in its origin, it is general in its development also. It is our observation, therefore, that the transference represents a state of universal unconsciousness, that it is the meaning not only of our private basis of social interchange, but that it is the basis as well of all our social institutions. This social transference dominates our courts, our clinics, and our academies. The home and the school are completely subjugated to this social image. Upon an analysis of man's religious impulse, we find it to have no other motive than the spurious promise of self-interest or favour represented in the phenomenon of transference. The fluctuating policies of government are traceable directly to the unconscious vacillations of this referred affect. Upon the insecurity of this unconscious transference rests the whole fabric of marriage, as upon it rest the relationships of whole nations to one another. In brief, through the unconscious reciprocity of this social image, it is the underlying mood of all our human relationships.[4] If I like or dislike, if I am confident or dismayed, it is transference. If my feeling is one of interest or boredom, if it is one of satisfaction or chagrin, it is transference. Whether I am irritated with a taxi-driver or whether, in my benevolence, I bestow charities upon the indigent, my mood is still one of transference. If I am a patriot or an anarchist, a socialist or an imperialist, believer or disbeliever, it is again transference. And if, in my dissatisfaction at finding my own image pursuing me at all times under this social obsession of transference, I turn to others with question and complaint, it is once more transference. It is the attitude of dependence, it is the referred affect, it is the mother image as it is reflected in the social image of one's self.

Due to this mood of dependence and its unconscious alternative of propitiation or redress (love or hate), the individual is constantly under the necessity to seek the cover of psychological concepts that are merely substitutive. Our philosophies, our ethics, our religious and educational formulations teem throughout with secondary social images that merely reflect this mood of transference or dependence. Nowhere is the individual's expression dependable in his relation to others because of this disparate mood that is incited at the very origin of his social relationships. In this situation, according to our group studies in analysis, our psychological concepts and intellectualisations represent replacements for the functional interrelationships natural to the individuals of the species. Accordingly, through the repression of the primary physiological mood of man, there is substituted in each individual an unconsciously projected defence affect, or transference, for which the function of analysis can only be its reabsorption and elimination by the individual organism.[5]

At the last meeting of the American Psychoanalytic Association, many questions were asked me regarding the principles and practice underlying the group method of analysis. There could be no doubt as to the sincerity and earnestness of the questions asked and I cannot but believe that the effort of response on my part was felt to be equally sincere. Nevertheless, the meeting, as a whole, failed to reach a common understanding. The positions held in our respective interpretations remained the same at the end as at the beginning of the enquiry. Such an ineptness in the efforts of understanding on the part of a scientific gathering seems to me quite inconsistent with its scientific aims. Thus, I welcome this opportunity to reconsider the seeming divergence of our ways.

As I see it, the difficulty lies precisely in the social image that constitutes everywhere the impediment in all human relationships. The very questions asked rested necessarily upon the opposite or disparate basis induced socially in the beginning of the life of every individual of us. As I look back, then, this rigid impasse to a common interpretation among us was inevitably bound up with the conditions of our universal social transference. The enquiry had to do with subjective data, that is, with feeling reactions or moods inherent in each of us. But, in dealing with subjective data, or data within oneself, questions which tend to be referred to another rather than applied to the subjective data themselves are questions which belong in every instance to the category of transference images.

In such circumstances, the technical procedure in our group or laboratory sessions has consisted in the effort to recall such subjective references back to their source within the individual and, by thus applying them directly to the subjective material at hand, or to the individual himself, to submit such references, together with their subjective involvement, to objective observation and analysis.[6] In the same measure, my own efforts to answer your questions from the basis of the opposite image or concept could only be, from the viewpoint of a social analysis, an evasion of such questions. It would mean adhering to the disparate mood or to an *image* of human relationships rather than, by analysing this image or mood, to recover the functional, phyletic basis of interchange that is the natural matrix of man's social relationships.

An analysis of the social mood cannot, of course, be reached by a discussion of its rationalisations. We are, of necessity, compelled to emphasise this circumstance in any presentation of our social technique. This means that, from a phyletic standpoint, we cannot meet the intellectual questions of the individual upon the mental basis which these questions assume. To the degree in which we enter into argument or intellectual discussion of concepts, we digress from our group technique and from an analysis of the mood which presents itself in a social form at the moment.

What is alone of interest from the basis of a laboratory or group analysis is the reaction of the individual to his immediate social environment. Our observation centres upon the physiological mood invariably present, not upon the psychological concept commonly superimposed. I know that to exclude intellectual debate is an offence not to be tolerated within the sphere of our social interchange. But it is precisely intellectual debate, conventional intolerance, and "social" interchange which are the proper materials of the group or phyletic basis of analysis. And so, where there are questions, I must, in consistency, refer them back to the mood that underlies them rather than credit them to the concept they contain. This is the accepted procedure of psychoanalysis in respect of the private fancy or image of the individual, and it is equally the procedure exacted of us when we attempt to analyse the images that pertain to the realm of our social phantasies. One's analytic technique toward one's individual patient does not consist in recourse to mere unchallenged social discussion, and no more may we rely upon unchecked social discussion in an analysis of our mass unconscious.

From a phyletic or group basis of analysis, then, conceptual questions regarding subjective data, whether the questions be practical or theoretical, are necessarily the expression of a social image, and these images in turn necessarily arise from the background of a disparate social mood. Our group position, on the contrary, is, as far as may be, the expression of a confluent physiological mood and its background is essentially physiological. Assuming this physiological background as our basis, it is the function of the group method of analysis to submit to examination precisely such psychological concepts or social images as have been commonly accepted by us as the legitimate material of our social interchange. This material, you see, must necessarily include the very questions with which the individual would approach an understanding of the group method.

As I use the term group in its phyletic meaning, so I am using the term physiological in an entirely phyletic sense. In this sense, the term connotes the instinctive interrelationships of the individuals of a species as represented in the organic integrations that constitute their common feeling and reactions. The reader is, no doubt, acquainted with the objective statement of this instinct of our primary racial solidarity as long ago set forth by Darwin. The more recent account of this racial principle described by Kropotkin in his thesis, *Mutual Aid*, is also doubtless familiar to everyone. In his recent work, *The Physiological Foundations of Behavior*, Professor C. M. Child also deals with biological integrations related to this same category. And, in simpler and more popular language, it is illustrated in passages of Herman Melville's account of his experiences among the natives of the South Sea Islands.[7]

As analysts of our own social reactions, however, our interest is not external, objective, or descriptive. It is internal and subjective. It deals with our own feeling reactions as social beings according to how we find these reactions immediately represented in our own immediate mood. For, in the findings of the group basis of analysis, the early introduction socially of an image of dependence or transference has occasioned a distinct conflict within the physiological personality of the social organism as a whole. Accordingly, there exists a social mood or reverie that is as truly based upon a system of unconscious images existing within the social personality as the system of unconscious images Freud discovered in the mood or reverie of the neurotic individual. After all, our group position is merely the extension and application to the group or phylum of this principle that is the accepted basis of the individual or ontogenetic method of psychoanalysis.

I hope I begin to make clear what I believe we shall come to feel is the essential identity of our psychoanalytic obligations of technique toward the social group or phylum and our obligations toward the analysis of our individual patients. I hope I begin to make clear that, where we are dealing with a social mood that is based upon an unconscious substitution of social images for reality, we may no more occupy ourselves with questions that represent intellectual concepts or transference images than we may entertain ourselves with an exchange of social concepts or transference images in dealing with the phantasy mood or transference of the individual patient.

This social image or transference is not, then, a sporadic phenomenon. It is by no means limited to the neurotic personality. It is the early and persistent prepossession of every individual living under the sway of our present social mood. If our group finding in this regard is correct, then the underlying occasion of the neurosis is not individualistic but social, and it behooves us to take into serious account its widespread social implication and apply to it a social technique of analysis comparable to that we have attempted to apply to our individual patients. In scientific consistency, there is demanded the mood analysis of our own repressed social mood. I do not think we need be surprised that there should exist among us a mood reluctance to accept a phyletic principle of analysis. Certainly, there has been no lack of reluctance on my own part. For this extension from an individualistic to a group basis of technique entails a fundamental reconstruction of the analytic process.

There is no question but that those of us who have applied over the years Freud's method in individual analysis have substantiated in every case Freud's basic postulate of the existence within the neurotic personality of a psychic conflict due to sexual repression. In our effort to uncover these repressions, we have been able to trace the manifold disguises of the unconscious into the endless substitutions and distortions first described by Freud, so that, as regards Freud's actual findings, there is no ground for disagreement among us. But careful observation would seem to demand that Freud's findings and our own substantiation of them need now to give way to a broader basis of enquiry. It would seem that, as isolated processes, these individualistic findings have served their usefulness and that the time has come for correlating such findings with a unitary principle of observation that possesses the scientific merit of universal applicability.[8]

In the somatic sphere of medical investigation, the ontogenetic study of disease processes consisted in discovering the various lesions occurring in the individual as indicated by the symptoms presented and in applying the treatment in accordance with these lesions. But when such disease entities became correlated under a general principle of science through the discovery of infective processes, and when through such discovery the micro-organisms responsible in the specific instance were cultivated and studied in detail, the outlook of the pathologist became revolutionised. Thenceforward, our interest has centred upon such measures as would safeguard the organism against the invasion of the germ demonstrated to be the cause of the disease in question. This discovery of the principle of infection meant the reversal of the entire method of pathology. It shifted the focus of medical interest from the individualistic symptom to the phyletic cause responsible for it.

An investigation of mental disease in its phyletic or group significance discloses a source of dissociation in the mental life as definite, as specific, and as universal as that which in the somatic sphere is found in the specific micro-organism traceable as the cause of infective processes. In the case of functional or phyletic disharmonies, the microgenic event to which these disorders are traceable is, according to our laboratory observations, nothing else than the moralistic, referred, or dependent attitudes we find in the transference—a transference early induced in the organism of the individual through the artificial imposition upon him of the social image of himself concomitantly with the opposite social images in which others are presented to him.

The individualistic method in psychoanalysis assumes that the conflicts discovered in the neurotic personality are the cause of his disorder. But, in a phyletic study of consciousness, these individual repressions are regarded as a result of a phyletic incident which antecedes this apparent ontogenetic cause. If this position is warranted, our treatment must be modified in accordance and, instead of remaining ourselves involved in an ontogenetic transference and inducing a like mood in our patients, every ontogenetic incident in a patient's unconsciousness must, like our own, be measured in the light of the social or phyletic transference in which he, as an individual, participates.

In its present unconscious social involvement, psychoanalysis is not the study of a neurosis; it *is* a neurosis. It is not an objective science applied to a subjective disease; it is a subjective reflection of the very disease it presumably submits to objective scientific study. And not psychoanalysis alone, but throughout the sphere of the subjective sciences, there remains to be recognised a transference mood that exists *socially* and that therefore underlies the processes of the observer as well as the processes which are to be observed.

If the social image and the disparate mood that underlies it are synonymous with the transference and its irreconcilable alternatives, and if this ambivalence and conflict are the basis of the neurosis, manifestly the sole function of psychoanalysis is the elimination of this dualistic image basis or transference and the re-establishment of the unitary physiological basis of function such as is the natural condition of the healthy phylum.

The reader is here reminded that this position is not a mere expression of my view. It should be understood that all that I am saying is the report of a laboratory or group finding with respect to my own processes and those of other individuals who have submitted themselves to the group analysis. Contrary to a frequent misinterpretation, *group analysis is not my analysis of the group, but it is the group's analysis of me or of any other individual of the group.* "Group" does not mean a collection of individuals. It means a phyletic principle of observation. This phyletic principle of observation as applied to the individual and to the aggregate is the whole significance of the group analysis.[9] Basing my work upon this phyletic premise, my whole endeavour has come to centre upon the effort to confront immediately the transference image, whether in the individual or in the group. With the extension of my work to fresh fields of contacts, it has been interesting to observe the quick response of the patient to an attitude in myself which, far from assuming the transference to be the *sine qua non* of analysis, regards the transference as precisely the major barrier to the freeing of the neurotic personality.

To sum up: the transference is nothing else than the mother image. Whether social or individual, the mother image cannot stand as reality to the organism. It can stand as reality only to the image of oneself. *For images and illusions are real only in so far as they are reciprocated by the images and illusions by which they are surrounded.* In a comprehensive view of our human phylum, there remains no other conclusion than that the social mind throughout comprises a systematisation of social images, and that society at large is, in fact, under the thrall of an unconscious social transference.

If this finding is correct, we have not as yet taken our position half seriously, half inclusively enough. Our obligation rests upon ourselves. There is no external aid we may call in to our support. That again is the transference and the mood of dependence. And so, I hope that my position does not seem inconsistent when, in response to the very earnest and valuable questions on the part of my colleagues generally, I am compelled to refer them to the same source to which I have had to turn for the answer to these same questions, which is to my own involvement in the social mood that underlies the psychological concepts or images with which this mood is commonly replaced. According, therefore, to the subjective finding of the laboratory or group basis, it is only by returning to the analysis of the social mood upon which our intellectualisations or social images ultimately rest that we may offset the prevalent tendency to image transference or mood dependence that is the unconscious basis of our social as of our individual personality.

Notes

1. Paper read before the third annual mid-year meeting of the American Psychoanalytic Association, New York City, 26 December 1926.
2. "The group method of analysis": to be published in a forthcoming issue of *The Psychoanalytic Review.*
3. "Social images versus reality": *Journal of Abnormal Psychology and Social Psychology, XIX*(3), October–December 1924.
4. "Our mass neurosis": *The Psychological Bulletin, XXIII*(6), June 1926; "Insanity a social problem": *The American Journal of Sociology, XXXII*(1), part 1, July 1926.
5. "The reabsorbed affect and its elimination", *British Journal of Medical Psychology, VI,* part III, 1926.
6. "The laboratory method in psychoanalysis": *American Journal of Psychiatry, V*(3), January 1926; "Psychiatry as an objective science": *British Journal of Medical Psychology, V,* part IV, 1925; "The need of an analytic psychiatry": *The American Journal of Psychiatry, VI*(3), January 1927.
7. "An ethnic aspect of consciousness": *The Sociological Review, XIX*(1), January 1927.
8. *The Social Basis of Consciousness: A Study in Organic Psychology* (Burrow, 1927a). International Library of Psychology. New York: Harcourt, Brace. London: Kegan Paul.
9. Led by this prevailing misapprehension, certain of my colleagues, adopting what they have supposed to be the group method of analysis, have assumed the role of analyst to a group of people!

PART III

GROUP ANALYTIC ESSAYS

Editors' note

During approximately the same period, that is, from 1924 to 1930, Burrow, with his co-workers, gradually developed the foundations of the theoretical–methodological structure of group analysis, the ascribing of which to Foulkes is clearly historically ungrounded, given the evidence in this third part of the essays.

Owing to the frequent confusion and misinterpretations about Burrow's work, we wish to emphasise that our selection criterion was to privilege those papers belonging to the first period, where it is possible to follow the origin and evolution of group analysis, and its key concepts of social images, social unconscious, social neurosis, transgenerational and transpersonal processes, along with the relativity of observation, the group analytic technique, and its specific therapeutic factors.

CHAPTER TWELVE

The laboratory method in psychoanalysis, its inception and development*

With the new basis of thought and procedure that emanated from the evolutionists, there was introduced into scientific method a new instrument for the determining of scientific processes. This instrument is the scientific laboratory. The distinction of the scientific laboratory is its precision of judgement with respect to the data under investigation. In order to understand the meaning of the laboratory as applied to our own subjective processes, we shall be helped if we will first demand of ourselves that we understand more clearly what is the meaning of the laboratory as applied to its commonly accepted objective materials—if we will ask ourselves just what the mind requires of itself and determine definitely what are its criteria in entering upon the method of the laboratory. Until we recognise the processes of mind that determine the function of this instrument of precision we shall not be able to adhere to the uncompromising criteria that everywhere characterise the discipline of laboratory procedure.

---

* Paper read before the Ninth Congress of the International Psycho-Analytical Association, Bad Homburg, Germany, 1925.

Paper to appear in its German version in the *Internationale Zeitschrift für Psychoanalyse*.

First published in *American Journal of Psychiatry*, *V*(3), January, 1926.

The laboratory presumes a basis of observation that rests upon a principle that is phyletic and inherent. In the absence of this phylogenetic basis there is no biological observation because there is lacking the underlying principle of all laboratory procedure. Through this principle, the laboratory establishes a method of comparison whereby the particular element of the species is seen in relation to its phyletic substrate. The study of comparative anatomy demonstrates that the elements of a species represent a phyletic continuum that forms a common basis for comparison throughout the elements of the species in question. Blood platelets are scientifically recognisable as blood platelets because of their structural identity or generic consistency. Likewise, the pathology of a structure or tissue is recognized as a deflection from the norm because of its divergence from recognised healthy elements. But, owing to habitual inadvertences of outlook traceable to man's personal inhibitions, there has not as yet been recognised within the mental or functional sphere the primary continuum that constitutes the substrate of individual life and that makes possible the recognition of pathological divergences. It has not been recognised that, under the conditions of our complex society, these divergences exist throughout the species as a whole.

Within the subjective sphere—the sphere of man's own inherent thought and function—Sigmund Freud was first to employ a laboratory technique through the application to consciousness of dynamic biological principles. The introduction of this dynamic factor marked the beginning of the scientific method within the unconscious sphere of our human behaviour. Thus, it was in the hands of Freud that the scientific instrument afforded by the method of the laboratory came to be utilised within the sphere of man's mental processes. But this innovation of Freud's within the subjective sphere, paralleling, as it does, principles long recognised by science in the objective sphere, has been socially opposed by obstinate inhibition on the part of the human organisms whose habitual prejudices, social as well personal, were necessarily affronted by this laboratory scrutiny. These inhibitions, contrary to our common interpretation, are by no means confined to those outside our psychoanalytic ranks. They are also operative among those comprising our own number.[1] Indeed, it is precisely within ourselves as psychoanalysts that the real impediment lies. And it is this impediment that has automatically diverted us from the original laboratory intention of Freud.

It is my position that because of this resistance intrinsic to ourselves, the indispensable instrument of science, namely the laboratory of scientific research, has yet to come into its rightful place among us. In order to arrive at a phylogenetic substrate within the mental sphere, we need to observe the unconscious from a social basis of technique that is analogous to the individual basis of technique originally applied by Freud to the individual neurosis. For, if we will observe the unconscious from a social basis, we shall find, I think, that there is the need for a laboratory study of consciousness in its social mechanisms that correspond to the study of consciousness in its individual mechanisms. We shall find that there is the possibility of a laboratory approach to distortions of consciousness existing socially that is identical with our approach to the mental distortions which, through Freud, we first learnt to recognise in the unconscious processes of the individual patient.

Through the development of Freud's thesis introduced into science the possibility of a laboratory method with respect to man's mental processes, psychoanalysis continued to be consistent with its medical tradition of the clinic. Having had its inception in the clinical approach, it was inevitable that psychoanalysis should adhere more and more to the therapeutic method of the clinic and depart to the same degree from method pertaining to the technique of the laboratory. As a result of this unperceived circumstance, the tendency has been for psychoanalysis to wander so far from its original basis of research as now to require very exacting processes of reconstruction if we are to restore it to the scientific postulates that originally underlay Freud's basic discovery. Sensing the need for a more encompassing procedure, my students and I began to centre our interest upon methods that would ensure a greater precision of a laboratory technique. With my associates, I came to realise the necessity of applying under conditions of actual laboratory or group analysis the methods which Freud had developed in the treatment of individuals. The outcome of our work has been the gradual recognition of the necessity to base the processes of our observation upon methods involving a social or consensual technique that is as definite of that of the laboratories of objective biology.[1] For, as the objective criteria of the laboratory reside in a consistent continuum or phyletic substrate comprising the species, so its subjective criteria are equally indispensable and reside equally in a subjective continuum that unites the subjective processes of the several observers. Consensual data are only recognisable through a consensual basis of sense impressions. Thus, it is becoming more and more evident that, in the absence of a social recognition of the need among us of this social instrument of precision, we are, as psychoanalysts, unconsciously lending our support to social dissociations that are as definitely unconsciously substitutions as the symbol substitutions which we have come to study clinically in the underlying displacements within the unconscious of the individual.

In a paper read before the American Psychoanalytic Association in 1917,[2] I attempted to establish a principle representing, in what I spoke of at that time as the "nest instinct" or the "preconscious", the primary subjective phase of man's mental life. This principle was posited with a view to the recognition of a biological phyletic continuum in relation to which might be compared not only individual correspondences but also their divergences in pathological reactions.

In its original position, this early principle of primary identification had significance merely as an accidental, isolated laboratory finding, and was limited in its application to the individual neurosis. As an isolated phenomenon it was, in its ontogenetic significance, necessarily applicable alone to an ontogenetic or individual basis of analysis. But, because of the evident approximation of this principle to that which is fundamentally organismic or phyletic, it quite inevitably led to wider phylogenetic bases of inference. It is interesting that, in ontogenetic bearing, this principle of primary identification has been fully substantiated analytically not only by my own studies of dementia praecox and adjacent disorders, but also by studies made by Dr L. Pierce Clark in the psychology of essential epilepsy and kindred manifestations.[3] Basing his observations on the principle of primary identification, Dr Clark has also definitely traced to this source the equally organic reactions embodied in the psychoneural regressions of the epileptic. But, as I have said, while the divergence represented in the individual neurosis is traceable to this principle of primary identification as the original substrate of mind, its application is adequate only to the individual analysis. But man is not an individual. His mentation is not individualistic. He is part of a societal continuum that is the outgrowth of a primary or racial continuum. As the individual finds his basis in an individual continuum with an ontogenetic matrix or maternal source, so the social organism has its basis in a continuum with a phylogenetic matrix that is societal or racial. It is my thesis that this racial continuum is the phylogenetic basis of man's societal life precisely as the individual's early continuity with the maternal organism—his primary identification with the mother—is the ontogenetic basis for his subsequent development as an individual. In brief, just as we may trace the mental life of the individual to a physiological source corresponding to this primary identification, so within our societal life we may trace man's common source to a principle of primary identification that is racial.

In recent years, the attempt has been made on the part of myself and a few students to establish a means for the practical recognition among us as individual organisms of this common substrate of feeling and reaction first posited theoretically under the symbol of the preconscious. Regarding this preconscious principle as the phyletic basis of individual mentation, it has been our practical endeavour to relate individual manifestations to this common racial principle shared among us and to study the pathological divergences of our various feeling reactions in the light of this common feeling continuum. The result has been the establishment of a practical laboratory of psychoanalysis in which a consensual agreement concerning the subjective material has rendered possible an exact observation of individual deflections precisely as the laboratory of structural biology has made possible the scientific observation of structural divergences from a commonly accepted phyletic norm. Under this laboratory discipline, reactions which, in accordance with the personal technique of psychoanalysis, are studied in private confidence from a necessarily private basis of observation, have come to be observed commonly among a consensus of individuals recognising and sharing among themselves a common basis of comparison. In this laboratory approach, the method of psychoanalysis no longer confines itself to the study and treatment of an isolated individual by another individual who, through his private function as an analyst, is no less isolated. But the social repressions common to the social consciousness or to groups of individuals, presumably united within the confederacy known as normality, come equally under the challenge of a scientific laboratory analysis.

As we have said, the criteria of the objective laboratory of biology reside in a structural basis among the organic elements that is phyletic and continuous. Concomitantly, the criteria of the subjective laboratory of biology reside in a condition of continuity that equally unites the processes of the individuals or elements comprising the several observers. But, in the subjective field, the individuals who observe are the object observed as well as the subjects observing, and just as the basis of observation in the objective laboratory resides in a homogeneity of objective sense impressions among the observers, so, in the subjective sphere, the test of accurate observation depends no less upon a homogeneous basis or continuity of the subjective sense impressions among the several observers. In this interpretation, the method of the laboratory becomes the method of consensual observation no less in the subjective than in the objective sphere. For this consensus of observation establishes the conditions for dependable scientific judgement in that it precludes the element of personal bias with respect to the data observed. In all subjective experiment, therefore, the requisite condition for its proper conduct is the elimination of this personal equation and its necessarily deterring influence upon processes that determine the observation.

By virtue of the inclusive basis afforded by this consensual laboratory approach, psychoanalysis might come to occupy the same broad relation to mental disorder that medicine elsewhere represents with respect to disorders within the structural sphere. It has been the merit of the laboratory study of tuberculosis or typhoid fever that these abnormal processes have now come to be envisaged in their social or collective implications. These disorders were formerly quite isolated personal conditions, calling only for isolated and personal treatment on the part of the individual physician. But, by virtue of the evolutionary and phyletic basis provided by the structuralists, with their instrument in the laboratories of histology and bacteriology, these disorders are now studied in their social significance and receive the recognition that makes possible their study and treatment from a social as well as from an individual basis of outlook.

The time has come when the laboratory method initiated by Freud through the principle he applied to the study of the individual neurosis must extend itself to the larger application envisaged by a laboratory study of the neuroses in their wider social implications. The neurotic is no more an isolated phenomenon than the tubercular. In both, the ontogenetic nature of their disorders has its counterpart in a phyletic substrate that is societal. Accordingly, the process of their therapeutic adjustment cannot be met upon a basis that is restricted to an ontogenetic source but must extend itself equally to a source that is societal and phyletic. With the recognition of the socially continuum or communicative nature of infectious diseases, there was made possible an inclusive laboratory study of the common source of these disorders and the tracing of this source to the common continuum of tissue represented in the healthy phylum. Correspondingly, with the recognition of the socially continuous or communicative nature of neurotic diseases and the tracing of their common origins through proper laboratory enquiry, there is made possible the recognition of the common source of these disorders within the sphere of consciousness.

Thus, after twelve years devoted to psychoanalytic work based upon the method of the personal analysis, it became apparent to me that the personal basis of the individual analyst is necessarily but the social counterpart of the presumably isolated reaction of the individual before him. I began to realise that no theory of the common or phyletic nature of neurotic processes could offset the quite contradictory ontogenetic basis of actual procedure whereby my patient became closeted with me, as it were, in our confidential contemplation of his private inadvertences. It became apparent that the ontogenetic basis upon which the personal analysis inevitably rests necessarily excludes the consensus of judgement that is coterminous with the phylogenetic principle of consciousness. In the absence of this consensual basis requisite to laboratory precision of judgement, the factor of the personal equation of the analyst necessarily operates unconsciously to inhibit more or less the direct and unprejudiced estimate of the data submitted.

It is this element of the personal equation which only a group or inclusive analysis is competent to challenge. Under its discipline, we shall find that, within the restrictions of the private analysis, this element of the personal equation unconsciously influences the personal judgement of the individual analyst. It is my position that because of this factor of the personal equation on the part of the analyst, the repression and the personal secrecy that characterise the patient's neurosis can never be completely eliminated as long as we confine ourselves only to the personal process embodying the confidential rapport between patient and analyst. From a more inclusive societal approach, such a type of rapport, with its necessarily individualistic limitation, may be recognised as an added factor in the repression and secrecy already dominating the unconscious of the individual patient.

In short, it is too often the snare of the private analysis, as it is too often the snare of marriage, under our present social system, that it unconsciously substitutes for the isolated neurosis of the individual a socially reciprocal relationship that is no less secret and repressed in its exclusiveness. This disclosure exposes a condition that is the embodiment of a social neurosis shared unconsciously by physician and patient, the mechanism of which consists in an unconscious pooling in a mutual situation of what had been the individually closed psychic compartment of each. It was the recognition of this mutual element of the personal equation that led to the gradual opening among my associates and myself of this secret and unconscious social situation.

The very natural culmination of such reflections as these was the quite spontaneous development of practical measures that led gradually to the establishment of a social or group method of analysis on the basis of a consensual laboratory technique. It might be of interest to mention briefly something of the actual situation that first led to our group basis of analysis. One of my patients, a student of unusual analytic insight and training, sensing the incongruity in the situation, challenged the discrepancy between my theoretical statements regarding our socially common basis of consciousness and the individualistic position which, as an analyst, I arbitrarily continued to maintain. I was straightaway caught up by his protest against the inconsistency of these conflicting positions and by the interest this recalcitrant attitude seemed to me to offer experimentally, though unconsciously I was still sceptical of its practical value. And so I reluctantly agreed to an arrangement whereby the student should become the analyst and I the analysand, it being presumed that the social basis I advocated only in theory would be adopted actually and without prejudice by him. The arduous months of this experiment served only to prove that the patient's opposition to the inconsistency of my personal method was actuated by an equally personal and inconsistent method on his part and that the theory of a social approach to individual consciousness was, from the unbiased point of view of the laboratory, no more actual in his case than in my own. This finding led to a further extension of my experiment, which consisted in the gradual development of a technique involving groups of individuals, first smaller groups and finally larger, the smaller groups consisting of as few as four, the larger of as many as twenty individuals. In such groups, there was abrogated entirely the distinction between analyst and analysand, each individual automatically becoming both. There was here presented a social continuum of affects, and the need was a common recognition of their social basis in our common societal phylum. The gradual result of our group enquiry was the reluctant exposure of social repressions that are as definite as the presumably personal repressions that have hitherto occupied us as individual analysts. This became the more apparent in the circumstance that individuals who have undergone an individual analysis because of their personal resistances and who represent presumably analysed personalities, are, when subjected to the more inclusive enquiry of a group analysis, still the victims of repressions having their seat in the collective repressions of our social life.

Perhaps the work of our group can best be described as the development of a social technique in the handling of problems which, being personal or ontogenetic, are equally social or phylogenetic. From the basis of a common societal accord, we have tried to secure conditions which permit an objective evaluation of the unconscious elements socially represented by each of us in his single isolation. The situation was, from the first, difficult even to envisage. The reason is, as I see it, that the individual, with all his personal subordination to the social system about him, is at the same time an integral and necessarily contributory part of this same unconscious social organism. At one and the same time, the individual is both victim and aggressor. He is at once both the aggrieved and the offender. And the effort on the part of our group to reunite these two artificially separated trends represented for many months an almost insurmountable difficulty in our work. In spite of its difficulties, the outcome of our group work has been the development of an analytic technique that grants to the individual a perspective upon these inhibiting social conditions and materially enlarges his outlook as well as his possibilities of function as an element in man's homogeneous social organism. We have been able to demonstrate that there exists a definite and as yet unrecognised confederacy of self protection and resistance throughout the social system that is as definite as those of the individual, and it has been shown that in this social consolidation of repression, we are all equally unconscious constituents. But it has become clear that, in spite of this mass fixity and its stolid resistance to self-enquiry, these processes are as susceptible to definite analysis and resolution as the equally stolid resistances we have learnt to recognise through our analysis of the reactions of the individual patient.

It is the authority of the laboratory that its basis is evolutionary and phyletic. In a broad phyletic encompassment, it may be said that through the application of the principles of biology to the objective or structural sphere, as demonstrated in the laboratory, science and evolution have become synonymous. It may be as truly said that within the subjective field of enquiry, the authority of all scientific investigation resides alone in the laboratory. Submitting to this authority, my associates and I have been forced to accept a phyletic basis as the structural continuum of consciousness in which individual men represent organically identical elements. Accordingly, our group work has endeavoured to envisage the artificial differentiations and dissociations comprising the neurosis from a principle which, being ontogenetic, is, of necessity, phylogenetic also. For it is obvious that in our complex society these artificial differentiations and dissociations have ruthlessly separated and distorted not only the single individual within himself, but the integral organism uniting all the individuals in their common societal consciousness.

I well recognise that this position frankly questions the completeness of our present psychoanalytic basis, that is, the frank acceptance of the fact that psychoanalysis has reached a definite impasse. I feel we might face the circumstance that psychoanalysis has been concentrating its efforts on improving methods of applying its principles rather than on the developments of the principles themselves. The approach presented in this paper, which recognises the individual not as an individual, but as part of a common societal organism, has, by actual experimental test, provided an instrument for the wider development of our essential psychoanalytic aims. The work of our group is not a theory of social values or a prescription for the betterment of social institutions. It is the definite analysis of social values and social institutions as they exist. This consensual approach is not a theory any more than the private approach to the neurotic individual is a theory. It is an investigation, and what we are insisting upon with respect to social groups is this recourse to investigation, not a theory of what social groups should be or might become. We can only reply to our critics as Professor Freud has, from the beginning, time and again replied to his critics. Said Freud, in effect, "Do not argue with me as to the nature of my findings but go directly to the source to which I have had recourse and where you may establish your own findings". For it was Freud's position that there exists something in human life that is definitely in need of investigation. This statement that Freud has applied over and over again to the individual needs now to be applied as insistently to the mass expressions of consciousness represented among these same individuals in their collective social life.

Notes

1. "Psychoanalytic improvisations and the personal equation": paper read at the Fifteenth Annual Meeting of the American Psychoanalytic Association, Richmond, VA, 12 May 1925.
1. "Psychiatry as an objective science": paper read at the Fifteenth Annual Meeting of the American Psychopathological Association, Washington, DC, 7 May 1925.
2. "The preconscious or the nest instinct": paper read at the Seventh Annual Meeting of the American Psychoanalytic Association, Boston, MA, 25 May 1917. This paper forms the nucleus of material that is being gathered into a book subsequently to be published. Preliminary reference to this principle was made in the "Genesis and meaning of homosexuality", a paper read at the Fourth Annual Meeting of the American Psychoanalytic Association, Albany, New York, 5 May 1914. Published in *The Psychoanalytic Review*, *4*(3), July, 1917.
3. Clark, L. Pierce, "A psychologic study of Abraham Lincoln", *Psychoanalytic Review*, *VIII*(1), January, 1921; "The narcism of Alexander the Great", *The Psychoanalytic Review*, *X*(1), January, 1923; "Some psychological data regarding the interpretation of essential epilepsy", *The Journal of Nervous and Mental Disease*, *61*(1), January, 1925.

CHAPTER THIRTEEN

Our mass neurosis*

Psychiatrists and psychoanalysts have as yet confronted but the half of their real problem. In confining their study to the individual's unconscious, they have entirely neglected the mass or social unconscious of which the individual is a part. This conclusion is not based upon abstract theory, but is the outcome of definite experiment in the study of social reactions through the analysis of individuals in groups.[1] Supplementing the analysis of the individual's complexes and repressions with sessions devoted to the collective analysis of the social mind, the view is experimentally warranted that nervous disorder and insanity are not restricted alone to the isolated individual, but that the actual presence of demonstrable disordered mental states exists unrecognised within the social organisations that form our present day civilisation.[2]

It is futile to attempt to remedy mental disease occurring within the individual mind as long as psychiatry remains blind to the existence of mental disease within the social mind. The invariable factor that characterises mental disturbance in the particular patient is the

* First published in *The Psychological Bulletin*, 23(6), June 1926.

presence of division or conflict within the personality. Experiments in the analysis of the social mind, as collectively represented in group assemblage, make clear the presence of this same inner discord and conflict within the mind of society as a whole. It is the paradox of mental disorder in our patients that repression and concealment are its telltale. Likewise, the examination of the expressions of the social personality indicates that concealment and repression are no less the secret witness of its disordered condition.

In dealing with the phenomena of the physical world, the relativists have introduced a wholly altered basis for conceiving of these phenomena. The static Newtonian system is found no longer tenable in the altered conception of Einstein. The aspect of the theory of relativity, however, that is perhaps of central significance, is its surrender of a position of unquestionable fixity or absolutism and its replacement by a system that posits relative values in respect to time and space.

There is, I believe, the necessity for a similar adjustment of our present evaluations in the sphere of consciousness. Like the Newtonian basis, the system that at present comprises the sphere of our human reactions is too circumscribed and static, it limits our observation of intrinsic data, and confines man's outlook to standards of measure that are arbitrary and imperial. As this rigidity, this autocracy of outlook, regarded in the larger survey, is the basis of our present system of consciousness, I should like in this study to make clear, if I can, just what I understand to be this unconscious absolute as compared with the more inclusive outlook of a relative basis of consciousness.[3]

It is the invariable condition of our present basis of mental exchange that every criterion of judgement within the affective sphere is dependent upon the personal predilection of the individual who judges. Within this systematisation of preferences that forms the background of experience, the judgement of the individual is not, as we suppose, the natural expression of a spontaneous idea, but it is the reflection of the social systematisation about him that he has unconsciously come to embody. Thus, the individual is not sponsor of the idea for which he is spokesman, but, rather, he is unconsciously sponsored by it. Instead of actuating his ideas, he is actuated by them. And not only the individual, but the collective personality is rendered equally servile to such unconscious systematisations.

Within this systematised consensus, every man's own judgement, however unwarranted, is rock-ribbed and unquestioned. Upon his personal basis of evaluation, his personal opinion is beyond challenge. John Smith may claim that he is the Emperor Napoleon, and there is no argument that can successfully assail his position. Within his own mental system, his judgement is entirely consistent and valid. His opinion is his criterion and his criterion is indisputable. Upon a social basis of analysis, however, it may likewise be shown that any individual living within our present social system of evaluations entertains a position that is no whit different from that of John Smith. Each of us maintains opinions merely by virtue of the assumed criterion of his own personal judgement. But such an absolute criterion of judgement necessarily presupposes an opposite term to which it stands contrasted. For every criterion is a standard of comparison, and a comparison necessarily presupposes a dual or contrasting basis of judgement.

I do not think we realise to what extent we are unconsciously driven by this vicarious alternation between two terms, both of which are mere projections of an arbitrary dualistic standard. This unconscious dualism is extremely significant. John Smith claims that he is the Emperor Napoleon in compensation for a secret sense of inferiority that places him at the extreme opposite pole to the conceptual standard represented by the Emperor Napoleon. But, in the light of an inclusive analysis, an analysis that takes account of the reactions of groups of individuals, it may be shown that this obsessive element of the comparative dominates our entire mental outlook. One finds that just as every individual is, upon an absolute or comparative basis, inevitably at odds with himself in his personal evaluations, so, upon an absolute or comparative basis, he is inevitably at odds with others in his social evaluations. This circumstance is one of such subtlety, however, that it is well-nigh impossible to realise its import. We have learnt from Einstein that a mathematical frame of reference that is fixed and unalterable is no longer valid from the viewpoint of relativity. Likewise, in the mental sphere, when the individual judges from a frame of reference that is comparative or fixed, he necessarily judges fixedly.[4] For, in the nature of a basis of comparison, the individual becomes, himself, the central point of fixation—the absolute standard of measure by which all observable phenomena are evaluated and compared. When John Smith states that he is the Emperor Napoleon, he entertains the secret alternative that other people *are not* the Emperor Napoleon. From his systematised basis of evaluation as fixed observer, he arbitrarily estimates as fixed the position of others as well as of himself. He does not realise that from a position of fixation he necessarily makes fixation a basic condition of the mental universe about him. He does not realise that when he judges from a position of fixed alternatives, he is but reflecting the position of fixed alternatives which first placed him as a child in the position of inferiority to his Napoleonic father.

This nip-and-tuck element expressed in the ambivalent processes underlying the absolutism of the individual neurotic are the familiar earmarks of his divided outlook. But if we will look at the social organism, we shall find that a similar pro-and-con attitude, that a like ambivalence of motive, also underlies *its* manifold processes. Just as the dogmatic affirmations of the neurotic personality are lacking in organic authority and express themselves in a division or conflict within the individual personality, so the insistent affirmations within the social mind lack the corroboration of biological unity as shown correspondingly in the division and conflict of judgement that underlie the expressions of the social mind. For, upon a relative or inclusive basis of analysis, it becomes clear that an essential division, an inherent discord, underlies the social unconscious that is comparable to the discord underlying the unconscious of the individual. And it is of greater significance still that the judgement of the individual rests invariably upon acquired inferences derived from this absolute position based upon the equally fixated alternatives of the social mind.

Nothing is as characteristic of the social consciousness as this division or conflict that is its basis. Its presence confronts us at every turn. It is present in our concept of good and bad, success and failure, hope and despair, rich and poor, aristocrat and proletarian, Jew and Gentile, Catholic and Protestant, Freudian and anti-Freudian. Indeed, the list of antagonists is infinite. One of our newspapers presented a prize contest for the best definition of a Republican and a Democrat. An answer sent in was as follows: "A Republican is a person who thinks a Democratic administration is bad for business. A Democrat is a person who thinks a Republican administration is bad for business. Both are right". The answer won the prize.

We have seen that either component of the individual's criterion necessarily contains the other. Whoever tends to feel his own importance entertains an equal conviction of his own insignificance. A criterion of goodness necessarily entails an alternative of badness. Also, if we will examine the above social comparatives,[5] we shall discover the rather startling circumstance that likewise neither element in any one of these alternatives may exist in the absence of the other. For, due to our present absolute basis, the advocates of a system are necessarily the unconscious adversaries of that system. A man who is moral is just in so far immoral. Whoever is a Jew is also a Gentile. In the degree in which an individual is a Catholic, to that precise degree he is also a Protestant. Those who are Freudians are self-convicted anti-Freudians, though we have been thus far adroit enough to avoid our dilemma on the plea of resistances. This brings us to the circumstance that is of most vital interest to the present study: *the advocates of a system based upon the ambivalent contrast of conflicting alternatives are no more accessible to argument than is John Smith with respect to the system that is his own ambivalent self-estimate.*

Every Roman Catholic knows absolutely that he is right, and, absolutely, he is right, since his criterion is absolute. . . . The Protestant also knows, of course, that he is right, and, of course, on the basis of his absolute criterion, he is equally so. For it is the unconscious merit of the absolute basis that it automatically makes right whatever is comprised within that basis. A basis, however, that makes tenable two such mutually opposite and exclusive positions as those of Catholic and Protestant is a basis of irreconcilable conflict. It is such a conflict that is the penalty of an absolute system of values, both personal and social. It is such a system that is the meaning of our present basis of consciousness.

It is the essence, however, of the absolute system that it does not see beyond its own system. This is its fixity. This is the fiction of its authenticity. For a division that is due to a basis of absolutism preserves its division by virtue of that self-same absolutism. . . . But again, an inclusive analysis shows us that each is in the precise position of John Smith who, possessing royal prerogative, is, like his Napoleonic father, justly heir to the imperial throne to which he lays claim. . . .

Urged by the impetus we have received from Freud, it has become objectively a quite simple matter to view with analytic exactness the conflict that is the basis of the neurotic personality. But, as yet, we have been led unconsciously to assume socially the position of onlooker in judging the mental conflicts of the neurotic individual. We have been led to assume a position socially that is not less absolutistic and arbitrary than the position assumed individually by the neurotic personality. It seems to me that it is now time that we lay aside our fixed and absolute position of mere detached observers, and that from a relative and inclusive position, we come to view the larger neurosis of the social organism that equally involves ourselves as elements within it—that we come to study with scientific disinterestedness the division and conflict which we ourselves embody as participants in the social personality, in order that, through an understanding of our social neurosis, we may reach a position of consciousness that permits a wider and more inclusive encompassment of life.

Freud struck strong against the establishment and the establishment has struck back strong in return. Freud's was a violent reaction against a violent condition about him. But, thus far, both sides have merely been antagonistic one toward the other. As long as such retaliative processes and mere counter-reactions are permitted to hold sway, we are merely marking time. There is not the possibility of progress toward larger and more inclusive outlooks. The establishment, having taken its stand, has declared that it is here to stay. Freud, having taken his, has declared no less stoutly that he is here to stay. But no system is here to stay. It is the here-to-stay attitude of mind that is precisely the fallacy of the system as it is the obstinate unreasoningness of all establishment. As long as there persists the mutual antagonism of two equally immovable positions, there remain only the unproductive friction and impaction of mere animosity and competition. While such comparative standards prevail, we may only clothe ourselves about with the outward gestures and symbolisms that are the mere disguises for growth. Though each disputant claims on the authority of his personal system that he is right, his personal system renders him, upon analysis, as undependable as John Smith. As long as our criterion rests upon the dual standard of an unconscious absolutism, we are embroiled in the inaccessible conflict of the absolute alternative. Under such a system, wherever there are two opposed opinions, necessarily both are wrong. Once more it is to revert to the ambivalent and comparative. It is again the two-edged criterion of all absolute measure.

There is required not that the Catholic's position be imposed upon the Protestant, or that the viewpoint of the Protestant be imposed upon the Catholic; neither is it required that between them they agree to the adoption of a common mean. But it is necessary that, through an analysis of the complexes of both, we resolve the absolute fixation determining the alternations within each.

What is needed is not to shift the direction of the alternative, but to eradicate the tendency to alternation. Although a patient's secret criterion of self-supremacy may be challenged by us in its fixation upon home and mother, he promptly finds an equally satisfactory lodgement in the ministrations of the psychiatric institute, or in the consultation room of the psychoanalyst. Though we rout a patient out of a depression, he still retains his secret criterion, either through the alternative of a frank elation or by means of the ever-handy alternatives offered in the unconscious subways of the social consensus.

Our dilemma, however, exists under conditions of such subtlety that, as I have said, it is well-nigh impervious to analysis. Its subtlety lies in the self-involvement of the thought processes responsible for it. For the inadequacy of our present mental system of evaluations is its failure to include in its envisagement the basis upon which we evaluate. On the contrary, a basis of relativity possesses the distinctive significance that it includes its own process within its own envisagement.

From these considerations, I have come to feel that a basis of relativity is as essential to an inclusive understanding of our human reactions as it is requisite to a comprehension of the data pertaining to physics or astronomy. I feel that a relative viewpoint is as essential to a clear understanding of the subjective processes within us as of the objective processes that surround us.

In a relativistic and inclusive comprehension of consciousness, an absolute system of criteria, with its personal basis of evaluation and its irreconcilable dualism and conflict, will be no more possible within the social personality than it will be possible within the individual. Just as we may view the individual from a relativistic position, so we may view the organism comprising our own social processes from a relative and inclusive viewpoint. From indications following several years devoted to an intensive study of processes dependent upon group or social reactions,[6] it seems to me a not too extravagant prediction that the basis of computation that has lately been replaced within the physical universe because of its absolutism and non-inclusiveness will also require to be surrendered for an equally inclusive basis of evaluations within the sphere of our conscious processes.

Notes

1. "Die Gruppenmethode in der Psychoanalyse": paper to appear in a forthcoming issue of *Imago,* Vienna, Austria.
2. "The laboratory method in psychoanalysis": paper read before the Ninth Congress of the International Psycho-Analytical Association, Bad Homburg, Germany, September, 1925. *American Journal of Psychiatry, 5*(3), 1926.
3. "A relative concept of consciousness", *The Psychoanalytic Review, 12*(1), 1925.
4. "Einstein's first great discovery was that there are many such systems of reckoning-many possible frames of space and time-exactly on all fours with one another. No one of these can be distinguished as more fundamental than the rest; no one frame rather than another can be identified as the scaffolding used in the construction of the world. And yet one of them does present itself to us as being the actual space and time of our experience; and we recoil from the other equivalent frames which seem to us artificial systems in which distance and duration are mixed up in an extraordinary way. What is the cause of this invidious selection? It is not determined by anything distinctive in the frame; it is determined by something distinctive in us - by the fact that our existence is bound to a particular planet and our motion is the motion of that planet. *Nature* offers an infinite choice of frames; *we* select the one in which we and our petty terrestrial concerns take the most distinguished position. Our mischievous, geocentric outlook has cropped out again unsuspected, persuading us to insist on this terrestrial space-time frame which in the general scheme of nature is in no way superior to other frames." "The Theory of Relativity and Its Influence on Scientific Thought", *The Scientific Monthly,* 1923, 16. Arthur Stanley Eddington, F.R.S.
5. In the psychological use of the term "comparative", I mean to convey the state of mind that is as definitely one of moral contrast as the state of mind involved in the use of the grammatical comparative is one of conditioned or mental contrast. The mother who counsels her child to be "a good boy" is really telling him to be *better than* other boys, or to be *better than* he was at some previous time. In brief, a standard of "goodness" is necessarily a standard of "betterness".
6. "Social images versus reality": *Journal of Abnormal Psychology and Social Psychology, 19*(3), 1924; "Psychiatry as an objective science": *British Journal of Medical Psychology, 5,* Part 4.

CHAPTER FOURTEEN

The group method of analysis*[1]

A paper that sets out with a paradoxical title can hardly be expected to invite one's confidence unless we can somehow get square with this initial misnomer. An analysis presupposes, of course, the isolation and examination of a part or element representing the structure of a system, combination, or group of elements. But, biologically, a group represents a synthesis and only its parts are susceptible of analysis, so that a group method of analysis is, of its nature, self-contradictory. One could as consistently speak of a synthetic method of analysis as of a group method of analysis. And yet, there is, in fact, the group material to be confronted and there is, as I see it, only the analytic method of confronting it. And so, in attempting to reconcile processes that are so obviously opposed (the one group or synthetic, the other individual or analytic), there is clearly some consistent explanation called for. It is this explanation for which it is difficult for me to find words. If, however, as far as may be, you will participate with me in this endeavour, I think that we may together arrive at some common interpretation that will reconcile this

*First published in *The Psychoanalytic Review, XIV*(3), July 1927.

seeming contradiction—a contradiction that has for a long time, I confess, been too little clear in my own mind.

I think we do not realise to what extent we have come to employ the term *group* or combination in an entirely artificial and conventional sense. The landscape gardener arranges a group of trees, the historian a group of chronological events. The educator will form a group of students, the sociologist a group of welfare workers. There may be a group of scientists, or iron workers, or artists. But such grouping is entirely external and arbitrary. There is no organic inherency uniting the several elements composing such groups. Where elements are assembled in such manner, what is really represented is but a collection or placing together of elements. On the contrary, when we come to speak of such a group as is represented in a colony of ants, let us say, or a herd of deer, or a tribe of primitive men, we are at once connoting an assemblage of elements that is grouped into one integral whole by reason of an inner organic bond common to the several elements of which it is composed. It is this type of group that unites the elements of the species. In such organic groups, the connecting link among them is an essential and instinctive one. It is not one that is separable by any arbitrary or external process of arrangement.[2]

The life of man today, in the midst of his complex civilisation, embodies still the organic bonds of this instinctive racial unity. The essential biology of the race is not in the least altered from that of the days of man's early primitive societies. Organic principles do not vary under the variations of external circumstance. Racial instincts do not wear out with time. But something has interposed itself unconsciously within the group life of man. Unlike the groups or colonies occurring within the lower orders, man's societal life has been arbitrarily affected by this unconscious factor and he has not been allowed to group or colonise in response to the natural behest of primary instinctive bonds. On the contrary, man has gathered or disposed himself in various forms of groupings and affiliations—social, political, economic, national, religious—that have been wholly superficial and utterly alien to him from the point of view of his instinctive group life. And so it is necessary that the synthetic and instinctive group life of primitive tribal man be very clearly distinguished from the collective or pseudo-group formations into which man has entered at the dictates of social and conventional tradition or authority.

Naturally, in a group that embodies but an arbitrary collection of individuals, the part or element within such an assemblage may, without jeopardy to organic instinct, be readily drawn aside and subjected to a process of isolation and examination—the process we know as analysis. Isolating the individual or part of such a conventional association of elements entails no organic breach—no more than would the disturbance of the landscapist's arrangement of trees or the school principal's distribution of pupils. But tearing the leaves or petals from their stalk in order to analyse them is a process that necessarily severs the part under examination from functional continuity with the organic whole of which it is a part. The continuity of the organism as a whole is instantly destroyed. So with the ants removed from their colony or the deer withdrawn from their herd. But, after all, the operation of this organic group law within the life of gregarious animals is not an observation restricted by any means to the biological expert. It is a circumstance of practical utility among all intelligent keepers of wild animals. Hagenbeck was not less familiar than Darwin or Kropotkin[3] with the significance of this organic principle uniting the individuals of a species. But, while we all tacitly admit that there is this tribal or racial instinct extending throughout and binding together the elements or individuals of a species, we have yet to recognise it within ourselves as *an organic principle of consciousness*. We have yet to see that this societal principal, observable in the spontaneous clusters of primitive man, exerts its instinctive and biological sway equally today within the life of civilised communities.

From these considerations, I have come to an altered outlook in my analytic work. I have come to the position that, with respect to the organism of man, an analysis, which presupposes the isolation and private examination of the individual elements apart from their instinctive racial congeners, leaves out of account the larger societal organism of which the individuals are a part and without which it is not possible for them to survive in their coherent unitary life. Such an isolated process of analysis, when applied to the individual of the species man, destroys the organic integrity of the organism as a group or race as truly as we destroy the integrity of the organism composing the flower when we isolate its petal or leaf in order to examine it apart from its structural continuity with the whole. The organic principle uniting the group or societal aggregate represents functional solidarity; the isolated element represents its disruption, so that the analysis of the individual element is contradictory to the preservation of the whole. In other words, the continuity of the group and the isolation of the individual are processes that are, of their nature, exclusive of one another.

In order to offset this inexorable breach as it operates within the system represented by our own psychoanalytic method, with its inevitable isolation of the single individual, the group of students with whom I have been working in association in the past years have undertaken, through a long and exacting experimental method, a process of analysis that takes account of reactions as they pertain to the species as a whole. This comprehensive scheme of analysis has the merit of leaving intact the material of our societal and instinctive group life, while at the same time it proceeds from this group background to examine analytically the social as well as the personal substitutions and repressions embodied in the arbitrary collective sum or pseudo-group represented in this selfsame societal organism.

In order to accept with scientific sympathy the analytic basis of this group technique, it is necessary that, as analysts, we forego, at least tentatively, certain personal and pseudo-group convictions, convictions that rest upon the artificial covenants of single individuals in their merely collective expressions rather than upon the organic bonds of their essential group biology. We need to rid ourselves of the idea that the neurotic individual is sick and that we psychopathologists are well. We need to accept a more liberal societal viewpoint that permits us to recognise without protest that the individual neurotic is, in many respects, no more sick than we ourselves. For we quite lose count of the circumstance that the neurotic, in his private substitutions and distortions, has merely failed to ingratiate himself in the collective confederacy of substitutions and distortions which you and I, with no less an eye to our self-protection, have had the cunning to subscribe to under the cover of our arbitrary, pseudo-group symptomatology. It begins to be clearer to me that only in this inclusive outlook shall we be prepared to take account of factors which otherwise are quite closed to us as social individuals thinking only of our social self-protection.

If we will make a disinterested survey of our psychoanalytic work upon its present personalistic and confidential basis of technique, a technique that concerns itself solely with the isolated element or individual, I think it must become evident that, from the point of view of science, our attitude is quite sadly in arrears. The esoteric practice of closeting a patient in our private consultation room in order to hear a story of ineptitudes and maladjustments that are due to social interpositions and substitutions common to the race and, therefore, identical with one's own, has, I think, nowhere its counterpart in any sphere of scientific procedure. We make no secret of the various physical anomalies to which man is subject. Cardiac and digestive disorders are willingly submitted to medical investigation. Likewise, diseases due to the abuse of our organisms, such as overeating, excess of alcohol, or even venereal disease, we accept quite openly in the clinic or laboratory. The reason is not far to seek. The individual no longer holds himself morally responsible for such conditions. Today, he no longer regards them as providential visitations. He does not think of them as in any sense reflecting upon his personal integrity. And yet, the no less organic distortions represented in our emotional and sexual inadvertences and pathologies we treat in a wholly moral and semi-religious manner, and, in compliance with the attitude of mind we now hold toward these conditions, we invite patients to meet us in secret conferences that are out of all relation to their medical and scientific significance.

Were we observing data presented in the chemical or biological laboratory, surely none of us would think of attempting to observe such processes in any other than in a consensual scientific attitude of approach.[4] Consensual observation is synonymous with scientific precision of technique. The noting of immediate data under conditions of observation that establish a correspondence of sense perceptions among the several observers is the acknowledged prerequisite of the laboratory criterion. And so, I think, we must come to see that it is only our unconscious social resistances that have all this while kept us psychoanalysts from adhering to the same basis of scientific procedure that has been the acknowledged criterion in every other sphere of scientific investigation. I think we must bring a social analysis to our own social resistances and gradually recognise that in the sphere of our mental observations we have adhered to an esoteric and imprecise basis of determination which we would not for a moment have employed regarding data pertaining to any other field of observation.[5]

In the laboratory or group work of my associates and myself, such factors as sexual fantasies, the unseemliness of family conflicts, the incongruities and deceptions that mark many of our social or pseudo-group contacts become the materials of our laboratory observation.

These ineptitudes, to which not only the moralist or preacher, but also the layman, generally holds himself, at least by implication, superior and which the psychoanalyst concedes mention of only behind closed doors, are openly presented and observed by us in sessions composed, at times, of as many as twenty people. After all, the point that we psychoanalysts have missed, because unconsciously we like to miss it, is not at all that an individual is a victim of sexual conflicts, but that *all individuals under our present social system of repression are equally the victims of equal sexual conflicts.* The reason that the nervous patient wishes to make so deep a secret of the inadvertences of his sex life is not at all because these matters are really private to him, but because society says to him "do not dare to presume that these matters are *not* private to you." And we psychoanalysts have unconsciously fallen in with the prevalent attitude of the social system that blindly bullies the so-called neurotic into inviolable self-concealment and isolation. And so, we invite in him this absurdly timorous and isolated attitude toward the social system because our own social attitude is equally timorous and isolated.

I have stated what seems to me the inadequate basis of the private method of analysis. In various writings, I have made as clear as I can the altered position to which I have been brought through the researches of my students and myself during recent years. It might seem to some that I have not placed sufficient emphasis upon the results of our work in the usual sense of an objective tabulation. But results in the subjective field cannot possibly have more than a theoretical meaning to those who, through circumstances, have felt obliged to leave entirely to others the task of securing these results. It is experimentally demonstrable that people who show most theoretical interest in the social processes which others have taken the pains to collaborate in understanding are precisely those who stand in greatest need of participating in the same group study of their own social processes. Therefore, I would remind the reader that the spirit of the mere onlooker at processes common to all of us as social beings is very far removed from that of the direct investigator of those processes as they may be witnessed within oneself, and that "results" must, of necessity, have a very different connotation according within or without. There have been results, very definite results, but the results people have in mind, who merely want to look at them, are results which imply something objectively pat and conclusive, like an experiment in chemistry, for instance, with its postulate and conclusion expressed in set terms of mathematical exactness. But the course and development of man's life is a process. It is a condition of continuous flow, of uninterrupted movement. It is not a static, fixed condition, so that, in the sense of a neat pharmaceutical remedy, obtainable upon application, one cannot speak of results as they pertain to the instinctive and evolutionary processes of man's growth.

The reader will readily understand, though, how much more thorough and effective is the result of an analysis that stirs to the bottom not only a patient's individual situation, but also whatever pseudo-group situation a patient finds himself a social participant in. This new process of analysis has the merit of uncovering complexes that are socially sustained under the covenant of the secret family cluster, as well as those occurring in the individual neurosis. Under these conditions, we have experienced again and again how much more readily the schizoid, for example, resting in his intrauterine lethargy, is roused from his dreaming inactions and learns to enter into the objective immediacy of the surrounding actualities; how much more radically the hysteric is ousted from his egocentric reveries and at length lends himself to the day's constructive demands; and, finally, with what greater despatch the cyclothymic surrenders his bi-dimensional mood alternatives in favour of an adaptation to life that represents a symmetrical, unitary effort. The result of this more encompassing programme, therefore, has assisted toward a rapid technique of restoration in our neurotic subjects and furthered the freeing not merely of individual, but also of mass reactions as a whole, whether represented in families or in other unconscious community clusters.

In summary, certain of the outstanding results among those of us who have been dealing at first hand with our own immediate reactions are as follows:

1. The disclosure socially of a universally unconscious social suggestion (the condition first recognised scientifically by Freud in its individual expression under the term "transference").
2. The phyletic dissolution of the bipolar fixation comprising the mother–child relationship such as underlies this social hypnosis or transference as represented in each individual.
3. The determination of the completely vicarious and socially unconscious reaction represented in the factor of "sublimation".

In addition, the following mechanisms have been observed and studied by us in their social setting:

1. The "vicious" alternative of the image fixation underlying the composite mother–child relationship as it exists within the personality of each individual, and the bipolar impasse of this image basis.
2. The social extension of this private image basis leading to the substitution unconsciously of social images for reality—"God", "love", "virtue", together with "marriage" and "family" regarded as "institutions". [6]
3. The social mechanism of projection as a universal manifestation and its gradual resolution into its ontogenetic source.[7]
4. The ambivalent irreconcilability of personal mood reactions within the "normal" as well as in the neurotic individual, and their compulsively alternating phases of good and bad, love and hate, praise and blame, as shown in the interreaction of these moods within the social milieu.[8]
5. The psychological identity of the pseudo-sexual images now commonly divided as "homo-" and "hetero-sexual", and the complete dissociation socially of both these components from man's societal or organic sex instinct.
6. The presence of distorted states existing in social clusters, such as paranoia, homosexuality, hysteria, and the like, but heretofore commonly regarded in clinical isolation as disease entities peculiar to the "neurotic" individual.[9]
7. The experimental evidence for *the principle of primary identification*[10] of the individual with the mother and the demonstration of a preconscious mode in its phylogenetic or societal significance that is comparable to this primary subjective phase of the infant psyche hitherto posited in regard to its ontogenetic basis.

The foregoing categories, I fully realise, cannot possibly be wholly clear to the reader in the absence of a laboratory background of experience in the study of subjective social reactions. Students of conditions that are the result of objective laboratory findings would not think of attempting to reckon with the processes leading to those findings in the absence of familiarity with the objective laboratory technique requisite to their understanding. But, because of the factor of social resistances involved in the study of subjective processes, those who have not as yet participated in the group study of these processes, notwithstanding their lack of training and experience, too commonly hold the subjective laboratory answerable for making a clear presentation of its findings. While the inadequacy of the preceding statements might be attributable in part to my own ineptness in formulating them, certainly the responsibility for the understanding of our methods and aims cannot rest wholly with me as long as the reader lacks familiarity with the processes and technique of the laboratory from which these results have sprung.

What the scientific enquirer is really interested to learn primarily, after all, are the advantages, if any, of the group method of analysis as compared with the restricted method that limits the analysis to conferences between the physician and his individual patient. First, it should be pointed out that the group method of analysis by no means excludes individual conferences between physician and patient. In point of fact, every patient's analysis begins with such personal interviews, and he is at liberty to return to them as his need demands. But it is of significance that such interviews do not rest upon the arbitrary and pseudo-group basis that presupposes only the neurosis of the patient while the physician stands as a mere onlooker in respect to it. The patient is at once expected to look at his own disorder as part of a neurosis shared very generally by a social community in which his physician is, along with him, also an integral part. From this organic group basis, composed thus of two persons, the patient later comes into conference with three or four individuals and gradually into the larger group conferences which might be composed of as many as eight to twelve. A significant aspect of these group sessions lies in the circumstance that the patient is, from the outset, observer as well as observed. He becomes at once a responsible student of our common human problems, personal and social. Besides, there is this further advantage in a patient's entering upon the group analysis. In his association with a group, whether as individuals or as a whole, quite apart from the analytic sessions, he becomes part of a societal plexus, as it were, along with people pursuing an interest common with his own. Still preserving these biological amalgamations inherent to his organism, he has the opportunity to form social relationships with more mature, more experienced students upon a basis that preserves throughout the day their mutually analytic aims. This means that the hysteric and paranoidal types have opportunities for social contact without being forced up against the vicarious accommodation of our socially galvanised pseudo-group adaptations. It means that the psychasthenic or precoid type of personality comes into group relationships which, while in no sense critical of his ingrowing habits of self-accommodation, do not permit him to regress into the privacy of his own introversion.

In the personal analysis, the consummation upon which the analysis depends from the outset is the transference. This must be brought about and preserved at all costs. *Keine Uebertragung, keine Psychoanalyse.* In our group procedure, this condition of a patient's dependence upon his physician is, from the outset, precluded. We know very well that the essence of the neurosis is the mother–child relationship, that this is the neurotic patient's unconscious impasse, that fixation is his unremitting quest. But, in the group, the mother–child relationship is from the very beginning submitted to consensual observation and study, and no surrogate for this relationship, such as obtains in the usual technique of analysis, is permitted to creep in unconsciously and defeat the real purpose of a psychoanalysis. I do not mean for a moment that there is not in each patient the tendency toward such a fixation or transference in the group situation. It is inconstantly present. But, under conditions of group association, naturally there is not the opportunity favourable to its secret lodgement and entertainment, as is the case in the private work involving months of solitary confinement with the individual analyst. What would be the individual transference in a private analysis becomes neutralised in the social participation of many individuals in their common analysis.

There is further inherent in the group method the opportunity for each student to see disinterestedly the elements composing his own neurosis as they are directly reflected to him in the neurosis of another. For, in a group analysis, the manifestations in another are repeatedly shown to be identical with one's own. This factor of our group method is of the greatest significance in its influence upon the central factor of resistance. I recall so well Freud's words at the Second International Psychoanalytic Congress in Nuremberg in the year 1911. It was in reference to a statement of Jung's. And I remember Freud's saying that the task of psychoanalysis lay not at all in the discovering of complexes, but in the dissolving of resistances. It is precisely here, it seems to me, that the group technique offers its most distinctive advantage. For the essence of resistance is undoubtedly one's sense of isolation in one's own conflicts. Where conditions allow the individual to recognise the common nature of his conflicts, naturally a sense of isolation is gradually resolved, and with it the resistances which are the backbone of his neurosis.

It must be remembered that our group work is still in its very beginning. There have been, in all, but four years of actual group analysis. The two years prior to that consisted simply of experimental variations upon the original analytic theme and in mere tentative adaptations of it. Naturally, with a method that is as young as ours and still in the process of its growth, other aspects are, from time to time, coming to light which yet remain to be tested in their fuller implication. But the outstanding interest of our work has been the realisation of what is man's commonly neglected societal or essential group basis and its challenge of our commonly accepted or pseudo-group amalgamations. From this essential group basis, the careful analytic study of the manifest content of our so-called social consciousness has revealed, and is daily revealing, latent elements in which there is no less contrast with our manifest social adaptations than that which Freud first discovered to be the contrast between the dream life of the individual patient and his actual or manifest adaptation as expressed in his daily life.

I do not wish to be understood as repudiating our conventional social forms of association. They undoubtedly have their place in the process of man's conscious evolution, precisely as our primitive societies had their place in the structural or organic sphere of our evolutionary scheme. I have in mind only to repudiate the substitutive factors whereby such external social groupings are made to replace the organic feelings and instincts that unite man as an integral colony, species, or race.

Persons who have become acquainted with our group method of analysis tend to think of it as an innovation in the psychoanalytic method. They seem to think that my thesis offers a departure from the original aims of Freud. I do not share their view. For this is to judge Freud upon wholly external and accidental grounds. It is to miss the internal significance of Freud's original direction of enquiry. In my interpretation, the group method of analysis is but the application in the phylogenetic sphere of the individual analysis as first applied by

Freud within the ontogenetic sphere.[11] In a just appraisement of the work of Freud, one must not fail to recognise the essentially laboratory spirit of procedure that was Freud's approach to the study of consciousness. From the very beginning, Freud attempted to replace personal prejudice with scientific observation. He observed what he saw in human consciousness not only as it exists in his patients, but also in himself, and he reported faithfully what he saw. This was the application to the field of consciousness of the same precision of laboratory technique that had hitherto characterised our scientific attitude of observation in respect to the biological sciences. In brief, Freud raised the study of consciousness to the sphere of the biological sciences. The result was an outrage to social sensibilities and the social mind, with all the weight of its traditional social unconscious, has opposed itself so compellingly to Freud's laboratory method that its extension to include the social organism was promptly intercepted.

Instead of receiving the support of a consensual group of co-workers, Freud was met by an unconscious resistance that was social and pertained to the collective, pseudo group reaction. He was alone in his position, and alone he was powerless to meet this reaction in its uncoordinated social form. This was inevitable. In the absence of a consensual societal group of co-workers, it was not possible for Freud's work to proceed to the inclusion of the generic social unconscious. Though it was inherent in the very nature of Freud's discovery that a consensual laboratory spirit of observation is alone competent to envisage the problems of consciousness, the social resistance with which Freud was confronted from the very beginning is still unrecognised and unresolved within our psychoanalytic ranks. It is the position of my associates and myself, working as a group, that the pseudo-group prejudices that are the unconscious basis of our social resistance will not be resolved until we have recognised that they are as definitely unconscious a manifestation on the part of the social mind as the individual resistances that are met in the individual analysis. The condition which our group investigations have led us to emphasise is that this resistance within the social mind can no more be resolved in the absence of a social analysis than in the absence of an analysis it is possible to resolve the private resistances of the individual patient.[12] In any other recourse, we become Freud's followers merely in the sense of collective, arbitrary, pseudo-group participants, and the spirit of the discoverer and of the laboratory becomes submerged under the mass weight of an imitative or competitive social unconscious. Far from being a departure from the essential significance of Freud's basic discoveries, the results that are now issuing from our group analysis are simply the results that, with Freud, were temporarily intercepted through an absence of a consensual collaboration on the part of his social congeners.

The sum of our findings resolves itself into this. The prevailing view that man is an individual is one that the psychopathologist needs to bring into serious question. Man is not an individual. He is a societal organism. Our individual analyses based upon differentiations, which, along with others of our kind, we have assumed to rest upon legitimate scientific ground, rest, in fact, upon very transient social artifices and lack the support of a true biological basis. Man's analysis as an element is his isolation as an element. And his isolation is an essential affront to an organic group principle of consciousness.

Notes

1. Paper read before the Washington Psychoanalytic Society, 14 November 1925. "Die Gruppenmethode in der Psychoanalyse", *Imago, XII* (1926), Heft 2/3. In the interval between the presentation of this paper in November, 1925, and its publication at the present time, investigations referred to in the text as being still in process have resulted in findings which call for certain modifications of the group method both in conception and in technique. With the group researches completed and the original laboratory organisation dissolved, the final description of the group basis remains to be written. It may be said, however, that the chief modification has been in the direction of greater emphasis upon the observation of *immediate material* with a proportionate disregard for reminiscent episodes.
2. "An ethnic aspect of consciousness": paper read at the mid-year meeting of The American Psychoanalytic Association, New York City, 28 December 1924.
3. P Kropotkin, *Mutual Aid*. Alfred A. Knopf, 1921.
4. "Psychiatry as an objective science": paper read at the Fifteenth Annual Meeting of The American Psychopathological Association, Washington, DC, 7 May 1925; *British Journal of Medical Psychology, V*, Part 4, 1925; "Psychoanalytic improvisations and the personal equation", read at the Fifteenth Annual Meeting of The American Psychoanalytic Association,

Richmond, VA, 12 May1925; *The Psychoanalytic Review*, *XIII*(2), April 1926.

5. "The need of an analytic psychiatry": paper read before the joint session of The American Psychiatric and The American Psychoanalytic Associations, New York City, 10 June 1926.
6. "Social images versus reality": paper read at the Fourteenth Annual Meeting of The American Psychopathological Association, Philadelphia, 7 June 1924; *The Journal of Abnormal Psychology and Social Psychology*, *XIX*(3), October–December 1924.
7. "The reabsorbed affect and its elimination": paper read at the Sixteenth Annual Meeting of The American Psychopathological Association, New York City, 11 June 1926.
8. "Our mass neurosis": paper read at the Fourteenth Annual Meeting of The American Psychoanalytic Association, Atlantic City, 3 June 1924; *The Psychological Bulletin*, *23*(6), June 1926.
9. "Insanity a social problem": *The American Journal of Sociology*, *XXXII*(1), Part I, July 1926.
10. "The genesis and meaning of homosexuality": paper read at the Fourth Annual Meeting of The American Psychoanalytic Association, Albany, New York, 5 May 1914; *The Psychoanalytic Review*, *IV*(3), July 1917.
11. "The laboratory method in psychoanalysis": paper read before the Ninth Congress of the International Psycho-Analytical Association, Bad Homburg, Germany, 1925; *American Journal of Psychiatry*, *V*(3), January 1926.
12. Just as no one has ever yet really understood the significance of the individual analysis except as he himself entered upon the individual analysis, so no one will by any process understand the group analysis except as he himself enters upon it. From the first, Freud emphasised the futility of knowledge *about* or *in regard to* psychoanalysis. Knowledge of psychoanalysis is not an intellectual process. Resistances, which are the barrier to an understanding of psychoanalysis, do not reside in the intellect. Only as one submits one's own feeling, personal or social, to the process of analysis does one truly come into an understanding of psychoanalysis in the only true sense of understanding—that is, into an internal acceptance of the significance of man's unconscious processes.

CHAPTER FIFTEEN

The basis of group analysis, or the analysis of the reactions of normal and neurotic individuals*[1]

Mental disorder is an industrial problem—a problem in how to get along. It is also an organic physiological problem—a problem in biological economy. The biological economy of an organism is the functional integrity of its parts. Mental conflict and insanity, industrial conflict, and crime are disorders of economy or of adaptation that lie within us as integral parts, not outside of us as detached onlookers. They present problems not of ourselves as isolated individuals, but of ourselves as a community. They are problems in community living, in how to get along with others. These problems are physiological and economic, biological and social.

Group or social analysis is the analysis of the immediate group in the immediate moment. A social group or community consists of persons each of whom is represented under the symbol he calls "I" or "I, myself". This proprietary symbol is socially accepted by the individuals of the group. It is the basis of their intercommunication. But the "I" that is socially accepted is socially elusive of analysis. The

* First published in *The British Journal of Medical Psychology, VIII,* Part III, 1928.

group composed of individual "I's" is equally elusive of social analysis. The sum of impressions symbolised as "I" would centre attention everywhere else than upon the sum of impressions thus symbolised. Group analysis is the objective analysis of this subjective symbol as represented in the immediate group in the immediate moment.

We have long grown familiar with the dual expressions of our neurotic patients, with their manifest or apparent content in contrast with their latent or repressed content as represented in dreams, in symptoms, and even in casual discourse. The group method of analysis has endeavoured to apply the same analytic principle to the manifestations of our casual social interchange and to discover in each expression of current social usage both the manifest and the latent content, the apparent and the repressed meaning. A statement is not taken upon its face value, but is subjected to the test of analysis in order to discover whatever unacknowledged content may be included in the overt expression. Where, ordinarily, an expression is accepted as quite *bona fide*, we now look for whatever reaction might run parallel to, and beneath, this manifest statement. No expression is considered complete in its surface aspect or content. But observation is directed toward whatever undisclosed proprietary motives might exist in contradistinction to our avowed statements.

The number of persons composing a group session has come to be limited, empirically, to about ten. As now arranged, the sessions are held once weekly and continue for one hour. The object of the group analysis is to give to the individual the opportunity to express himself in a social setting without the inhibitions of customary social images. By the social image, I mean that deflection of attention that shifts the individual's focus of interest upon his awareness of himself in respect to others' awareness of him. I mean the duplicate or self-reflected image that constantly attends him in the mental and social standard he has of himself. This factor of a shift of attention has significance for us as being fundamental in the structure of the latent social content, for it would appear that, by virtue of this social or duplicate image, each one of us tends to enact a given role, to portray a certain character or part in the social scheme of things, and it is the object of the group technique of analysis to enable the individual to express himself as he is—as he himself thinks and feels when utterly divorced from, and unsupported by, this social image of himself.[3]

In addition to the opportunity afforded each student or patient to give expression to himself apart from his social image or self-reflection, there is the opportunity for him to observe and to demonstrate in other students of the group any expression that might carry with it this latent import of the social image. In this way, each student has the opportunity to bring to observation the latent social content discoverable in the manifest content of any other student. In this function, he brings to evidence latent social tendencies not otherwise brought to observation. In his function toward the social analysis, each student, like the psychoanalytic patient in respect to his own symptoms or dreams, discovers latent social reactions in which he must otherwise, like the patient, remain an unconscious proprietary participant.

Upon bringing to light the manifestations of the latent social content, it would seem that these manifestations consist of feelings that would tend to place each individual opposite to, and in a relation of, transference or moralistic dependence upon every other individual.[4] In his latent social manifestations, the patient or student appears to be acutely sensitive to the impression he creates upon others. He is at all times at pains to reconcile his impression or image of himself with the image or impression that others entertain in regard to him. This marked deflection of attention toward concerns that are irrelevant to the immediate enquiry, this preoccupation with his appearance or behaviour with respect to those about him, is shown to be the outstanding expression of the latent social content.

And so it would appear that a condition of self-consciousness or of preoccupation with this duplicate social image is characteristic of this latent social mood. This acutely self-conscious, moralistic attitude is plainly correlated with the moral feelings of one's early home environment. It makes connection with the earliest impressions of the family and especially of the parent–child relationship. For this fictitious social image is substituted in the childhood of each of us. Each of us is early initiated into this manifest or symbolic content of the social consciousness and, under the symbol of the "I", one's very self becomes a symbol in this manifest social expression. For each of us is made aware of his image or appearance in relation to those about him. Each is made aware of his image in the light of the image others have of him. Our place, our position among others is reckoned wholly in terms of this social image or manifest content, and in the memories of our own childhood we may trace its ancestral descent. As the student becomes more and more skilled in the technique of observation afforded by group analysis, he is enabled to demonstrate again and again the intervention of this quite irrelevant social image and to indicate its generic place in the latent social content common to the group or community.

Let us take an instance in which a patient or student voices some complaint, offers an opinion or asks a question—instances typical of the manifest social content. The opinion, the complaint, or question is not regarded in its apparently direct meaning, not any more than the symptom or dream of a patient, and it does not, therefore, receive a direct answer. Instead, one looks into its latent content, into the elements that might have prompted the question. One looks for whatever is proprietary and irrelevant. Who is the person asking the question? What is his background? Why has he asked this particular question? What will he do with the answer? Why does he direct it to this or that particular person? What is that person's especial relation to him, or what relation would the questioner like to assume toward the person addressed? I do not mean that the student is literally confronted on every occasion with these specific demands, but they will indicate the general background against which our statements are tested. Perhaps some gesture accompanies the question, some expression of rigidity, a disclosure of uncertainty not implicit in the question itself, a fear perhaps, a suspicion; or there might be some effort of propitiation, some indirect plea for sympathy and anticipation of dependence. Perhaps the question discloses a note of competition, or criticism, or indicates some irritation. All these and many more such physiological accompaniments and latent intimations are material for analysis. For the repeated observation of the interreactions of individuals in groups indicates that there is never the absence of such accompaniments, and that such accompaniments are never without their conflicting symbols or images in contrast to the manifest content of the spoken word.

This over-evaluation in each individual of the self-image symbolised as "I", this image of oneself which one tends to carry about with him, comparing himself with the mental image he carries of others and which others carry of him, is again and again brought to open group awareness. But always emphasis is upon the common, socially pervasive character of what the individual presumes are quite privately cherished and secretly guarded images, so that the immediate recourse of the isolated individual to elaborations of the self-image called "I", or "I, myself", is viewed not as specific to the individual, but as generic to the group, and not to any particular group, but to the community as a whole. The patient's invariable effort, therefore, to obtain attention upon himself because of what he calls his particular manifestations, clinging to them avariciously as though they were some incommodity or illness quite private to him, is consistently neutralised by distributing our group attention upon these same conditions as actually demonstrated in the group as a whole.

This feature of group analysis I should especially like to emphasise. Under no circumstance does the procedure consist in the analysis of the individual by another individual or individuals. Whatever manifestation a student might present, in no circumstance is he made answerable for it as though it were a reaction particular to him. Whatever it might be, the manifestation is viewed as the expression of a latent content that is common to the group as a whole. Under no circumstance is the reaction of anyone regarded as isolated or separate. Neither does the group as a whole mean any particular group as differentiated from another group, but by "group" is meant the social constellation generally, with its ramifications throughout the community at large, the immediate group being but a constituent of this larger unit.

Perhaps the most interesting feature of group analysis is its tendency to break down certain categorical demarcations in the field of mental pathology, particularly the differentiation between normal and neurotic reactions. As far as our observations have progressed, it would seem that, from the basis of the group enquiry, there is no difference whatever between the social images of the neurotic and social images as they occur in normal individuals. The origin and mechanism of their development would seem to be identical in both, so that from the position of the group basis of observation, the discrimination between the neurotic and the normal becomes an artificial one. Not only is the normal as completely a prey to the images comprising his latent social content, but he is quite as inaccessible to a rational attitude toward these private images occurring in himself as the neurotic is inaccessible to a rational view of these images as they occur in him. It is repeatedly observed in actual experimentation that individuals who may take a quite objective attitude toward the social images of others are utterly inaccessible to all approach when these same images are operative within themselves. In this lack of insight, there is no difference between the reaction of the normal and of the neurotic. This identity between social repression existing in normality and the individual repression observable in the neurotic has naturally led to an altered evaluation of neurotic processes as well as to an altered technique in the effort to cope with them.

As one attempts to account for this phenomenon of the social image, one is faced with the necessity of very radical modifications of approach. These modifications are in the direction of more generic backgrounds—backgrounds that are not theoretical, but actual, not historical, but experimental and immediate. Mental disorders come to be seen as the product of racial inadvertences of growth rather than as individual anomalies.[5] As elsewhere in biology, a phylogenetic basis of interpretation becomes essential in correlating ontogenetic findings, and mechanisms illustrative of the intersocial reactions of individuals as a community or race have made imperative a consideration of the origin of man's interreactions as a community or racial organism.[6]

Among the processes which mediate the functioning of the social organism must be included those physiological balances of tension and release which place the individual in conscious relationship to his environment—the process we know as attention. The chief instrument employed by man in the process of attention is the social symbol or image expressed in the spoken word. This instrument or image adopted by the race serves as sign or token of a common content of meaning. In this common meaning, there is comprised the manifest content of the social consciousness.

In the evolution of man, however, and in his emergence toward higher processes of integration, it would seem that this manifest content of consciousness became vitiated, and that the image or symbol represented in the spoken word too often lost its primarily common meaning. Apparently, with the introduction of the moralistic image of self, that is, the image or symbol expressed in the individual's "good" or "bad" appearance or behaviour and its private advantage or disadvantage to the individual, his attention became deflected from a socially common meaning or function to a private interest or wish. Instead of mediating always a common content of meaning, these social symbols were made to serve at times wholly personal, proprietary ends, so that, in addition to the common content of meaning, there is introduced a personal, proprietary content. While the manifest content of the spoken word remains intact as a common symbol, in so far as it has become influenced by this personal image, a wholly arbitrary and private meaning necessarily attaches to it.

In this miscarriage of the social image and in the deflection of attention it entails, the social organism has been seriously affected in its intrinsic economy. As psychopathologists, our interest has centred chiefly in those symbolic distortions and image substitutions which Freud first traced in the manifest content of the neuroses. But, in our social images or meanings, there are deflections of attention which indicate a wider social impairment. It is this maladjustment among us socially which, it is felt, a group or social analysis contributes to repair.

While, then, it is the function of psychoanalysis and of psychiatry to deal with impressions and images in persons who are mentally ill or definitely ill-adapted socially, group analysis occupies itself with social images or with images shared among people generally, regardless of whether they are designated as neurotic or normal. It places an emphasis upon the latent content of consciousness as it underlies our manifest social interchange, rather than restricting its enquiry to the reminiscent materials of consciousness as they occur in the isolated expressions of the neurotic or insane individual.

For many years, it was my daily experience in personal analyses to pursue diligently the secret phantasies and symbolic irrelevancies of the individual unconscious, hunting them out from their remotest crevices with meticulous painstaking. And there is no doubt that the entertainment afforded my patients in our mutual search for various clues or associations was, in many cases, sufficiently diverting to constitute what is commonly called a cure. It is true that the individual patient feels that his neurosis, his sense of unworthiness and chagrin, his depression and pain, is caused by unsavoury, irrelevant preoccupations and inept tendencies that characterise him alone. He goes to his physician to receive treatment for a condition peculiar to himself—a condition in which he feels himself isolated from others. And so it was not unnatural that in its development from psychoanalytic traditions, the group method of analysis tended at first also to lay stress upon the habitually repressed, reminiscent material of the individual's unconscious.

In group analysis, however, the patient is made witness to the situation wherein these irrelevancies and secret excursions constitute a latent tendency that characterises equally the social group about him. It becomes gradually plain to him that his adoption of a code of symbols possessing only a private latent meaning is a general social condition. He discovers that the common manifest meaning of current social usage is quite as unstable as the manifest content of his restricted personal code. Accordingly, the deflections of attention shown in the substitutions and irrelevancies, the symbolisations and conversions of the neurotic patient are interpreted as being but special manifestations of a deflection of attention existing throughout the social organism.

This interpretation has led to an increasing emphasis upon the factor of the social image as an inducement to the substitutions occurring in individuals of both the neurotic and normal reaction. With the gradual maturing of the group method, the cherished reminiscences and private ruminations of the individual have come finally to be wholly disregarded. In their stead, the latent social content of consciousness, revealed beneath the manifest material represented in the habitual opinions and discussions of social interchange, have become the sole material of analysis. The only concern that occupies the group analysis is the immediate interrelationship socially of the members composing it, as expressed in the symbols of their momentary interchange. It is our group finding that, in resolving these social images of common group adoption, there follows the automatic restoration of group function in common social activities. For it is the interruption to this co-ordination of function within the social organism that, in our view, is the sole occasion for those states of proprietary symbolisation or introversion expressed in the regressions of the neurotic individual.

The reason, therefore, for this enquiry into latent manifestations existing socially—that is, in normal as well as in neurotic persons—is the evidence that the social image of self-awareness, characteristic of the group or community, tends to obstruct the activities of individuals in their natural group interfunctioning; further, that those ingrowths toward secret self-satisfaction which we find to be clinically characteristic of the neurotic personality result secondarily from this wider social obstruction.

It is the daily experience of the psychopathologist that a parent brings an ill son or daughter to him for diagnosis and advice. This situation is placed in a very different light if, quite unknown to themselves, the parent of the patient and the household generally are, along with the physician himself, preserving unconsciously among them a social form of repression, and if, upon analysis, this social repression is shown to be the real cause of the more intense reaction expressed secondarily in the patient. As it bears upon the structure and outcome of mental disorder, it makes a very great difference whether the individual patient is from infancy a constitutional neurotic, or whether the barriers to the natural interfunctioning of individuals, as these barriers exist in the social cluster comprising the family, have from childhood obstructed the patient's natural feelings of intercommunication and have forced his attention into the regressive symbols of phantasy and dream.

A programme, therefore, which would seem to me a valuable adjunct to our present endeavours on behalf of neurotic and insane patients, would be one which placed upon groups of the community the responsibility of insanity as a social or community problem. Through this programme, the community would endeavour to bring its own latent processes and social images to objective group observation as a generic group condition. In such groups, there would not be the situation in which certain individuals would study other individuals as presumably different in constitution from themselves, but in which all individuals would be equally responsible for the study of a constitutional condition common to all. Such a programme would, I should think, begin among groups composed of the more thoughtful element of the community. It would begin first of all, perhaps, among groups like ourselves, whose interest is precisely in the field of psychopathology.

And so, if I may suggest that procedure which would seem to me of value in meeting the conflicts of the individual and the community, conflicts expressed in mental disorder and insanity, in industrial disorders and crime, it would be a programme which most closely affects the interreactions existing among ourselves as components in an economic social organism. This programme, in freeing us from the restrictions of latent social images and repressions, would more and more place ourselves and the community at large upon a common basis of intercommunication and function. In so doing, it would render psychopathology less a psychological theory of human interrelationships and make possible the immediate expression of those interrelationships in their physiological actuality.

Notes

1. Paper read on the occasion of the Fifteenth Anniversary of the Phipps Psychiatric Clinic, Johns Hopkins Hospital, 30 April 1928.

   Naturally, a paper having to do with the adaptation of groups or communities as it bears upon the interreactions of individuals as social integers suggests at once those factors of integration which Dr Meyer has for so long emphasised. This position is one with which Dr Meyer has, for a period of more than twenty years, so fully identified himself that it is a familiar theme to those of us who have been associated with the Phipps Clinic and with his fundamental conceptions. My only excuse for returning to these factors on this occasion is the circumstance that, for several years, I have, in association with others, been daily occupied with the practical observation of these interreactions as they are found to occur under the experimental conditions of actual group setting.
2. "Social images versus reality": *The Journal of Abnormal Psychology and Social Psychology, xix*(3), October–December 1924.
3. "The problem of the transference", *The British Journal of Medical Psychology, VII*, Part II, 1927.
4. "On a social approach to neurotic conditions", by Hans C. Syz, M.D. *The Journal of Nervous and Mental Diseases, LXVI*(6). December 1927.
5. *The Social Basis of Consciousness*. London: Kegan Paul, Trench, Trubner; New York: Harcourt Brace.

CHAPTER SIXTEEN

The autonomy of the "I" from the standpoint of group analysis*

With your permission I should like, in the moment, to approach the problems of our human conduct from a background that calls for the tentative adoption among us of a basis of observation that is, individually, neither yours nor mine according to our habitual acceptations. This might seem to you a strange proposal. But my hope is that, in proportion as it appears strange to you upon a casual view, it may prove the more interesting in its application as a direct method of experimentation. And so I am taking the liberty of inviting you to participate with me in a purely experimental adventure.[1] In the absence of certain preliminary experience such as provides the better facility for our undertaking, I must ask your utmost patience in my effort to initiate you into this quite fresh basis of endeavour.

As our procedure will deal with the reactions of human beings in their personal and social relationships as experienced also by ourselves, we shall be assisted if, preliminary to our enquiry, we shall

* Paper read at the Seventeenth Annual Meeting of the American Psychoanalytic Association, Cincinnati, Ohio, 31 May 1927. First published in *Psyche*, *VIII*(3), January 1928.

recall certain biological considerations first brought to the attention of science through the investigations of Darwin. I have in mind the observations of Darwin respecting the interreactions of the individuals of a species in their group or societal function. You will recall that, contrary to popular assumption, Darwin did not base his principle of the survival of the fittest entirely upon the special equipment of the individual. He based it also upon this instinct of racial solidarity which, operating within the species as a whole, tends to unite and preserve the individuals composing it as a concerted biological unit or group.[2]

As I have referred in other papers to this principle relating to the physiological interreactions mediating the group life of the species, there is no need to enlarge upon it here.[3] I have referred to it many times as a conceptual premise. The present reference to this instinctive substrate of man's interreactions as it operates within social communities is made because of the pragmatic background it affords for an undertaking that rests upon a group or societal standpoint of investigation.

Proceeding now to our direct enquiry, we shall find, I think, that a gathering of individuals such as we represent here, each constituting a separate social "I", offers a convenient foil against which we may observe certain specific data respecting the "I" not possible of observation from the standpoint of the individual "I" itself. Such a social or group situation in which it is permitted to discount the authority of this commonly unchallenged "I"—unchallenged, I mean, in its habitual private values—affords, in my experience, an entirely new background for computing our human evaluations and, incidentally, discredits many of our habitual personal and social inferences. "Knowing" is found to be not the knowing it is commonly conceded to be on the mere authority of the "I" that "knows", and "feeling" not so dependable a feeling as has been assumed on the purely personal premise of the individual who "feels". For, quite automatically, each individual is influenced more or less by a private criterion, which, without his awareness, he preserves quite apart from other individuals.[4]

In so far, then, as the individual "I" has come to embody a separate mood tone with respect to every other "I", we are confronted socially with a situation that only a stabilised and disinterested mood approach is competent to observe and estimate accurately. As this basis of observation menaces customary submission to established images, personal and social, it naturally does violence to prevailing prepossessions. But we shall, of course, discount this tendency as far as possible in the interest of the experiment upon which we are entering. It is the very premise of our experiment that a stabilised mood basis shall replace the normal criterion of the individual "I" in the sphere of feeling and of knowing, and that this generally accepted criterion shall be empirically discarded in favour of uniform standards of measurement in the sphere of our subjective human reactions.

It is exceedingly important that we be prepared to accept a completely fresh basis of observation if we are to be adequately orientated toward our present experimental procedure. It is important to realise that the object that challenges our enquiry is nothing less than the entire background of our personal and social habituations. Naturally, to envisage one's entire medium offers difficulties, for it is inevitable that habituation should obscure the medium habituated. Obviously, if a fish should become suddenly capable of conscious observation, the last thing it would observe would be the water in which it swims. Its own medium is too much a part of itself to become an object of its own contemplation. The very fact that the water presses close against the visual sense organ and is in constant contact with the fish at every point on its surface would preclude the possibility of the water becoming an impression of which the fish could be made aware. It would be necessary first to remove the fish from its habitual environment in order that it should obtain an objective view of the watery medium in which it had previously been accustomed to move.

In the same way, I think it may be shown that there are contacts belonging to man's social medium that impinge upon him too closely and too constantly on every side to afford him impressions of which he is aware. He moves in and amid these contacts, but they are too much part of himself to become an object of his consciousness. He reacts to their influence without knowing to what he reacts or why. He responds constantly to the impressions of the social medium about him and constantly receives responses from it in return, but always that which is himself and that which is the medium about himself are merged into one another too imperceptibly to make it possible that the social medium of which man is a part should become an object apart from himself.

By "social medium", I mean the medium of mental interchange that everywhere exists among human beings and that makes possible their understanding of one another through the adoption of commonly accepted symbols of images. The social medium of which I am speaking represents states of mind which exist solely by virtue of an agreement in terms that has come to be socially adopted among people; as, for example, the names of the objects surrounding them or of the sensations perceived within them. In addition to the state of mind corresponding to the symbol or image of any single object, there are states of mind that reflect a whole system of images or symbols such as the highly complex agreement in terms or images embodied in our various social institutions. Government, for example, is a state of mind created socially by the adoption of certain covenants or systems of images on the part of the individuals subsisting under it in their collective capacity. The social medium, therefore, of which I am now speaking, refers specifically to those consciously adopted and agreed symbols which mediate the quite purposive and sophisticated adaptations of man in social communities.

It is of vital importance that we keep carefully in mind the distinction between the biological group principle which unites the individuals of a species and constitutes man's instinctive societal bond and the highly complex system of intercommunication that constitutes the social medium of civilised man today; the one representing an instinctive or organic racial principle based upon physiological interreactions, the other representing a wholly sophisticated and peripheral manner of adaptation mediated upon a level of socially agreed images.

The result of careful studies of individuals in groups, observed on the basis of the agreed terms which unite the individuals composing such groups, has led to the discovery of an unconscious social factor with which we need very seriously to reckon. This factor, far from giving to the terms of common adaptation a common signification, tends to invest them with images or connotations which possess for each individual a wholly private and arbitrary meaning. Accordingly, an object or sensation might mean one thing to one individual and quite another to some other individual. Or it might take on a meaning for the same individual at one time which is wholly contradicted at another. "Property" or "home", for example, assumes a quite different meaning according to whether it is my property or home, or some one else's. And even "*my home*" has one connotation when the members composing it are quite agreed respecting the wisdom of my general management of it and quite another when there is not so marked a consensus within the household as to the merits of my jurisdiction over it.

It is true that certain social images of common acceptation would seem to possess a quite permanent meaning, as, for example, an axe, a boat, a house, or a ball of yarn, and it is not to be denied that the meaning or symbols for such objective entities are less liable to corruption than the more subjective designations or agreements that have come to exist socially among us. It is with reference to these subjective symbols that there is the need for serious reckoning. For the observation of social groups has made it apparent that, in respect of man's subjective interpretations, there is lacking a unanimity of accord in the images or symbols possessing a supposedly common meaning. Not only this, but, like the manifest symptom or dream image of the neurotic patient, this outer unanimity of agreement is found to serve merely as a diplomatic code or gesture beneath which each individual reserves the right to an interpretation that rests entirely upon his private feeling with respect to it. Closer investigation points to the circumstance that the person called "I" possesses unanimously a *feeling*—or *mood*—prerogative that is wholly arbitrary and private to him and that this private assumption has come to colour and distort his relationship to the social medium about him in such manner that he is no longer capable of viewing it as an object of disinterested observation apart from himself.

Let us consider more closely this "I" and its autonomies. Let us consider it in its subjective prerogative and compare the same reaction as observed in its objective evaluation. I wish, indeed, that in the interest of experiment it were possible suddenly to create subjectively, among those of us composing the present group, conditions of observation similar to those obtaining objectively when, in a lecture illustrated with lantern slides, one shows, for example, certain tissue conditions as they are demonstrable in anatomical or histological sections. The darkened room merges the audience into a common obscurity as far as their customary social perceptions of one another are concerned and automatically obliterates those features which mark the personal differentiae existing among them, while the speaker himself is wholly effaced or becomes at most but a moving shadow that passes momentarily across the screen.

In the absence of conditions as favourable to a clear, unobstructed subjective demonstration of man's biology as the conditions obtainable in a lecture illustrative of his objective biological features, let us at least, through what power of imagination we may summon, render ourselves as far as possible quite oblivious of our customary differentiae and so dispel momentarily the attitudes of mind habitual to our adopted social medium. By abrogating in this way the mental symbols or social images that habitually mediate our external agreement with one another, we shall find ourselves automatically thrown back upon an internal basis that more nearly approximates man's primary racial co-ordination. In this way, we are better enabled to obtain a common ground for evaluating those images or symbols that too often interpose obstacles to clear observation.

It is this group principle of co-ordination that represents the group basis of analysis, as it is the images of common interchange sponsored by the social medium that represent the material to be analysed. We should understand, however, at the outset that the social medium is represented quite as completely in the single individual as in a group of individuals, precisely as the instinctive group principle of man is embodied as fully in the single individual as in the group. In the sphere of the social medium, images that are social are necessarily personal also, just as in the sphere of man's instinctive life his phylogenetic basis is ontogenetic as well. In my private analysis, I do not cease to adhere to a group principle of analysis because there is only one individual to be analysed, no more than in the sphere of biology I should cease to adhere to laboratory principles of observation because I happened to be alone in a laboratory when studying my material.

In the laboratory of subjective processes or in group analysis, it is the reactions of the subject or of the "I" which become the material under examination. Turning, then, to the "I" (that is, to each of us and to his isolated autonomies), we find such reactions as the following, along with the undisputed authority they claim, to be quite general and of common social acceptance. "I don't like John"; "I just can't stand a crowd"; "I guess I know what I want"; "I possess the best parents in the world"; "I possess the truest religion and the only country worth while"; or, "My children possess exceptional talent"; "My automobile is the best the market puts out"; or, "John likes *me* and he is a nice fellow"; "That man is not favourably disposed toward me and I have no use for him"; "That autoist came near to running over and killing me and he ought to get twenty years"; and so on *ad infini-*

tum. All quite usual affirmations based upon private images and connotations, every one of which may be flatly and quite as authoritatively contradicted by another individual or "I" who happens to be under the influence of an opposite system of images or prejudices.

If we will alter the habitual form of the statement and, instead of the above subjective premise, we will substitute a more objective statement of the same proposition, our formula would run: "The 'I' says *it* does not like John", or, "The 'I' claims that *its* country is the best of all countries", or, "The 'I' guesses that *it* knows what *it* wants". In this mere shift of the mood emphasis from subjective to objective, a totally different proposition results. In other words, standing, as one habitually does, inside of the "I", one may easily maintain a view that one would not think of maintaining were one to place himself, for a moment, outside of the "I" and observe its processes quite objectively. When I do not like John, that settles the matter. It is the finish of John from *my* standpoint, or the standpoint of "I". Some one else, however, overhearing my statement in regard to John and being subjectively quite disinterested in respect to both of us, might quite naturally question my judgement and the private prerogative upon which it rests.[5] The drivers of two taxicabs that have inadvertently collided will hurl epithets at one another which express in no unequivocal terms the subjective view maintained by each with respect to the other. Yet, to the bystander who has witnessed the accident from the objective position of the detached observer, the subjective autonomy of both drivers is as patent as it is absurd.

You observe that the separate "I", when speaking in its subjective sovereignty (when I, for example, say that I do not like so and so), necessarily assumes that the presumable object of its dislike is somehow to be held accountable—that if *I* do not like John, *John* must do something about it. But discarding all subjective prerogative in the matter and viewing the same formula with objective disinterestedness (what was "I" becoming "the I"), one could not accept this view. One would say that here are two terms not in agreement, but that it is impossible to say that one of them should be invariably held accountable and that the other should invariably hold it accountable. Such a view would be manifestly absurd. And yet what very different reactions we habitually obtain from individuals according to whether the images and connotations composing the social medium are subjectively or objectively apprehended by them!

Upon closer view, the first observation that strikes us is that the separate "I" that "does not like" some particular individual, and which never questions the rightness of its separative judgement in regard to that individual, is quite as often counterbalanced by the attitude of another, separate "I", which, contrariwise, *does* like that same individual and which is quite as assured in turn of the rightness of *its* separate judgement toward him. It also appears to be a universal law of the social medium that a person who adopts an autonomous attitude opposite another person, automatically induces in that person an equally autonomous and opposite attitude toward himself.

A further interesting phenomenon coming under repeated observation of persons in groups plainly indicates the social character of the autonomy expressed by the individual. It indicates how inseparably the autonomous reaction of the individual is bound up with the autonomous reactions of the social medium about him. Under repeated experiment, certain tendencies among the individuals of a group are found to be quite automatic. For example, it is found that their collective emotions form a spontaneous cluster, as it were, about the emotional mood of any one individual in accordance with the unconscious sympathy of the group in the autonomy expressed by him, and, conversely, that they form an emotional cluster opposite him if his autonomous position happens to be irreconcilable with their own—a social mechanism identical with that just noted in regard to the single individual. The formation of these clusters is apparently wholly irresistible, and repeated observation renders their occurrence quite predictable.[6] It would seem that these cluster formations possess all the fatality of chemical combinations. Indeed, such reactions represent actual social reflexes and are as uncontrollable as the spasmodic reflex to be observed in the compulsive tic or anxiety reaction of an individual patient. As fear is the underlying motive to these reactions in the individual, so a collective, social fear appears to underlie these reactions within the group. What happens, evidently, is this: the individuals who automatically align themselves with another individual's autonomous position are unconsciously constrained to do so because of the protection this temporary agreement seems to offer their own autonomies. So, what is true of the individual, with his separate "I", is equally true of a society composed, as it is, of a collection of such separate "I's", a circumstance that has been observed in social groups again and again in the cluster reactions just cited. Accordingly, where one finds one person claiming, upon a purely private premise, that his religion is the best of all religions, one finds a whole community of persons proceeding upon this same private premise. Yet again, this proposition is invariably offset by a counter proposition that is equally sponsored by the social medium. Or, where one finds half a nation of people quite convinced that theirs is the most representative and upstanding of all political parties, one also finds half a nation of people stoutly denying this proposition of the first faction and claiming the same prerogative for their own party and always on the basis of an authority that rests its security upon quite as autonomous a premise.

This social situation is a wholly subjective one, and, accordingly, only a quite objective observation of the social medium, whether represented in an individual or in a group, can adequately disclose the extent to which individuals are dominated by social images possessing no other authority than the private claim of the individual. Neither can we realise anywhere, perhaps, so adequately as in the actual social group the tenacity with which these spurious values cling to one. There may occur a social agreement among many members of such a group with respect to this or that opinion or judgement, but, upon analysis, it is found to rest (like the opinions of individuals regarding their common political party) upon an agreement that represents collectively the subjective autonomy of the "I".

Our economic, religious, and political views, then, would seem to rest not upon the covenants of an accepted ethic with respect to one another, but upon quite proprietary possessive claims, which, being private and covetous, rest upon subjective pre-possessions that are completely lacking in objective authority. It would appear that there is no economic system, that what we call our economic system is really a proprietary system.

If our social medium of images and covenants really rests upon opinions which lack the foundation of sound racial or economic principles and which are liable to the constant vacillations of subjective presuppositions, it might be worth while to enquire how far the age-old conflicts that constantly beset our national, political, and economic life are traceable to such social images and covenants. It might be well to discover whether these cherished talismans merit the sincere assent of the individuals who are supposedly bound by them, or whether they are not really devoid of validity because of the private right of interpretation secretly exercised by them, both in their personal and in their collective function.

This mechanism of autonomy, as I have elsewhere attempted to point out, has its inception in the very earliest impressions received by the child from the social medium surrounding him as sponsored by the mother. There is perhaps nothing so subversive of harmony and growth throughout the entire social scheme as the attitude of parents who, in their own autonomy, imbue their children with an unconscious attitude that is equally autonomous. It is such projections of parental autonomy that are really answerable for the agitations today that centre around the so-called problem of the child. It is not the child that is the problem, but the parent, and it is precisely the parent's autonomy that causes him to find pleasanter entertainment in what he calls the problem of his child than in what he refuses to call the problem of himself and his autonomies. What is true of the arbiters of the home is equally true of the vicarious arbiters appointed by the home. Our schools represent an autonomy that exists upon an even larger scale than that of the home. In the attitude of the church, the university, and the world of business, the situation is the same. And it is not possible to find a solution to the problems of human adjustment in our courts of law, because our courts of law rest upon subjective opinions or affects that are also based in each instance upon the inaccessible autonomy of the "I", either individual or collective.

As psychoanalysts, however, our interest is pre-eminently in neurotic personalities and in those conflicts which impose barriers to their realisation of a unified sex life. It is precisely in its influence upon the sex life that the autonomy of the "I" merits most uncompromising challenge. As seen against the background of a group principle of analysis, I have been convinced that the subjective prerogative of the separate "I" is the all-important obstacle to the healthy adaptation of man and woman in their mutual sex function. Social images that are mutually accepted by two individuals in their external adaptations, but with which they are not in accord with their internal evaluations, cause an obstruction to their natural sex function and necessarily lead to unassimilable image constructions and to the inverted elaboration of autoerotism. These image-formations can only preoccupy each to the exclusion of the other, except as their private images become mutually self-gratifying upon a purely peripheral, narcissistic plane. But a union based upon a sexual accord that is nothing else than the reflex social cluster of two individuals in response to mere autonomous social images is not a biological sex union.

Freud has shown—and we have all been a witness to the accuracy of Freud's thesis—that the neurosis represents the thwarted expression of the life of the individual, and that, concomitant to this obstruction in the individual's life, he is preoccupied with endless phantasy constructs represented in symbols which are invariably traceable to distortions in his instinctive sex life. But what is the constant and universal cause of this repression? To what does the system of images comprising the phantasy world of the neurotic owe its existence? We know, of course, that the neurotic is not in contact with the actualities of his environment. We know this from our repeated analysis of his repressed unconscious trends. But why is he not in contact with the actuality of things? Why is he repressed? To say that the individual's early environment and the over-zealous interest of the mother were the chief factors contributing to the subsequent development of his neurosis is very true, *but an environment that represses is itself also repressed*. The individual who becomes neurotic in response to his social environment is reacting to an environment that is equally neurotic.

Through the technique of group analysis, I have had the opportunity to witness in their immediate social contact just such social groups as normally compose the environment of childhood. I have had the opportunity to observe in their social setting just such phantasy constructs and symbolic distortions as occur in the individual neurotic. As it has been found that these social phantasies of immediate daily analysis possess the same content as the wish-fulfilments disclosed upon the analysis of the individual's dream, and as these social images have been traced in every instance to the circumscribed phantasy system that is each individual's subjective autonomy, my conclusion is that the instigation of these two identical processes—the social image and the individual dream—is due to an identical cause: to the autonomy of the "I" and to its indisputable right to interpret the universe in terms of its private delectation.

It is not true that the neurotic dreams only in the dissociated images of the sleeping state. The neurotic is dreaming throughout all of his day. It is not true that his dream is built of the impalpable fabric of phantasies only. In the casting of his images, he employs no less the solid materials of daily actuality also. Nor is it true that the medium out of which the neurotic weaves his images of unreality, sleeping and waking is any other than the medium that forms the tissue of man's images generally. Accordingly, the analysis of the motives that operate in support of the separate "I" and its autonomy is an analysis of the causes that lead to the construction of both the dream imagery of the individual and of the waking imagery of the collection of individuals composing the social milieu.

This process, however, cannot rest upon theory, and neither can it rest upon the authority of my statement. Again we need to return to conditions that provide a basis of objective scientific experimentation. Only conditions of disinterested observation can serve us if we are really to observe these sporadic manifestations represented in the private affect as sponsored by the individual's subjective autonomy.

A biological group, observing the reactions of an individual to the social group medium about him, will discover that the unfailing symptoms of the personal autonomy is the reaction of protest and of disavowal that is invariably elicited at the least suggestion of examination into it. This often demonstrates itself in the prompt recourse of the individual to obscure the reaction calling for immediate observation. This he will do through an effort to cover his autonomous reaction with intellectual substitutions. Or, failing this recourse, he will, through the very autonomy of his efforts, fall straightaway into the autonomous affect he is seeking to circumvent. In this situation, if there is a sufficiently strong emotional cluster to rally to his support, as we have frequently seen occurs, the individual's autonomy straight way acquires the social authority necessary to avert an objective enquiry into his processes. Thus, through this autonomous social reflex, the individual succeeds in withdrawing again into the shell of his private autonomy. In brief, in one's biological group integrity, it is possible to observe that the individual in his single or collective persona is quite incompetent to take part in a scientific evaluation of his own subjective processes. We find that, like the fish in respect to its impinging medium, the very closeness of the social medium precludes the individual's objective observation of it.

As I have said, an objective examination of the social medium of which we have all become subjectively so close a part, tends at first to offend accustomed prepossession and, naturally, I have no wish to impose this experimental procedure upon others. But, having found it of incalculable assistance to myself in my scientific outlooks, and having found it of great practical service to my patients, I have taken the liberty of offering it here for whatever value it might seem to you to possess.

To sum up: Freud has, through the principle and method of psychoanalysis, provided us with an instrument and a technique for probing amid the tissues of man's mental life and exposing to view mechanisms and reactions hitherto unsuspected by students of medicine and biology. Where there had previously existed only an anatomy of the mind, there now exists a histology of the mind. Where formerly the study of the emotions was restricted to macroscopic structures only, there has now been opened to us the study of emotional processes in their minutest microscopic details. Such has been the contribution of the method of psychoanalysis as discovered by Freud.

We must come to see, however, that an analysis of a particular symptom or individual has as its scientific aim the discovery of the universal cause that will synthesise our understanding of *all* symptoms and of *all* individuals. It appears to have been forgotten that the ultimate object of analysis is not analysis but synthesis, that analysis is only a means of which the end is a synthesis of our analytic findings. In the bacteriological technique invented and applied by Pasteur and Koch in their effort to discover disease germs, many discoveries were made regarding the minute cell structures which came under their examination during the process of their enquiries. But they were not, on this account, led to lose sight of the primary purpose of their enquiries. It was Koch's effort to discover and to establish beyond question the specific and universal cause that would synthesise our understanding of tuberculosis and enable us to deal intelligently with its manifold symptoms and processes. Perhaps the most interesting of the disclosures incident to the discovery of the bacillus of Koch is the fact that this germ resides practically universally in the tissues of healthy individuals, as well as in those who are manifestly victims of the disease.

A group analysis has afforded evidence that there is a microgenic incident responsible for the neuroses and that this incident resides in the mental constitution not only of the neurotic individual, but of all individuals. It has afforded evidence that the manifold proliferations of this microgenic incident may be traced to a universal phyletic source which can be uncovered only through a synthesis of our understandings of the social medium with its basis in the autonomy of the "I". It is inevitable that the private individual in his private prerogative should tend to adhere to an individual method of analysis that leaves unchallenged the private autonomy of the analyst. But an unchallenged autonomy, as viewed objectively, is of the essence of dogma and fundamentalism. The advance of the biological sciences began with the abrogation of dogmatic fundamentalism and with the adoption in its stead of evolutionary principles that opened scientific investigations to the consensual method of the laboratory. An advance in the biology of the mental sciences must likewise be paralleled by an equal adoption of laboratory methods of observation and by an enquiry into our human processes that uncovers completely the pathological incident residing in the subjective autonomy of the "I".

* * *

It is stated in a note at the end of this paper that this presentation was intended as an opportunity of initiation of my psychoanalytic *confrères* into the principle and procedure of group analysis. The experiment was sociologically significant. The members had made a request, in all sincerity, for this opportunity to participate in a group analysis. There could be no question of the entire good faith in which my colleagues had sought a closer understanding of the group method. But it was inevitable that their interest should rest upon a purely theoretical basis that when there came the critical issue and when from "theory" there was launched a direct mood challenge of habitual mood situations as they exist socially, this opportunity was found most unwelcome and was met with solid group resistance. The only response elicited was characteristic of group reactions elsewhere. From the standpoint of group analysis, the meagre response voiced by the meeting rested precisely upon the autonomous basis of the "I" and, obviously, without the least suspicion on the part of the Association of the autonomous mood basis represented by its response. A social mood-cluster stood unconsciously as a solid phalanx against the least hint or suspicion that might reflect upon its habitual group-mood. This is scientifically interesting, and I feel that it is vitally important from the point of view of our mass needs organically as well as sociologically.

This impasse to the acceptance of an objective approach to man's social mood has demonstrated itself again and again during the past seven years in similar group situations. This is not a circumstance peculiar to one particular group. It is characteristic of all observable groups. The conclusion is inescapable that there resides within the unconscious social processes of man a mood habituation that is utterly inaccessible to us on the basis of our present social mood. It is evident that there exists a state of mind which, by common social consent, automatically resists all attempt at a social self-enquiry. If this is true, it becomes further evident that there is required some fundamental reconstruction within the mental constitution of society throughout. For this widespread social resistance points inevitably to the presence of an attitude of *transference*, or unconscious dependence, that exists socially among us as definitely as there exists this unconscious dependence in the attitude of the child toward the parent or of the patient toward the analyst.

The mood-impasse occurring at the meeting at which this group experiment was attempted has served still further to crystallise the feeling long dormant with myself and my associates (as in our own group work we have experienced this same social rigidity within ourselves) that a technique must be opened to society generally such as will allow it to take responsible care as a social unit of its own unconscious social processes.

How far the insidious influence of an arbitrary autonomy masquerades under the credentials of stabilised authority has not begun to be suspected by us in any analytic sense. It has not begun to be suspected how far this purely private and uncontrolled mood presumption dominates our entire social life. The sexual repression that Freud has so rightly emphasised in individual neurotics is, I am convinced, quite secondary to this more general mood interdiction within the *social* instinct of man. The pathological effect of this arbitrary social mood in repressing man's natural societal instinct is traceable throughout our social institutions everywhere. It is the position of group analysis that the concurrence between this widespread social repression and the general increase socially of insanity points to a definite causal relationship. For a society thus dominated is unthinkingly dominated. It is a society that is a prey to unconscious repression as definitely as the individual neurotic is a prey to unconscious repression.

Discussion, argument, and speculation will not avail. This is mere rationalisation and evasion. The light understanding of this widespread social condition calls for the application of scientific method. This means the method of the laboratory. It means the scientific recourse to a technique that makes possible the observation of the physiological processes that mediate the behaviour of human beings in their social interreactions. Such a procedure calls for the development of controlled methods and criteria whereby we may discriminate with objective precision between the pseudo-physiological reactions that are artificially dictated by an autonomous social mood and those physiological interreactions that are the natural expression of societal man.[7] We have need to face the circumstance that there must somehow be awakened a *unitary social responsibility* toward what is now the *collective social mood* of man with its unconscious transference between individual and individual. To attempt to face the problem of the individual neurosis or transference in the absence of serious reckoning with man's mass neurosis or transference is to miss the real problem of our human pathology.[8] A broader basis than that maintained by our present psychiatric criteria is urgently demanded. In New York State alone, for example, according to a report quoting the State Commissioner of Mental Hygiene, the increase in the number of insane patients for the year ending June 30, 1927 was more than double the average yearly increase for the previous ten years. According to the same report, there are in the hospitals of New York State 47,514 insane patients, and so rapidly is insanity on the increase that these hospitals are today forced to house 10,000 inmates in excess of the capacity of these institutions. It is amazing that science could for so long have looked on idly at this appalling disparity between the methods obtaining in the field of mental illness as compared with the progress of its methods in the structural field of medicine. Only some very obstinate obstruction to man's capacity of self-observation as a social unit could, all this while, have allowed him to accept with complete impotence the steady increase, in our social communities, of mental illness as compared with the overwhelming decrease of disease in the structural sphere.

We are an immediate witness to the clearly demonstrable mood-obstructionism existing socially within groups coming under analytic observation, and this even among scientific groups, such as our own, whose function is precisely the study and analysis of pathological mental states. Such a situation, together with the situation existing socially with respect to insanity at large, or to mood-reactions occurring within the community, is, I feel, an ominous tell-tale of the serious need in which we stand for reconstructing our psychiatric and psychoanalytic foundations.

There have been seven years of intensive study and analysis on the part of my laboratory associates and myself of social processes as they habitually exist within so-called normal groups. If this study is in the least deserving of scientific consideration, the situation before us calls for the recognition of our mass responsibility and for an unflinching stock-taking of processes existing socially among ourselves as elements in a mass neurosis.

Notes

1. I have been repeatedly asked by members of the American Psychoanalytic Association to afford them an opportunity to witness a session of group analysis. I had always to explain that a social analysis of its nature demands participation in its process. Naturally a social analysis admits of no outsider. There is no extra-social individual, no non-participant in a neurosis common to the social organism. This, however, was not unnaturally interpreted as an evasion on my part. So, not wishing to seem inhospitable, I offered this group presentation, which, as I stated before reading my paper, was a recourse intended to afford opportunity to the Association of converting the meeting directly into a group analysis.
2. "Those communities", wrote Darwin, "which included the greatest number of the most sympathetic members would flourish best, and rear the greatest number of offspring" (*The Descent of Man,* 2nd edition, p. 163). See also P. Kropotkin's *Mutual Aid,* A. A. Knopf.
3. *The Social Basis of Consciousness,* London: Kegan Paul, Trench, Trubner, 1927, New York: Harcourt Brace; "An ethnic aspect of consciousness", *The Sociological Review, XIX*(1), January 1927; "The laboratory method in psychoanalysis", *The American Journal of Psychiatry, V*(3), January 1926.
4. This mood-bound habituation within the social organism is, I feel, the biology of the tendency reflected in the intellectual habit of "word-magic" so clearly described by C. K. Ogden. For these linguistic tendencies within the race disclose emotional implications which are shown in group analysis to possess deep social significance.
5. Pirandello has attempted to illustrate the situation in his clever dramatic sketch "Right you are if you think you are". But Pirandello's sketch is not so much a play as it is the projection in play form of the author's own

unconscious participation in the same mechanism he feign [*sic*] would disclose. Pirandello's thesis would appear in a very different light were it submitted to examination from the standpoint of group analysis. The truth is it is really concealing under the symbol of actuality the very actuality it is supposedly disclosing. The playwright is practically asking us to observe with him how wrong other people are who are right, when all the while this is again but an attitude of equal rightness and autonomy on the part of the would-be observer! Only a group analysis offers the background for the observation of just such self-enveloping autonomies with their complete inaccessibility to the individual "I" and its "rightness". In truth, what the playwrights are perpetrating these days with their naïvely "psychological" image-juggling is only matched by the equally naïve achievements of their image-bejuggled audience!

6. "The heroic role—an historical retrospect", *Psyche, VI*(25), July 1926.
7. "Biological foundations and mental methods": paper read at the Seventeenth Annual Meeting of the American Psychopathological Association, Cincinnati, Ohio, 3 June 1927.
8. "The problem of the transference", *British Journal of Medical Psychology, VII*, July 1927.

CHAPTER SEVENTEEN

So-called "normal" social relationships expressed in the individual and the group and their bearing on the problems of neurotic disharmonies*[1,2]

I

This audience is probably aware that anything I might have to say on the relatedness of the two sciences of sociology and psychiatry will be presented from the background of the group or phyletic approach to the individual neurosis.[3] As a physician and psychiatrist, my work has confronted me with problems having definite sociological implications, but, needless to say, as a technician, I am a complete stranger to the science of sociology, so that, in accepting an invitation to present a paper before this sociological group, I hope you will appreciate something of the limitations of my position. I must ask, too, that you bear patiently with me in the presentation of a thesis that must, of necessity, be limited to only its broadest aspects and which, therefore, might seem too sweeping in theory and programme. But when I recall that sociology as a science is committed to a programme that deals with nothing less than those principles which underlie our entire human society as a condition in evolution, I feel confident that

*First published in *American Journal of Psychiatry*, X(1), July 1930.

an audience of sociologists can hardly be inhospitable to a phyletic approach to our common human problem.

By the group or philetic method of analysis is meant a method that attempts to explain the reactions expressed in the relationships of individuals to one another and to the social group upon a physiological basis of interpretation. As human beings, we are, by nature, primary physiological. We have become psychological only secondarily and by adoption. As elements of a species, we were originally organisms interrelated by common instincts and feelings long before the day when, as members of civilised society, we became related to one another through a medium of agreed images and symbols. Amid the overwhelming impetus of our present-day interrelationships based upon these social images and symbols, man has become wholly preoccupied with the sphere of his later adoption, that is, with the sphere expressed in the language and customs that pertain to his more recent psychological adaptation. Accordingly, the sphere of his physiological origin, with its basis in those native instincts and feelings that knit the elements of the species into a continuous organic whole, are now, apart from mere intellectualisation and theory, quite neglected or wholly forgotten. I should like to return to this original basis of man's interrelationships and to the consideration of a mode of consciousness that is primary and physiological in contradistinction to the secondary psychological consciousness that now mediates our intercommunication in the form of the spoken language or social symbol.

It may be said that sociology stands midway between psychiatry and the broad unclassified field of human activities generally, between the science that has to do with mental disorders and the problems of everyday life—problems of getting on, of making a living. Setting aside the broader, technical meanings of sociology, the problems of the sociologist are problems in inter-individual efficiency, in social economy and industry. The development of my work as a psychiatrist into what I have called group analysis has been such that I find myself faced with two fields of activity seemingly remote from one another—that of the psychiatrist as a specialist and that of the lay individual as a social being surrounded by all manner of problems of living, such as those subsumed under the science of sociology. In brief, it has become the function of group analysis to combine and relate the field of psychiatry and the field of the everyday industry of man. For the basic principles of the group approach to neurotic disorders imply an inescapable economic and industrial meaning. May I, then, suggest that in an enquiry into the relation of the individual to the group, we are straightaway launched upon a consideration of a sociological psychiatry or, more specifically, upon a consideration of an industrial psychiatry.

I am using the word industrial to imply the broad field of the inter-individual reactions of the layman as against the specialist and his professional position. In speaking of group analysis as combining and unifying the field of the psychiatrist as specialist on the one hand, and the everyday field of human industry as the field of the layman on the other, the union I refer to will not be comprehended in the ordinary terms of agreement. For the union I have in mind between the field of psychiatry and the field of industry is one of *physiological* synthesis. But to speak of a physiological synthesis in a social or inter-individual sense calls for a preliminary statement in explanation of the phylogenetic basis upon which this synthesis rests.

The organism of man, as a phylum, race or society, is composed of individual elements that have basically an identical structure throughout. In their biological composition, they represent the same substance, muscle for muscle, bone for bone. This continuity, which is shown throughout the species in its structural features, has its counterpart in a basic *identity* of instincts and feeling reactions. But with man's attainment of the faculty of abstraction and his use of the symbol or of language, there was automatically invented a totally new medium of continuity. With the emergence of the symbol and of language, there arose a form of social continuity and interchange in which the elements or individuals of the species now depended for their agreement among one another precisely upon the *differences* in the meaning or content connoted by the symbols or abstractions employed by them.

In this situation, in which there is introduced an intercommunication between individuals through the medium of abstraction or of the symbol, the set of reactions which is brought into play inter-individually is very different physiologically from the set of physiological reactions which existed inter-individually among us before the introduction of the abstraction or symbol. In the process through which part of an object is selected to represent the whole object through the medium of the sign or symbol, it is only the external projective senses—the sense of vision and the auditory sense, together with the laryngeal sense or the sense of articulation—that are brought into operation, so that communication is now mediated inter-physiologically among the elements of the species through an inter-cerebral continuity or chain of contact that is abstractive or part-functional. Through this developmental achievement, man established a vast system of mental or symbolic intercommunication which is secondary and psychological, and which is physiologically wholly distinct from the original intercommunication that existed between individual organisms in the primary reaction of the organism as a whole. This disparity between the two systems of reactions existing in our human communities—between the primary physiological and the secondary psychological system—has not been clearly recognised, and, consequently, in our efforts toward the adjustment of human relationships, personal and social, we are unconsciously subject to the utmost confusion in determining those expressions that belong to men's interchange as instinctive societal organisms on the one hand and as abstractive social individuals on the other.

It is a practical circumstance worthy of note that group analysis had its actual beginning in the work of a small community composed partly of physicians and professional persons and partly of lay students of different avocations. In this small nucleus, there was offered a sociological setting in which the factors represented in psychiatry and those represented in the lay or industrial community were united in a co-operative analysis.

I should especially like to make clear at the outset, however, that the method of group-analysis is not so named because the procedure is carried on by groups of people. This circumstance is really wholly accidental and subsidiary. "Group" merely means the integral or inclusive method characteristic of the laboratory as it relates the function of the individual organism to the community or species as a whole. As the method concerns the species as a whole or the interreactions of individuals as components of the race or phylum, in order to avoid a needless confusion of meaning, I have recently substituted the term "phyloanalysis" to replace the original term "group-analysis". The meaning of "group" in the collective sense should be carefully distinguished from "group" in its integral or inclusive meaning. The former applies to the imitative automatisms of our secondary, psychological adaptations, the latter to the spontaneous physiological reactions of the organism as a whole, such as are the basis of man's conscious, creative individuality. The group method, then, or phyloanalysis, attempts to study the sensations and reactions of the individual as the expression of reactions and sensations which are continuous throughout society as a unitary social organism. Phyloanalysis as a laboratory basis implies a phylogenetic premise or, more specifically, it implies a *physiology of affect considered as a racial phenomenon.*[4]

II

Science is the study of observable phenomena through objective methods of investigation. Phyloanalysis views all subjective disturbance or mental disease arising from psychogenic causes as the absence of the application of an objective method in dealing with subjective phenomena. But it regards this inadequacy as characterising equally the mental habits of normal groups as of pathological subjects. Its scope, therefore, is phyletic and its method is applicable to the processes of society at large. It should be emphasised that, like the science of bacteriology or any other science, phyloanalysis is primarily a method of observation and adjustment; it is not primarily a cure. To make clear what I mean: the remedy for religious obsession does not lie in any form of so-called curative agency. Religious obsession—I am speaking, of course, of symbolic religion—is a disease inseparable from its symbolic religious premise. The elimination of religious obsession, with its symbolic, subjective prepossessions, is effected only through the introduction of a method that is not subjective and symbolic but is biological and objective. When we examine phyloanalytically the industrial or social mind in its so-called normal activities, we find that its processes rest not upon objective observation, but upon symbolic prepossessions and beliefs.[5] It is important, then, to keep in mind that in the present thesis we are dealing no less with normal than with neurotic symbols and that the position of the social image or normal symbol is of basic significance in this study.

I hope that this preliminary effort of explanation is of assistance. The matter of terminology in dealing with the relation of the individual to the group is important, but at the moment I can expect hardly more than to attempt to make clear, if possible, the few basic terms that are inseparable from our topic. By *phyloanalysis*, then, I mean the observation of the integral elements represented in the individuals of the species as typical of the function of the species as a whole. By the words *industry* and *industrialism*, I mean the everyday world of the layman in his inter-individual, living-making reactions, as these reactions refer to society as a unitary organism. And by the term *physiological*, I mean man's subjective, inter-individual reactions, as these reactions may be correlated under a general principle of sensation represented in the feeling continuity of man's organism as a race or phylum.

Let me make still clearer, if I can, my meaning of the term physiological. In his study of the emotions in men and animals Darwin[6] has indicated the general physiological basis of emotional reactions. The fascinating thesis presented in the James–Lange theory of the emotions served further to clinch the biological method of attack with its prior emphasis, you recall, upon the organic reaction. The heart does not beat faster because we are frightened, but we are frightened because the heart beats faster. We do not weep because we are sad, but we are sad because we weep. This is not a trick of logic. It is bedrock physiology. For the biological concomitant of the emotion experienced subjectively as grief (whether prior or synchronous is not here to the point) is represented in physiological reactions and release—muscular, visceral, vaso-motor—which, in their general character and distribution, are specific to the emotion of grief. If you will note the external features expressive of this physiological reaction, it is clear that this reaction is by no means confined to the shedding of tears. The whole physiognomy is distorted with muscular spasm, the chest is contracted, the muscles of the abdomen and the shoulders show convulsive movements, and the whole picture presents a regressive appearance. But, *in its essential physiological expression, the reaction is uniform and consistent.*

The *mental concomitant* of the grief reaction, on the other hand, that is, the symbolic, social expressions arising from the secondary psychological system, are *infinitely varied and arbitrary*. Let us suppose that a man has lost his wife to whom he is devoted. Under these circumstances, there may be presented any one of a whole series of reactions corresponding to his social or psychological response. He might withdraw into retirement, he might get drunk, he might become angry at the undeservedness of his fate, he might endow a hospital, he might seek diversion in Havana, he might take unto himself another wife, or he may up and shoot himself. In fact, he might adopt all these reactions and many more.

Or let us take the situation of the psychiatric patient presenting a depression. One patient will explain his state of mind on the ground that he has lost interest in his work, another that his wife no longer loves him, another that he has an incurable disorder, another explains it on the ground of his moral unfitness and of wishing only to destroy himself, another that his children are starving, another that he thinks he has committed an unpardonable offence, and so on *ad infinitum*. These reactions of different individuals are like the different reactions of the single individual who has lost his wife. That is, they are *varied and unpredictable* in their expression.

III

Let us consider these social and biologic implications in their more intimate aspects. You will recall that in the primary physiological reaction of fear cited by Darwin—the fear expressed by man or beast in the jungle—these reactions were in the nature of a protective reaction to the organism. The taut, hard muscles, the stiff, erect hair, were the expression of a defence mechanism. So, in man, similar reactions, together with the blanched anaemic surface, were all reactions calculated to conserve the life of the organism against attack. Thus, the reactions of fear cited by Darwin are, both for the individual and for the race, conservative organic reactions. They are expressions that belong to the primary physiological system of the organism.

There is, however, another expression of fear, which I should like to describe—an expression of fear which is human and social and which belongs solely to the secondary psychological system of our inter-individual reactions. This fear-reaction invites an attitude of suspicion and antagonism, of disaffection and resistance, of unproductive competition or sentimental dependence in both the individual and the community. In our industrial interrelationships, this secondary fear reaction serves useful biological aim. It does not operate to protect either the individual or the group in its industrial or social expression but, on the contrary, is an obstruction to those economic and industrial processes which may serve for the survival of civilised man.

We shall be helped by an examination of this secondary psychological mechanism in its elemental source within the individual, for it is here that there is disclosed the symbolic and pseudo-industrial nature of this reaction. The first movements of the child toward his environment arise from the primary physiological system, that is, they arise prior to the individual's adoption of language or the secondary psychological system. These primary movements of the child in its relation to the community and to its objective environment are a species of industrialism. They are activities of investigation and of adaptation such as will, with accumulated experience, fit him eventually for making his living in a socially interrelated scheme of enterprise and activity. It is noteworthy, though, that the individual's first movements represent the unchecked expression of the primary organism as a whole. *It means that man's first industrial impulse arises from the primary physiological system.*

Concomitant, however, with his growth and with the widening of his excursions of investigation, the child meets with certain interdictions from the social community about him. The community speaks from its secondary psychological system. It encroaches upon the child's primary movements through inculcating certain precepts and through encouraging him toward certain actions which the community calls "right" and it discourages his tendency toward other movements which the community calls "wrong".[7] That is, the child is taught to fear to do "wrong" or to fear not to do "right". Please observe that it is not the interdiction to this or that act to which I am calling attention. The animals, as we know, promptly intercept certain tendencies of reaction in their young. But they do so on the basis of their natural physiological communication, not through the interposition of a symbolic or secondary psychological system.[8]

If we will examine the physiological situation occurring in the child, we shall see that what takes place is something like this: first, there is an extraneous check upon the infant organism which inhibits its spontaneous expression as a whole. Physiologically, the child's reaction becomes limited to a cerebral plane of reactions. The tension of the organism becomes abstractive, delimited, discriminative. That is, following this check, the child is admonished to *hear* what is *said* to him and to *look* and *see* what action will be approved by the community whose code of behaviour is derived from the secondary psychological system of symbols and language. In this procedure, emphasis is placed upon the organism's part-physiology to the exclusion of the whole or primary physiology of the child—upon the ocular, auditory, and laryngeal part-functions to the exclusion of the whole organism. This check or impediment to the primary or whole physiological impulse of the child is cumulative throughout the course of his growth and development as an element in a social and industrial community. As this check or impediment affects all individuals in their primary industrial activity, it affects the activity of the industrial community as a whole. Here, you see, is presented a condition that is physiological and which at the same time bears directly upon man's social economy. It is thus a socio-physiological condition.[9]

We have seen that there is physiologically but one grief reaction, and that this reaction is unified and constant, while psychologically the expressions of grief are infinite in their variety. In the same way, there are psychologically an infinity variety of induced social fear reactions occurring inter-individually, but man's social fear as variously expressed in his inter-individual reactions likewise possesses only one basic and consistent reaction physiologically. In other words, the expressions of fear arising from the secondary psychological system, in response to which one must *see* what is socially approved before acting, are entirely arbitrary, variable, and unpredictable. Yet, as is the case with the manifold reactions of depression or grief, there exists an underlying physiological concomitant to these manifold social fear expressions which is unified and constant and which lends itself to scientific observation and adjustment.

This reaction of right and wrong, this reaction of social fear, is of enormous complexity and variability in its mental content. Its social ramifications are infinite in extent and in their varying modifications. Like the patients whom we have cited with their various mental explanations, or the normal individual in his grief, the social individual may interpret this emotion of right, or fear-conduct in all manner of ways. In reference to himself, he might feel that it is right that he live up to certain professional standards, that it is right that he make certain donations to charity, that it is right that he be faithful to his wife, that he observe the various civic ordinances, that he attend services in his particular church, and so on and so on. He has also definite feelings of right with respect to the conduct of others. He has feelings of what constitutes right conduct in his wife and his children, as to what they should do and should not do. He has feelings of what is right in the conduct of his employees, his servants. But again, like the neurotic patient, *his various mental accounts of this emotional right are infinitely varied, while the physiological concomitant to these mental expressions is unitary and consistent.*

In the efforts of the physician to remedy the emotional disturbances occurring in the mentally ill patient and in the efforts of sociologists and educators to remedy the various social, political, economic, and industrial conflicts occurring within the community and throughout the nation, the remedy has always been applied to the disharmonies occurring in the secondary psychological system, to the *manifest content of consciousness*[10] as expressed in the various arbitrary and unconscious expression of the individual and the community. On the other hand, the group or phyletic procedure, abrogating the various inconstant and arbitrary *mental* reactions that occur in neurotic and normal individuals, addresses itself directly to the inherent *physiological* situation. For the physiological substrate is constant; the mental account is inconstant. The physiological substrate is specific and invariably concerns the intrinsic relation of the individual to himself and to others of the community in their basic interreactions; that is, this substrate is not only specific and physiological, it is socio-physiological.

It has been the finding of the laboratory of phyloanalysis that the neurosis, whether individual or social, has to do with the habitual substitution of this secondary psychological system for the primary, physiological system of man's reaction and with the consequent blocking and distortion of his essential feeling-life. It is its finding that the neurosis of man is due to the unconscious encroachment of a wholly symbolic, pseudo-industrial system of reactions upon the system of physiological interrelationships that represents man's true industrial economy.

Further, it is the experimental finding of the group or phyletic method of study that it is possible to approach the emotional factors operative in our inter-individual or social relationships only as we approach their direct physiological expressions as experienced subjectively by the individual in his immediate reactions to his immediate group setting. To do this, it is necessary to discount the infinite and unending variety of social fear-expressions that are the mere emanations of the secondary psychological system, expressions which can only release in the ever-present and obsessive tendency to social and intellectual discussions, and approach directly the primary and basic physiological reaction of social fear as it underlies these manifold superficial expressions.

This does not mean that more emphasis is placed upon physiology and less upon psychology. On the contrary, phyloanalysis tends more and more to obliterate the empty distinction between "physiological" and "psychological" as separate part-expressions, just as, happily, it also obliterates the tedious and phantastic part-expressions represented in the opposed positions of structuralist and functionalist. And this it does through emphasising the reaction of the *whole organism in its function as a whole.* As yet, we have not felt the random and socially uneconomic nature of our secondary psychological procedure—of our obsessive pursuit of the arbitrary, symbolic, "mental" symptom. Man's powerful mental or symbolic habituations are such that he has failed to realise that in this recourse he is pursuing adventitious images and symbols and that these images, however current socially and psychologically, are quite secondary to a basic socio-physiological situation. If, in the biological evolution of man, he has unwittingly placed over-emphasis upon a part-development, upon his social, symbolic, or abstractive, development, our recourse in lifting the burden of this negative one-sided situation consists in turning to the seat of the major distortion, to man's subjective physiology or to his affective experiences as a race or phylum.

The discrepancy existing between those reactions which rest upon the continuity of basic instinctive feelings and those reactions which rest upon acknowledged differences of sensation, as symbolically agreed among different individuals, represents an inter-physiological situation among the elements of the species in their relation to one another. Only a physiological approach to such physiologically divergent behaviour patterns makes possible an analysis and resolution of this conflict, whether it appears in the neurotic and isolated individual or in the social and industrial group, whether in the personal neurosis and insanity of the single individual or whether in social crime and in international war.

The technique of phyloanalysis, then, is adapted to the specific function of differentiating between these two major programmes of reaction as they occur within the individual and the community. It is its function to afford a means through which individuals and groups may learn to differentiate between reactions that are organic and reactions that are symbolic, between reactions that tend to preserve the health of the individual and of the species and reactions which, in their cerebral or symbolic function, tend only to foster conflict and disorder in the individual and the community. The sensations recorded in various visceral, muscular, and vaso-motor tensions and strains are characteristic and specific to each system of reactions. These subjective sensations are as susceptible to objective observation as other perceptible phenomena in the objective world. But in the absence of an objective discrimination between these two contrasting systems, as subjectively perceptible in the internal balances and tensions pertaining to each, the society of man confuses its feeling reactions and interrelations throughout and, under the form of mere symbols of secondary adoption, places upon itself economic and industrial burdens which are wholly artificial and symbolic and which, therefore, lack a basis of scientific observation and control.

IV

In conclusion, let me say that, in principle, the method of analysis that is phyletic is not in any sense new. It was employed by Darwin fully seventy years ago in his biological analysis of structural forms, but, even with Darwin, the method was merely an emphasising and correlating of principles more or less vaguely apprehended by man from time immemorial, that is, principles bearing upon the intrinsic continuity between the part and the whole within the organic sphere. Neither is the application of the biological or phyletic method in the sphere of human conduct new. In my very first acquaintance with the teaching of Adolf Meyer some twenty years ago, what impressed me was the fact that here was the application of definite principles of biology to mental and social disharmonies. In Meyer's study of the individual patient, it was not the individual alone that he saw before him, but a socially integrated situation that related the individual to the community as a whole.[11] The entire impetus of the school of psychiatry that originated with Meyer and is represented in the work of MacFie Campbell, of Kirby, Henderson, MacCurdy, Syz, and others lies precisely in the generic and inclusive inferences derived from the specific data under observation. Even in my very earliest acquaintance with the field of psychiatry, which I owe to Stewart Paton, the method rigidly enforced by him was distinctly that which related the biological growth and development of the individual to principles inherent in the species. Likewise, throughout the work of all of our modern psychiatrists—the work of White, Jelliffe, Brill, Clark, Kempf, Sullivan, Wholey, and others—one sees always this firm adherence to intrinsic biological principles. So, with regard to principles, I can claim nothing new for the scientific principle represented in phyloanalysis.

When, under the stimulus, of Meyer, I undertook the study and the application of psychoanalysis to the problems of individual adjustment, it was inevitable that I should apply to the analytic field, with its latent manifestations of man's consciousness, the same underlying principles I had learnt from Meyer. But even the specific development of my analytic work from these principles and its insistence upon the subjective nature of the problem in hand does not allow me to make any claim for its originality. I did not discover the specific method of group analysis, as employed by me now for many years. This innovation was due to quite accidental and incidental social causes, which, however, must be understood to be definitely traceable to the biological principles that I had learnt from my predecessors in the field of psychiatry.

This specific incident and its social development had its setting primarily in the social relationship of the two individuals represented, on the one hand, by myself and, on the other, by my assistant, Mr Clarence Shields, and it had to do specifically with the relationship between the two individuals from the point of view of their industrial or economic interreactions. The association of my assistant and myself in a joint social analysis was subsequently augmented through the participation of others, students and patients, normal and neurotic, professional as well as lay individuals. Here, the stage was set for a significant sociological development, because it presented in miniature the social situation represented in both the normal community and in the individual neurotic.

This research project, beginning with the symbolic analysis of the single individual and extending to the phyletic analysis, first of two persons and then to groups of ten and twenty, finally developed into efforts of adjustment of inter-individual problems which, more and more, manifested themselves as inseparable from the processes and problems of the community at large. At the same time, the increasing recognition on the part of certain members of the community of the continuity between their industrial situation and the industrial conflict expressed in the neuroses and in insanity have coalesced into a research setting that unites our objective problems and our subjective conflicts toward a common synthesis and solution.

Concomitantly with the increasing poignancy of this industrial and social situation, there has been slowly forming a community organisation that, under the name of The Lifwynn Foundation, attempts to mark the beginning of an industrial community psychiatry. Abrogating the manifold suggestions and symptoms which comprise the manifest content of man's social consciousness, the organisation represented in The Lifwynn Foundation[12] strives through its laboratory approach to our subjective problems to bring to recognition those destructive reactions which comprise man's latent social affects. These latent social affects of man are not only the embodiment of those conditions which bear directly upon the normal relationships of the individual and the social group from the point of view of the neurosis; they represent a socio-physiological condition that forms the crux of man's social disharmonies generally.

The problem, then, for sociologists, as for psychiatrists, is that of distinguishing clearly between the system that is secondary, psychological or symbolic, and the system that is primary, physiological and phyletic. Phyloanalysis traces to the confusion between these two systems the serious havoc in the emotional life of the individual expressed in the neuroses and in insanity, and, through the controlled observation of the interreactions observable in social groups, phyloanalysis has arrived at findings which give indication that such social disorders as occur among us economically and industrially in the sinister outbursts of crime and of war are likewise traceable to the disparity existing socially between these two systems of man's organism. We have need, therefore, to see that man is faced with a conflict that is characteristic not only of the isolated neurotic, but that is endemic to society at large, and that only a radical social approach to this social disharmony may effect an adjustment of our individual, community, and national disorders.

Notes

1. Read before the Section on Sociology and Psychiatry, at the twenty-fourth annual meeting of the American Sociological Society, Washington, DC, December 30, 1929. Published with acknowledgment to *The American Journal of Sociology*.

2. I would like to make very clear that the terms *industry* and *industrialism* as they occur in this paper are not used in the specialized sense in which the industrialist employs these terms. What is here meant is the quite primary physiological industry or industrialism of the race of man in his ordinary interests and activities. The word *occupational* has been suggested, but, for the physician, this carries definite psychotherapeutic connotations which quite preclude its application here. If in my sense of the term I seem to be stretching unduly a quite fixed usage, I hope I may be pardoned this transgression, as in the present study no other term seems to express my meaning half so adequately.
3. Other writings by the author in a similar trend may assist the reader in understanding the present thesis, so that, where it seemed apt, reference has been made to these earlier studies.
4. "The physiological basis of neurosis and dream—a societal interpretation of the sensori-motor reactions reflected in insanity and crime", *The Journal of Social Psychology*, *I*(1), February 1930.
5. "Biological foundations and mental methods", *The British Journal of Medical Psychology*, *VIII*, Part I, 1928; "The autonomy of the 'I' from the standpoint of group analysis, *Psyche*, *VIII*(3), January 1928.
6. Darwin, C., *The Expression of the Emotions in Man and Animals*, London, 1873.
7. "The social reaction of right and wrong—a biological approach to criminal behavior": paper read before the Section on Legal Psychology, The Ninth International Congress of Psychology, held at Yale University, 3 Sept 1929.
8. *The Social Basis of Consciousness*, New York: Harcourt Brace, 1927, pp. 51–61.
9. "The basis of group-analysis, or the analysis of the reactions of normal and neurotic individuals", *The British Journal of Medical Psychology*, *VIII*, Part 3, 1928; Syz, Hans C., "On a social approach to neurotic conditions", *The Journal of Nervous and Mental Disease*, *66*(6), December 1927; Syz, Hans C., "Remarks on group analysis", *American Journal of Psychiatry*, *VIII*(1), July 1928.
10. Freud, Sigmund, Die Traumdeutung, Leipzig and Wien: Franz Deuticke, 1900.
11. Meyer, Adolf, "The problems of mental reaction-types, mental causes and diseases", *The Psychological Bulletin*, *V*,(8), August 1908; Meyer, Adolf, "The dynamic interpretation of dementia praecox", *The American Journal of Psychiatry*, *21*, 1910; Meyer, Adolf, "The contributions of psychiatry to the understanding of life problems": address delivered at the celebration

of the One Hundredth Anniversary of Bloomingdale Hospital, 26 May 1921; Meyer, Adolf, "Inter-relations of the domains of neuropsychiatry", *Archives of Neurology and Psychiatry, VII*(3), 1922.

12. The term foundation generally implies an organisation that is financially maintained through munificent endowment. The Lifwynn Foundation, however, is one whose resources consist solely in the affiliated efforts of its participants, whether with or without financial revenue, to establish a nuclear community process in industrial integration and social growth.

REFERENCES

Abse, D. W. (1990). Trigant Burrow and the inauguration of group analysis in the U.S.A. Talk for Dorothea Dix Hospital, Raleigh, North Carolina. September, 20, 1990. Reworked version of: Trigant Burrow and the inauguration of group analysis in the U.S.A. *Group Analysis*, 1979, *12*: 218–229.

Ackerman, N. (1964). Foreword. In: T. Burrow, *Preconscious Foundations of Human Experience* (pp. v–xvi), W. E. Galt (Ed.). New York: Basic Books.

Alexander, F., Eisenstein, F., & Grotjahn, M. (Eds.) (1966). *Psychoanalytic Pioneers*. New York: Basic Books [reprinted New Brunswick, NJ: Transaction, 1995].

Ancona, L. (1983). I fondamenti della gruppoanalisi (The basis of group analysis). In: F. Di Maria & G. Lo Verso (Eds.), *Il piccolo gruppo. Verso una fondazione epistemologica* (The Small Group. Toward an Epistemological Foundation) (pp. 69–88). Rome: Bulzoni.

Ancona, L. (1996). Psicoanalisi e gruppo-analisi a confronto (Psychoanalysis and group analysis. A confrontation). *Gli Argonauti*, *18* (68): 29–47.

Ancona, L. (2007). Personal communication (audio-recorded) to E. Gatti Pertegato, 16 March 2007.

Anderson, S. (1919). *Winesburg, Ohio*. In: *Enciclopedia Europea*, 1976, Vol. I. Milan: Garzanti.

Anderson, S. (1921). *Seeds*. In: *The Triumph of the Egg* (pp. 21–24). New York: B. W. Huebsch.

Anthony, J. (1971). The history of group psychotherapy. In: H. I. Kaplan & B. I. Sadock (Eds.), *Comprehensive Group Psychotherapy* (pp. 4–31) Baltimore, MD: Williams & Wilkins.

Babini, V. P. (2009a). *Liberi tutti. Manicomi e psichiatri in Italia: una storia del Novecento* (All Free. Mental Hospitals and Psychiatrists in Italy: A History of the Twentieth Century). Bologne: Il Mulino.

Babini, V. P. (2009b). Psichiatria in tre movimenti (Psychiatry in three movements). *Psicoterapia e Scienze Umane, XLIII*(4): 463–490.

Basaglia, F. (Ed.) (1968). *L'istituzione negata. Rapporto da un ospedale psichiatrico* (The Denied Institution. Report from a Psychiatric Hospital). Turin: Einaudi [reprinted Milan: B. C. Dalai, 2010].

Behr, H. (2004). Commentary on "Two early experimenters with groups" by R. D. Hinshelwood. *Group Analysis, 37*(3): 333–338.

Behr, H. (2011). Why is the past important in group analysis? *Group Analysis, 44*(4): 454–465.

Behr, H., & Hearst, L. (2005). *Group-Analytic Psychotherapy. A Meeting of Minds*. London: Whurr.

Bender, L. (1979). Paul Schilder's contribution to group therapy. In: L. R. Wolberg & M. L. Aronson (Eds.), *Group Therapy. An Overview* (pp. 1–9). New York: Stratton Intercontinental, Medical Book Corporation.

Berne, E. (1963). *The Structure and Dynamics of Organizations and Groups*. Philadelphia, PA: Lippincott.

Binswanger, L. (1944). *Il caso Ellen West*. Milano: SE, 2001.

Binswanger, L. (1955). La concezione eraclitea dell'uomo. In: *Per un'antropologia fenomenologica. Saggi e conferenze psichiatriche* (pp. 91–124). Feltrinelli: Milano 1970, 3rd edn, 2007.

Binswanger, L. (1956). *Ricordi di Sigmund Freud*. Rome: Astrolabio, 1971.

Binswanger, L. (1965). *Delirio. Antropoanalisi e fenomenologia*, E. Borgna (Ed.). Padua: Marsilio, 1990.

Bion, W. (1961). *Experiences in Groups and Other Papers*. London: Tavistock.

Bollas, C. (1987). *The Shadow of the Object*. London: Free Association Books. [reprinted New York: Columbia University Press, 1989]. Quoted in: Mitchell, S. A. (1993).

Borgna, E. (1990). La fenomenologia husserliana e l'ontologia heideggeriana in Ludwig Binswanger (Husserl's Phenomenology and Heidegger's Onthology in Ludwig Binswanger). In: L. Binswanger (1965), *Delirio. Antropoanalisi e fenomenologia* (pp. vii-xxviii). E. Borgna (Ed.). Padua: Marsilio, 1990.

Borgna, E. (1994). La storia dolorosa e straziata di Suzanne Urban (Suzanne Urban's sad and lacerating story). In: L. Binswanger (1952) *Il caso di Suzanne Urban* (pp. 9–21) . E. Borgna, & M. Galzigna (Eds). Padua: Marsilio.

Borgogno, F., & Calorio, D. (1976). Fondazione dell'analisi di gruppo. L'opera di Trigant Burrow (The foundation of group analysis. Trigant Burrow's work). *Psicologia e Lavoro, XI*(42): 25–51.

Brill, A. A. (1913). The conception of homosexuality. *Journal of the American Medical Association, 61*(5): 335–340.

Brown, D. (2001). A contribution to the understanding of the social unconscious. *Group Analysis, 34*(1): 29–38.

Brown, D., & Zinkin, L. (1994). Preface. In: D. Brown & L. Zinkin (Eds.) (1964). *The Psyche and the Social World.* London: Routledge.

Burnham, J. C. (1946–1950). *Dictionary of American Biography,* Suppl. Four. New York: Charles Scribner's Sons.

Burnshaw, S. (1970). *The Seamless Web.* New York: George Braziller.

Burnshaw, S. (1984). Introduction. In: T. Burrow (1984), *Toward Social Sanity and Human Survival* (pp. vii–xiv), A. S. Galt (Ed.). New York: Horizon Press.

Burrow, T. (1909). *The Determination of the Position of a Momentary Impression in the Temporal Course of a Moving Visual Impression. The Psychological Review,* Monograph Series, Vol. XI, No. 4.

Burrow, T. (1911). Freud's psychology in its relation to the neuroses. *American Journal of the Medical Sciences, 141:* 873–882.

Burrow, T. (1913). Psychoanalysis and life. Unpublished. Read before the New York Academy of Medicine, October 14th, 1913. By courtesy of Alfreda Sill Galt, president of the Lifwynn Foundation, Westport CT, to Edi Gatti Pertegato, April 1993.

Burrow, T. (1914a). Character and the neurosis. *Psychoanalytic Review, I*(2): 121–128.

Burrow, T. (1914b). The psychoanalyst and the community. *Journal of the American Medical Association, 62*: 1876–1878.

Burrow, T. (1917a). The genesis and meaning of "homosexuality" and its relation to the problem of introverted mental states. *Psychoanalytic Review, 4*: 272–284.

Burrow, T. (1917b). Notes with reference to Freud, Jung and Adler. *Journal of Abnormal Psychology, 12*: 161–167.

Burrow, T. (1918). The origin of the incest-awe. *Psychoanalytic Review, V*(3): 243–254.

Burrow, T. (1924). Social images versus reality. *Journal of Abnormal Psychology and Social Psychology, 19*(3): 230–235.

Burrow, T. (1925a). A relative concept of consciousness. An analysis of consciousness in its ethnic origin. *Psychoanalytic Review*, *12*(1): 1–15.

Burrow, T. (1925b). Letter of 3/4/1925 to S. Freud. In: *Trigant Burrow Papers*. New Haven, CT: Yale University Library, Manuscript and Archives, & in Burrow, T. (1958), *A Search for Man's Sanity. The Selected Letters of Trigant Burrow*, W. E. Galt (Ed.). New York: Oxford University Press.

Burrow, T. (1925c). Letter of September 5, 1925 to Hans Syz. In: Burrow, T. (1958), *A Search for Man's Sanity. The Selected Letters of Trigant Burrow* (pp. 110–111), W. E. Galt (Ed.). New York: Oxford University Press.

Burrow, T. (1926a). The laboratory method in psychoanalysis, its inception and development. *American Journal of Psychiatry*, *5*(3): 345–355.

Burrow, T. (1926b). Psychoanalysis in theory and in life. *Journal of Nervous and Mental Disease*, *64*(3): 209–224.

Burrow, T. (1926c). Our mass neurosis. *Psychological Bulletin*, *23*(6): 305–312.

Burrow, T. (1926d). Psychoanalytic improvisations and the personal equation. *Psychoanalytic Review*, 1926, *XIII*(2): 173–186.

Burrow, T. (1927a). *The Social Basis of Consciousness*. New York: Harcourt, Brace, International Library of Psychology.

Burrow, T. (1927b). The group method of analysis. *Psychoanalytic Review*, *XIV*(3): 268–280.

Burrow, T. (1927c). The problem of the transference. *British Journal of Medical Psychology*, 1927, *VII* (part II): 193–202.

Burrow, T. (1927d). Speaking of resistances. *Psyche* (London), *7*(3): 20–27.

Burrow, T. (1927e). Letter to D. H. Lawrence. Florence, Italy; February 7, 1927. In: Burrow, T. (1958), *A Search for Man's Sanity. The Selected Letters of Trigant Burrow* (pp. 163–164), W. E. Galt (Ed.). New York: Oxford University Press.

Burrow, T. (1927f). Letter to D. H. Lawrence. Florence, Italy; December 21, 1927. In: Burrow, T. (1958), *A Search for Man's Sanity. The Selected Letters of Trigant Burrow* (pp. 195–196), W. E. Galt (Ed.). New York: Oxford University Press.

Burrow, T. (1927g). Letter to D. H. Lawrence. Florence, Italy; September 9, 1927. In Burrow, T. (1958), *A Search for Man's Sanity. The Selected Letters of Trigant Burrow* (pp. 184–187), W. E. Galt (Ed.). New York: Oxford University Press.

Burrow, T. (1927h). Letter to Leo Stein, December 29, 1927. In: Burrow T. (1958), *A Search for Man's Sanity. The Selected Letters of Trigant Burrow* (pp. 196–197), W. E. Galt (Ed.). New York: Oxford University Press.

Burrow, T. (1928a). The elements of group analysis. Unpublished. In The Trigant Burrow Papers, the Manuscript Department, Yale University Library, New Haven, CT.

Burrow, T. (1928b). The basis of group analysis, or the analysis of the reactions of normal and neurotic individuals. *British Journal of Medical Psychology*, *8*(3): 198–206.

Burrow, T. (1928c). The autonomy of the 'I' from the standpoint of group analysis. *Psyche* (London), *8*(3): 35–50.

Burrow, T. (1930). So called 'normal' social relationships expressed in the individual and the group, and their bearing on the problems of neurotic disharmonies. *American Journal of Psychiatry*, *X*(I): 101–116.

Burrow, T. (1931). Letter to Goodwin B. Watson. March 21, 1931. In: Burrow, T. (1958), *A Search for Man's Sanity. The Selected Letters of Trigant Burrow*, W. E. Galt (Ed.). New York: Oxford University Press.

Burrow, T. (1933). A phylogenetic sudy of insanity in its underlying morphology. *Journal of the American Medical Association*, *100*: 648–651.

Burrow, T. (1934). Letter of June 18, 1934 to Leo Stein, Florence, Italy. In: Burrow, T. (1958), *A Search for Man's Sanity. The Selected Letters of Trigant Burrow*, W. E. Galt (Ed.). New York: Oxford University Press.

Burrow, T. (1935). Neuropathology and the internal environment: a study of the neuromuscular factors in attention and their bearing upon man's disorders of adaptation. *Human Biology*, *7*: 74–94 [reprinted in: T. Burrow (1937). *The Biology of Human Conflict: An Anatomy of Human Behavior Individual and Social*. New York: Macmillan].

Burrow, T. (1937a). *The Biology of Human Conflict: An Anatomy of Human Behavior Individual and Social*. New York: Macmillan.

Burrow, T. (1937b). The law of the organism: a neuro-social approach to the problems of human behavior. *American Journal of Sociology*, *42*: 814–824.

Burrow, T. (1941). Kimograph records of neuromuscular (respiratory) patterns in relation to behavior disorders. *Psychosomatic Medecine*, *3*: 174–186.

Burrow, T. (1942). Letter to F. J. Hoffman, The Ohio State University, October 2, 1942. In Burrow, T. (1958), *A Search for Man's Sanity. The Selected Letters of Trigant Burrow* (pp. 442–443), W. E. Galt (Ed.). New York: Oxford University Press..

Burrow, T. (1943). The neurodynamics of behaviour: a phylobiological foreword. *Philosophy of Science*, *10*: 271–288.

Burrow, T. (1945). Electroencephalographic recordings of varying aspects of attention in relation to behavior (with William E. Galt). *Journal of General Psychology*, *32*: 269–288.

Burrow, T. (1948). Letter to Stanley Pargellis. The Newberry Library, Chicago. January 22, 1948, In: Burrow, T. (1958), *A Search for Man's Sanity. The Selected Letters of Trigant Burrow*, W. E. Galt (Ed.). New York: Oxford University Press.

Burrow, T. (1949a). Letter to Thomas Sancton of September 28, 1949, New Orleans. In: Burrow, T. (1958), *A Search for Man's Sanity. The Selected Letters of Trigant Burrow* (pp. 580–584), W. E. Galt (Ed.). New York: Oxford University Press.

Burrow, T. (1949b). Letter to William Phillips. The University of Chicago. March 4, 1949. In: Burrow, T. (1958), *A Search for Man's Sanity. The Selected Letters of Trigant Burrow* (pp. 558–560), W. E. Galt (Ed.). New York: Oxford University Press.

Burrow, T. (1950). *The Neurosis of Man. An Introduction to a Science of Human Behavior*. New York: Harcourt, Brace [reprinted New York: Philosophical Library, 1953].

Burrow, T. (1953). *Science and Man's Behavior*, W. E. Galt (Ed.). New York: Philosophical Library.

Burrow, T. (1958). *A Search for Man's Sanity. The Selected Letters of Trigant Burrow*, W. E. Galt (Ed.). New York: Oxford University Press.

Burrow, T. (1964). Introduction. An unreckoned element. In: W. E. Galt (Ed.), *Preconscious Foundations of Human Experience* (pp. 1–6). New York: Basic Books.

Campos Avillar, J. (1990). Un prototipo di modello gruppale per la psicoanalisi: dal 'gruppo a due' fino ai 'gruppi di due più n persone' (A prototype of group model for psychoanalysis: from the 'group of two' to the 'groups of two plus n people'). In: G. M. Pauletta (Ed.), *Modelli psicoanalitici del gruppo* (pp. 65–87) (Psychoanalytical Models of Group). Milan: Guerini & Associati.

Campos Avillar, J. (1992). Editorial note. In: T. Burrow (1932), *The Structure of Insanity: A Study in Phylopathology*. London: Kegan Paul, Trench, Trubner.

Cheney, D., & Seyfarth, R. M. (2007). *Baboon Metaphysics: The Evolution of a Social Mind*. Chicago, IL: Chicago University Press.

Corbella, S. (1988). La terapia di gruppo (Group Therapy). In: A. A. Semi (Ed.), *Trattato di Psicoanalisi*. Vol. I, *Teoria e Tecnica*. (Treatise of Psychoanalysis. Vol. I, Theory and Technique). Milan: Cortina.

Corbella, S. (2004). Il gruppo: ponte tra individuo e società (The group as a bridge between individual and society). *Gli Argonauti, XXVI*(103): 383–402.

Corbella, S. (2006). Un atzeco e il mototaxi. Il gruppo come possibile modello relazionale (An Aztec and the motortaxy: the group as a possible relational model). *Rivista Italiana di Gruppoanalisi, XX*(3): 81–102.

Corbellini, G., & Jervis, G. (2008). *La razionalità negata. Psichiatria e antipsichiatria in Italia* (The Denied Rationality. Psychiatry and Anti Psychiatry in Italy). Turin: Bollati Boringhieri.

Crocket, R. (1999). The Ingrebourne Center and Trigant Burrow: a personal perspective. *Group Analysis, 32*(2): 285–287.

Cuomo, G. (1996). Fabrizio Napolitani. Un profilo (Fabrizio Napolitani. A Profile). *Rivista Italiana di Gruppoanalisi, XI*(1): 11–21.

Cuomo, G. (2006). Ricordando Fabrizio Napolitani (Remembering Fabrizio Napolitani). *Rivista Italiana di Gruppoanalisi, XX*(1): 157–162.

Cuomo, G. (2009). La funzione della 'dramatis persona' nella gruppoanalisi (The function of the 'Dramatis Persona' in Group Analysis). *Rivista Italiana di Gruppoanalisi, XXIII*(1–2): 115–123.

Cuomo, G. (2010). Personal communication to E. Gatti Pertegato of 26 February 2010.

Dalal, F. (1998). *Taking the Group Seriously.* London: Jessica Kingsley.

Dalal, F. (2001). The social unconscious: a post-Foulkesian perspective. *Group Analysis, 34*(4): 539–555.

Darwin, C. (2008). *Evolutionary Writings,* J. A. Secord (Ed.). Oxford: Oxford University Press.

De Maré, P. B. (1972). *Perspectives in Group Psychotherapy: A Theoretical Background.* London: Allen & Unwin.

Di Maria, F., & Formica, I. (2009). *Fondamenti di Gruppoanalisi* (The Foundations of group analysis). Bologna: Il Mulino – Manuali.

Edelman, G. M. (2006). *Second Nature. Brain Science and Human Knowledge.* New Haven, CT: Yale University Press.

Enciclopedia Europea (1976). Vol. II. Milano: Garzanti.

Ettin, M. F. (1992). *Foundations and Application of Group Psychotherapy: A Sphere of Influence.* Boston, MA: Allyn and Bacon [reprinted 2nd edn London: Jessica Kingsley].

Ferenczi, S. (1913). Entwicklungsstufen des Wirklichkeitsinnes. Internationale Zeitschrift für Psychanalise, I. Jahrgang, Heft 2. Marz.

Ferenczi, S. (1916). *Contributions to Psycho-analysis,* E. Jones (Trans.). Boston, MA: Gorham Press.

Foulkes, S. H. (1946). On group analysis. *International Journal of Psycho-analysis, 27*: 46–51.

Foulkes, S. H. (1948). *Introduction to Group Analytic Psychotherapy.* London: Heinemann [reprinted London: Karnac, 3rd impression, 1991].

Foulkes, S. H. (1961). The position of group analysis today with special reference to the role of the Group-Analytic Society (London). Extracts from an address given to the Group Analytic Society, on 31 January 1955. *News and views*, n.1 Reprinted in: S. H. Foulkes, *Selected Papers. Psychoanalysis and Group Analysis* (pp. 146–150). London: Karnac, 1990.

Foulkes, S. H. (1964). *Therapeutic Group Analysis*. London: Allen & Unwin.

Foulkes, S. H. (1973). The group as matrix of the individual's mental life. In: R. L. Wolberg & E. K. Schwarz (Eds.), *Group Therapy: An Overview* (pp. 211–220). New York: Intercontinental Medical Books.

Foulkes, S. H. (1975). *Group Analytic Psychotherapy. Method and Principles*. London: Gordon & Breach [reprinted London: Karnac, 1986, second impression, 1991].

Frank, L. K. (1948). *Society as the Patient*. New Brunswick, NJ: Rudgers University Press.

Freud, S. (1896b). Further remarks on the neuro-psychoses of defence. *S.E., 3*: 159–186. London: Hogarth.

Freud, S. (1913j). The claims of psycho-analysis to scientific interest (Part I). *S.E., 13*: 165–173. London: Hogarth.

Freud, S. (1921c). *Group Psychology and Analysis of the Ego. S.E., 18*: 67–143. London: Hogarth.

Freud, S. (1923b). *The Ego and the Id. S.E., 19*: 3–66. London: Hogarth.

Freud, S. (1926). Letter to Burrow of May 3, 1925. In: *Trigant Burrow Papers*. New Haven CT: Yale University Library, Manuscript and Archives.

Fromm, E. (1990). *L'inconscio sociale. Alienazione, idolatria, sadismo* (The Social Unconscious). Milan: Mondadori, 1992. *Die Entdeckung des gesellschaftlichen Unbewußten: zur Neubestimmung der Psychanalyse.*

Fromm, E. (1991). *I cosiddetti sani. La patologia della normalità* (The Pathology of Normality). Milano: Mondadori, 1996.

Galt, A. S. (1974). Letter of December 9, to Dr. Ralph Crowley, New York City.

Galt, A. S. (1984). Editor's note. In: *Trigant Burrow, Toward Social Sanity and Human Survival: Selections from His Writings* (pp. 1–2), A. S. Galt (Ed.). New York: Horizon Press.

Galt, W. E. (1953). Foreword. In: T. Burrow, *Science and Man's Behavior* (pp. 1–3). New York: Philosophical Library.

Galt, W. E. (1964). Editor's Preface. In: T. Burrow, *Preconscious Foundations of Human Experience* (pp. xvii–xxi), W. E. Galt (Ed.). New York: Basic Books.

Galzigna, M. (1994). Binswanger e la struttura della presenza (Binswanger and the structure of the presence). In: *Il caso di Suzanne Urban* (pp. 23–54). Padua: Marsilio.

Gatti Pertegato, E. (1987). *Dietro la maschera – Sulla formazione del Sé e del falso Sé* (Behind the Mask. On the Formation of True and False Self). Milan: Franco Angeli, 1994, 4th revised edition.

Gatti Pertegato, E. (1994a). Sulle tracce di Trigant Burrow alla ricerca della matrici della gruppoanalisi (On the tracks of Trigant Burrow. Searching for the matrix of group-analysis). *Rivista Italiana di Gruppoanalisi, IX*(1): 9–24.

Gatti Pertegato, E. (1994b). Trigant Burrow tra Freud e Foulkes: la fondazione della gruppoanalisi e trasformazioni epistemologiche della psicoanalisi (Trigant Burrow between Freud and Foulkes: the foundation of group-analysis and epistemological transformations of psychoanalysis). *Rivista Italiana di Gruppoanalisi, 9*(3–4):7–44.

Gatti Pertegato, E. (1999). Trigant Burrow and unearthing the origin of group analysis. *Group Analysis, 32*: 269–284.

Gatti Pertegato, E. (2001a). Il contributo di Trigant Burrow alla psicoanalisi: dalla pulsione alla relazione (Trigant Burrow's contribution to psychoanalysis: from instinct to the relationship). Seminar held at IGAR, Group Analytic Institute, Rome, 12 May.

Gatti Pertegato, E. (2001b). Dalla psicoanalisi alla gruppoanalisi (From psychoanalysis to group analysis). Seminar held at IGAR, Group Analytic Institute, Rome, 9 June.

Gatti Pertegato, E. (2001c). Introduzione. Le dinamiche della psicoterapia di gruppo e la sua applicazione di L. Wender (pp. 13–15). *Rivista Italiana di Gruppoanalisi, XV*(1): 17–25. Introduction. The dynamics of group psychotherapy and its application by L. Wender. *Journal of Nervous and Mental Disorders* (1936), *84*(1): 54–60.

Gatti Pertegato, E. (2005). Le "Otto Proposizioni" della gruppoanalisi di Trigant Burrow: il ruolo dei processi transgenerazionali e transpersonali nel conflitto e nella psicopatologia (Trigant Burrow's "Eight Propositions" of group analysis: the role of transpersonal and transgenerational processes in conflict and psychopathology). Seminar at IGAR, Group Analytic Institute, Rome, 6 May.

Gatti Pertegato, E. (2009a). Riscrittura della storia della gruppoanalisi. E la teoria? Part I: La lunga e sofferta elaborazione della gruppoanalisi. Censure, appropriazioni e distorsioni storiografiche (The rewriting of group analysis' history. And its theory? Part I: The long and suffered elaboration of group analysis, censorships, appropriations and historiographic distortions). *Rivista Italiana di Gruppoanalisi, XXIII*(1–2): 81–100.

Gatti Pertegato, E. (2009b). Riscrittura della storia della gruppoanalisi. E la teoria? Part II: Foulkes e la teoria della gruppoanalisi. Ambiguità e contraddizioni (The rewriting of group analysis' history. And its theory? Part II – Foulkes and the theory of group analysis. Ambiguities and contradictions). *Rivista Italiana di Gruppoanalisi, XXIII*(1–2): 101–113.

Gatti Pertegato, E., & Pertegato, G. O. (1995). Rimozione di Trigant Burrow nell'opera di S. H. Foulkes e sua riscoperta nel movimento analitico di gruppo (Burrow's removal in Foulkes' work and its rediscovery in the analytic movement of group psychotherapy). *Rivista Italiana di Gruppoanalisi, X*(2): 101–121.

Gatti Pertegato, E., & Pertegato, G. O. (2003). La gruppoanalisi nelle istituzioni Psichiatriche. Presentazione dell'articolo di P. Schilder (1936) (Group analysis in Psychiatric Institutions. Introduction to the article by P. Schilder (1936). The analysis of ideologies as a psychotherapeutic method, especially in group treatment). *Rivista Italiana di Gruppoanalisi, XVII*(1): 75–78.

Gatti Pertegato, E., & Pertegato, G. O. (2006a). Burrow's concept of wholeness versus divisiveness: in the individual, in society and scientific world. Presentation at Lifwynn Conference: "Science, Philosophy and Embodiment: Pathways to Wholeness". New York University, 25–27 July.

Gatti Pertegato, E., & Pertegato, G. O. (2006b). La scoperta della prima struttura teorica della gruppoanalisi: le "Otto Proposizioni" di Trigant Burrow e la natura sociale dell'individuo, del conflitto e della psicopatologia (The discovery of the first theoretical structure of group analysis. Burrow's "Eight Propositions" and the social nature of the individual, of conflict and psychopathology). *Rivista Italiana di Gruppoanalisi, XX* (3): 135–153.

Gatti Pertegato, E., & Pertegato, G. O. (2009). *Dalla psicoanalisi alla fondazione della gruppoanalisi. Patologia della normalità, conflitto individuale e sociale.* (From Psychoanalysis to the Foundation of Group Analysis. Pathology of Normality, Individual and Social Conflict). Milan: IPOC.

Gatti Pertegato, E., & Pertegato, G. O. (2010). The role of social images in conflict and pathology of "normality". Presentation to Lifwynn Conference & C. G. Jung Foundation: "Dream, Dialogue and Embodied Wholeness", New York University, October 29–31.

Gay, P. (1988). *Freud: A Life for Our Time.* New York: Norton.

Gibran, K. (1932). *The Wanderer. His Parables and His Sayings.* New York: Knopf.

Gilden, L. (1999). Trigant Burrow's group analysis. *Group Analysis, 32*(2): 255–265.

Gruen, A. (1992). *The Insanity of Normality*. New York: Grove Press.

Hinshelwood, R. D. (2004). Two early experimenters with groups. *Group Analysis, 37*(3): 323–333.

Hopper, E, (2001). The social unconscious: theoretical considerations. *Group Analysis, 34*(1): 9–27.

Hopper, E., & Weinberg, H. (2011). *The Social Unconscious in Persons, Groups, and Societies. Volume 1: Mainly Theory*. London: Karnac.

Hrdy, S. B. (2009). *Mothers and Others*. Harvard: Belknap.

Huxley, A. (Ed.) (1932). *The Letters of D. H. Lawrence*. London: Heinemann [reprinted 1956].

Jones, E. (1955). *The Life and Work of Sigmund Freud*, vol. 2. London: Hogarth Press.

Jones, E. (1959). *Free Associations: Memories of a Psychoanalyst*. London: Hogarth Press.

Kandel, E. R. (2005). *Psychiatry, Psychoanalysis, and the New Biology of Mind*. Washington, DC: Psychiatry Publishing.

Kempf, E. J. (1921). *Psychopathology*. St. Louis, MO: C. V. Mosby.

Lawrence, D. H. (1921). *Psychoanalysis and the Unconscious*. New York: Thomas Selzer.

Lawrence, D. H. (1927a). Letter to Burrow of 3rd August 1927. In: A. Huxley (Ed.). *The Letters of D. H. Lawrence*. London: Heinemann, 1932 [reprinted 1956, pp. 687–689].

Lawrence, D. H. (1927b). Letter to Burrow of 13th July 1927. In: A. Huxley (Ed.), *The Letters of D. H. Lawrence*. London: Heinemann, 1932 [reprinted 1956, pp. 685–686).

Lawrence, D. H. (1927c). A new theory of neuroses. *The Bookman*, New York, November [reprinted in: M. Rosenbaum & M. Berger, 1963].

Levenson, E. (1983). *The Ambiguity of Change. An Inquiry into the Nature of Psychoanalytic Reality*. New York: Basic Books.

MacCurdy, J. T. (1922). *Problems in Dynamic Psychology*. New York: Macmillan.

Mazzotta, F. (2009a). Trigant Burrow: vita e opere di un pioniere del lavoro analitico con i gruppi (Life and work of a pioneer of the analytic approach to groups). Dissertation discussed on 6/11/2009 with Prof. Maurizio Gasseau, at the Faculty of Psychology, University of Turin.

Mazzotta, F. (2009b). Personal communication to Edi Gatti Pertegato of 10/01/2010.

McDougall, J. (1985). *Theaters of the Mind: Illusion and Truth on the Psychoanalytic Stage*. New York: Basic Books [reprinted New York: Brunner/Mazel, 1990]. Cited in Mitchell S. A. (1993).

Merton, T. (1955). *No Man is an Island*. New York: Harcourt, Brace [reprinted Boston, MA: Shambhala Library, 2005].

Migone, P. (1995). Le origini della gruppoanalisi: una nota su Trigant Burrow (The origin of group analysis. A note on Trigant Burrow). *Rivista Sperimentale di Freniatria, CXIX* (3): 512–517.

Mitchell, S. A. (1993). *Hope and Dread in Psychoanalysis*. New York: Basic Books.

Modell, A. H. (1984). *Psychoanalysis in a New Context*. New York: International Universities Press.

Montesarchio, G. (1993). Leonardo Ancona racconta se stesso (Leonardo Ancona talks about himself). Interview by Gianni Montesarchio. *Attualità in Psicologia*, EUR, *8*(41): 89–103.

Mullan, H., & Rosenbaum, M. (1971). *Group Psychotherapy: Theory and Practice*. New York: Free Press of Glencoe.

Muller, H. J. (1943). *Science and Criticism*. New Haven, CT: Yale University Press. Quoted in: Burrow, T. (1984).

Musatti, C. L. (1977). *Trattato di Psicoanalisi* (Treatise of Psychoanalysis). Turin: Boringhieri.

Napolitani, D. (1981). Struttura 'gruppale' della psicoanalisi e analisi del gruppo (The 'group' structure of psychoanalysis and group analysis). In: C. Ravasini (Ed.), *Le frontiere della psicoanalisi* (The psychoanalysis' frontiers) (pp. 89–136). Milan: Franco Angeli.

Napolitani, D. (1987). *Individualità e gruppalità* (Individuality and groupness). Turin: Boringhieri [reprinted Milan: IPOC, 2006].

Napolitani, D. (1994). Editoriale (Editorial). *Rivista Italiana di Gruppoanalisi, IX* (1): 3–6.

Napolitani, F. (1961). Report on a psychiatric therapeutic community self-administrated by patients, Montreal, June. In: *Proceedings of the Third World Congress of Psychiatry*, Toronto University Press/McGill University Press.

Napolitani, F. (1962). Experiment einer Psychotherapie der Psychosen, Durchgefuehrt in einer Durch Patienten Selbstverwalteten Abteilung. In: Krager, 1963, *Biblioteca Psichiatrica*, Basilea: (Experiment of psychotherapy of psychoses in a department self-administrated by patients).

Napolitani, F. (1985–1986). Nota previa per un'introduzione storica alla COIRAG (A previous note for a historical introduction to COIRAG). *Rivista Italiana di Gruppoanalisi*, *I*(1–2): 131–143.

Nitsun, M. (2001). Towards a group-analytic approach to individual psychotherapy. *Group Analysis*, *34*(4): 473–483.

Oberndorf, C. (1927). History of the psychoanalytic movement in America. *Psychoanalytic Review*, *XIV*: 281–297.

Oberndorf, C. (1953). *A History of Psychoanalysis in America.* New York: Grune & Stratton.

Parmegiani, F., & Zanetti, M. (2007). *Basaglia. Una biografia* (Basaglia. A biography). Trieste: Lint.

Pauletta d'Anna, G. M. (1990). Introduzione. La psicoanalisi e il gruppo: evoluzione di un difficile rapporto (Introduction. Psychoanalysis and the group: evolution of a difficult relationship). In: G. M. Pauletta D'Anna (Ed.), *Modelli Psicoanalitici del gruppo* (Psychoanalytical Models of Group) (pp. 15–62). Milan: Guerini e Associati.

Pianigiani, O. (1990). *Vocabolario etimologico* (Etymologic Dictionary) (3rd edn), D. Meldi (Ed). La Spezia: Melita Editori.

Pigott, C. (1990). *Introduction a la psychanalise groupale* (Introduction to Group Psychoanalysis). Paris: Appsygé.

Pines, M. (1981). The frame of reference of group psychotherapy. *International Journal of Group Psychotherapy, 31*(3): 275–285.

Pines, M. (1991). The matrix of group analysis. An historical perspective. *Group Analysis, 24*(2): 99–109.

Pines, M. (1999). Forgotten pioneers: the unwritten history of the therapeutic community movement. 1998 Maxwell Jones Lecture – Henderson Hospital, 26th June 1998. *Therapeutic Communities, 20*(1): 23–42.

Pines, M. (with Tubert-Oklander J., & Hernández-Tubert, R.) (2011). A conversation with Malcolm Pines: Part Two. *Group Analysis, 44*(1): 3–26.

Pisani, R. A. (2000). *Elementi di gruppoanalisi. Il gruppo piccolo e intermedio* (Elements of Group Analysis. The Small and Median Group). Rome: Edizioni Universitarie Romane.

Pontalti, C. (2008). Ricordando Leonardo Ancona (Remembering Leonardo Ancona). *Gruppi, X* (2): 7–11.

Read, H. (1943). *Education Through Art.* London: Faber & Faber. Quoted in: Burrow, T. (1958), p. 173.

Read, H. (1949). To be or not. 6 Opinions on Dr. Burrow's *The Neurosis of Man. The Tiger's Eye*, October: 115–117.

Read, H. (1958). Foreword. In: Burrow, T. *A Search for Man's Sanity. The Selected Letters of Trigant Burrow*, W. E. Galt (Ed.). New York: Oxford University Press.

Reber, A. S. (1985). *The Penguin Dictionary of Psychology.* New York: Penguin.

Redl, F. (1980). Group emotion and leadership. In: S. Scheidlinger (Ed.), *Psychoanalytic Group Dynamics. Basic Readings* (15–68). New York: International Universities Press.

Roazen, P. (1975). *Freud and His Followers*. New York: Knopf [reprinted New York: Da Capo Press, 1992].

Roazen, P. (1995). La storiografia della psicoanalisi (The historiography of psychoanalysis). *Psicoterapia e Scienze Umane, XXIX*(4): 51–78.

Rosenbaum, M. (1975). Introduction. In: Foulkes, S. H. *Group Analytic Psychotherapy. Method and Principles*. London: Gordon & Breach [reprinted London: Karnac, 1986, second impression, 1991].

Rosenbaum, M. (1986). Trigant Burrow: a pioneer revisited. *Group Analysis, 19*(2): 167–177.

Rosenbaum, M. (1992). Trigant Burrow: a seminal thinker. *Lifwynn Correspondence, II*(2): 9–13.

Rosenbaum M., & Berger M. (1963). *Group Psychotherapy and Group Function*. New York: Basic Books.

Rossi Monti, M. (2006). Bleuler Eugen. In: F. Barale, M. Bertani, V. Gallese, Mistura S., Zamperini A. (Eds.), *Psiche. Dizionario storico di psicologia, psichiatria, psicoanalisi, neuroscienze* (Psyche. Historical Dictionary of Psychology, Psychiatry, Psychoanalysis, Neurosciences). Turin: Einaudi.

Ruitenbeck, H. M. (1966). *Freud and America*. New York: Macmillan.

Sabourin, P. (1985). Postfazione (Afterword). In: S. Ferenczi, *Diario clinico*. Milan: Cortina, 1988.

Scheidlinger, S. (Ed). (1980). Introduction. In: *Psychoanalytic Group Dynamics. Basic Readings* (pp. 3–4). New York: International Universities Press.

Scheidlinger, S. (1987). Trigant Burrow: a pioneer revisited. (Commentary to article by M. Rosenbaum). *Group Analysis, 20*(1): 73–76.

Schilder, P. (1936). The analysis of ideologies as a psychotherapeutic method, especially in group treatment. *American Journal of Psychiatry, 93*(3): 601–615.

Semi, A. A. (1988). *Trattato di Psicoanalisi. Teoria e tecnica*. Vol. I (Treatise of psychoanalysis. Theory and technique. Vol. I). Milan: Cortina.

Siegel, D. J. (1999). *The Developing Mind: Toward a Neurobiology of Interpersonal Experience*. New York: Guilford Press.

Slavich, A. (1968). Mito e realtà dell'autogoverno (Myth and Reality of the Self-Administration). In: F. Basaglia (Ed.), *L'istituzione negata. Rapporto da un ospedale psichiatrico* (pp. 179–201) (The Denied Institution. Report from a Psychiatric Hospital). Turin: Einaudi. [reprinted Milan: B. C. Dalai, 2010].

Stein, L. (1927). Psychoanalysis psychoanalyzed. *The New Republic*, December 14, 1927. Quoted in: Burrow, T. (1958), p. 172.

Stephan, R. (1949). Editorial. *The Tiger's Eye.*
Sullivan, H. S. (1972). *Personal Psychopathology*. New York: Norton.
Swick Perry, H. (1971). Introduction. In: H. S. Sullivan, *Personal Psychopathology*. New York: Norton.
Syz, H. (1957). Trigant Burrow's thesis in relation to group psychotherapy. In: J. Masserman & J. L. Moreno (Eds.), *Progress in Psychotherapy* (147–155). New York: Grune & Stratton.
Syz, H. (1961). Problems of perspectives against the background of Trigant Burrow's group-analytic researches. *International Journal of Group Psychotherapy, 11*: 143–165.
Tubert-Oklander, J., & Hernández-Tubert, R. (2011). A conversation with Malcolm Pines: Part Two. *Group Analysis, 44*(1): 3–26.
Tuttman, S. (1986). Theoretical and technical elements which characterize the American approaches to psychoanalytic group psychotherapy. *International Journal of Group Psychotherapy, 36*(4): 499–515.
Van Schoor, E. P. (2000). A sociohistorical view of group psychotherapy in the United States: the ideoogy of individualism and self-liberation. *International Journal of Group Psychotherapy, 50*(4): 437–454.
Vegetti Finzi, S. (1990). *Storia della psicoanalisi* (History of Psychoanalysis). Milan: Mondadori.
Verdecchia, A. (2004). Commentary on Gary Winship's "The Democratic Origins of the Term 'Group Analysis', Karl Mannheim's 'Third Way' for Psychoanalysis and Social Science". *Group Analysis, 37*(4): 556–558.
Weiss, E. (1970). *Sigmund Freud as a Consultant*. New York: Intercontinental Medical Books.
Wender, L. (1936). The dynamics of group psychotherapy and its application. *Journal of Nervous and Mental Disorders, 84* (1): 54–60.
Winnicott, D. W. (1950). Aggression in relation to emotional development. In: D. W. Winnicott (1958). *Through Paediatrics to Psycho-analysis* (pp. 204–218). London: Tavistock [reprinted London: Hogarth Press, 1975, 1977, 1978, 1982, 1987].
Winnicott, D. W. (1954). Mind and its relation to the psyche-soma. In: D. W. Winnicott (1958), *Through Paediatrics to Psycho-analysis* (pp. 243–254). London: Tavistock [reprinted London: Hogarth Press, 1975, 1977, 1978,1982, 1987].
Winnicott, D. W. (1960). Ego distortion in terms of true and false self. In: *The Maturational Processes and the Facilitating Environment* (pp. 140–152). London: Hogarth Press, 1965, sixth impression 1985.
Winship, G. (2003). The democratic origins of the term 'group analysis', Karl Mannheim's 'third way' for psychoanalysis and social science. *Group Analysis, 36*(1): 37–51.

Wolberg, L. R., & Aronson, M. L. (Eds). (1979). Preface. In: *Group Therapy. An Overview*. New York: Stratton Intercontinental, Medical Books.

Wordsworth, W. (1807). Ode: Intimations of Immortality from Recollections of Early Childhood. In: *Poems, in Two Volumes*. London: Longman, Hurst, Rees, & Orme.

Yalom, I. D. (1970). *The Theory and Practice of Group Psychotherapy*. New York: Basic Books.

INDEX

www.ingramcontent.com/pod-product-compliance
Ingram Content Group UK Ltd.
Pitfield, Milton Keynes, MK11 3LW, UK
UKHW022206190926
475702UK00003B/233

* 9 7 8 0 3 6 7 1 0 0 9 9 5 *